Modernity and the Pandemic

Modernity and the Pandemic: Decivilization, Imperialism, and COVID-19 applies the tools of critical social theory to make sense of the COVID-19 crisis and presents a critical sociological analysis of aspects of the political and community response to the pandemic.

The book focuses on key themes integral to a sociology of pandemics in the "global" age. Firstly, Creaven argues that cultures of individualism and consumerism, and of pervasive and deeply entrenched social inequalities (that is, *decivilization*), significantly weaken the cause of public health by weakening the compliance of people with state-mandated non-pharmaceutical interventions (including and especially physical distancing rules) and encouraging vaccine hesitancy. Secondly, Creaven examines how interstate competition and imperial politics have undermined an effective global policy response to the COVID-19 pandemic. Policy failure with regard to the management of the pandemic is interpreted as being rooted in the dominance of neoliberal ideology and governance in the politics of international relations, particularly in the politics of the leading state actors, by protecting corporate interests at the expense of public health, and in the constraints imposed on state actors by the competitive dynamic of multinational capitalism in the "global" age.

Modernity and the Pandemic will appeal to scholars in the humanities and social sciences with interests in neoliberalism and its social, cultural, and epidemiological impacts.

Sean Creaven is Senior Lecturer in Sociology and Criminology at the University of the West of England, UK. His research interests include the sociology of modernity and postmodernity, sociological theory, critical theory, Marxism and post-Marxism, critical realism, and criminological theory. He is the author of *The Pandemic in Britain: COVID-19, British Exceptionalism and Neoliberalism* (Routledge, 2023), *Against the Spiritual Turn: Marxism, Realism, and Critical Theory* (Routledge, 2010), *Emergentist Marxism: Dialectical Philosophy and Social Theory* (Routledge, 2007), and *Marxism and Realism: A Materialistic Application of Realism in the Social Sciences* (Routledge, 2000).

The COVID-19 Pandemic Series

This series examines the impact of the COVID-19 pandemic on individuals, communities, countries, and the larger global society from a social scientific perspective. It represents a timely and critical advance in knowledge related to what many believe to be the greatest threat to global ways of being in more than a century. It is imperative that academics take their rightful place alongside medical professionals as the world attempts to figure out how to deal with the current global pandemic, and how society might move forward in the future. This series represents a response to that imperative.

Series Editor: J. Michael Ryan

Titles in this Series:

COVID-19 in Brooklyn
Everyday Life During a Pandemic
Jerome Krase and Judith DeSena

The Pandemic in Britain
COVID-19, British Exceptionalism and Neoliberalism
Sean Creaven

Women and COVID-19
A Clinical and Applied Sociological Focus on Family, Work and Community
Edited by Mariam Seedat-Khan and Johanna O. Zulueta

State-Society Relations around the World through the Lens of the COVID-19 Pandemic
Rapid-Test
Edited by Federica Duca and Sarah Meny-Gibert

Contagion Capitalism
Pandemics in the Corporate Age
Sean Creaven

Modernity and the Pandemic
Decivilization, Imperialism, and COVID-19
Sean Creaven

Modernity and the Pandemic
Decivilization, Imperialism, and COVID-19

Sean Creaven

Routledge
Taylor & Francis Group

LONDON AND NEW YORK

First published 2024
by Routledge
4 Park Square, Milton Park, Abingdon, Oxon OX14 4RN

and by Routledge
605 Third Avenue, New York, NY 10158

Routledge is an imprint of the Taylor & Francis Group, an informa business

© 2024 Sean Creaven

British Library Cataloguing-in-Publication Data
A catalogue record for this book is available from the British Library

ISBN: 978-1-032-56796-9 (hbk)
ISBN: 978-1-032-56798-3 (pbk)
ISBN: 978-1-003-43720-8 (ebk)

DOI: 10.4324/9781003437208

Typeset in Times New Roman
by Deanta Global Publishing Services, Chennai, India

This book is dedicated to Margaret Archer (1943-2023), in appreciation of her outstanding contribution to the development of a humanistic critical-realist social science in times that have never been more needful.

Contents

Foreword

Modern culture is arguably a consumer culture and, where it isn't, is certainly on the road to becoming so. Consumer culture, in turn, is nearly always a corporate-controlled culture and one that seeks to emphasize (at a cost) individuality. As individuals and nation-states "modernize" and increasingly come to accept consumption as not a necessity, but rather a way of life, they also become increasingly individualistic and under the direct control of corporate influence.

There are more reasons to be concerned about the above than there are pages in this volume available to explore them, but of central concern here are the ways in which "our" modern culture has been responsible for individualized responses to the ongoing collective global health crisis of the COVID-19 pandemic. Responses to social issues, especially those related to health, necessitate a sense of shared community that runs counter to the more individualized emphasis of many (most?) other aspects of the lives of many in the privileged (and even not so privileged) spheres of society.

One of the great contributions of Creaven's work is that it demonstrates how, rather than something exceptional, the impact of the COVID-19 pandemic, as well as the responses to it, should have almost been expected. In other words, they are the direct result of the current configurations of modern society rather than anything "exceptional". Thus, while we have tended to paint the pandemic as a "once in a generation event", and it certainly was to some degree, we should also understand the ways in which it was an (il-)logical outcome of contemporary social, largely corporatized, internationalized, structures.

Creaven's detailed analysis of the above brings forth the kinds of insights necessary to not only help better understand the impact of the COVID-19 pandemic, but also to understand a multitude of other health, social, cultural, and political issues facing the world today. More than just an analysis of the pandemic, the insights in the following pages represent a truly global, truly social analysis of culture today.

J. Michael Ryan
Series Editor, *The COVID-19 Pandemic Series*
June 2023

Preface

The purpose *of Modernity and the Pandemic: Decivilization, Imperialism, and COVID-19* is to present a sociological analysis of aspects of the political and community (people) response to the novel coronavirus outbreak.

With regard to the political response, the focus here is on state policymaking in addressing the pandemic, as this has been constrained and facilitated by the structures and processes of the interstate system and of international corporate capitalism. Analysis here purports to interpret the inadequacies of state policymaking with regard to COVID-19 not only as the result of neoliberal ideology and the protection of corporate interests but also of the constraints imposed on state actors by interstate competition and imperial rivalries on the world stage.

With regard to the public or "people" response, the focus here is on variable levels of compliance at the societal-community level with public health protection policies and norms (especially those of national lockdowns, non-pharmaceutical interventions or NPIs, and mass vaccination), which partially undermined the effectiveness of these responses in saving lives and defending public health. The analysis here interprets such weaknesses of public response as resulting from decivilizing mechanisms integral to corporate-driven processes of modernization and "globalization" in the capitalist world economy. These drivers are, as I will argue, much more consolidated in the developed world, in high-income countries, and especially in the North Atlantic zone (the West or Global North), where consumerism and the culture of wholly individualized rights and entitlements are most entrenched.

In pursuit of these goals, this book addresses two key themes that are arguably integral to a sociology of pandemics in the corporate age.

- Firstly, the impacts of cultures of individualism and consumerism, and of pervasive and deeply entrenched social inequalities (that is, decivilization), in weakening the compliance of people with non-pharmaceutical interventions (NPIs) and in encouraging vaccine hesitancy that would protect communities from pandemics such as COVID-19.
- Secondly, how the primacy of interstate competition and imperial power politics over interstate cooperation in international relations has, at the time of writing, undermined an effective global policy response to COVID-19.

The book was more or less completed as a whole first draft in the period from the start of April 2020 up until October 2021. It has since then been finalized at various points last year up until more or less the present. Finalization, for the most part, entailed supporting the analysis by drawing on additional, later, sources. But this also involved a degree of updating, particularly with regard to the state of play with the international vaccine rollout, public compliance with NPIs under circumstances where governments withdrew from legally mandating them, and persisting vaccine hesitancy amongst substantial minorities worldwide. The analytical and conceptual elements that apprehend these events have not required significant modification.

Nonetheless, since the COVID-19 crisis is ongoing and will be with us for some time to come, this does render the present work's coverage of pandemic events, and of analysis linking to these, as inevitably time-limited or time-specific. For perhaps years to come, accounts of the pandemic in global political economy and in contemporary society and culture must be highly provisional and radically incomplete. This is certainly the case for this book.

Modernity and the Pandemic will hopefully appeal to scholars of sociology, philosophy, and politics with interests in neoliberal ideology, global political economy, and their manifestation in social, political, and cultural life.

Sean Creaven
7 May 2023

Acknowledgements

This book is one of a trilogy concerned with sociologizing the COVID-19 pandemic, all of which were written in draft form in the period from April 2020 to October 2021. Consequently, the arguments and analysis of this present volume, like those of the others, benefited especially from my dialogue (or was it monologue?) with specific colleagues and students at the University of the West of England (UWE). The students in question were those who were studying my third-year option module, "Contemporary Critiques of Modern Society", in its "virtual year", in those COVID-stricken times. The colleagues in question were especially Andy Mathers, Ian Walmsley, and Jack Spicer, but also on isolated occasions Maria Stadnicka and Lita Crociani-Windland. I thank them for tolerating my musings and for their input.

I also owe a particular thank you to J. Michael Ryan, series editor of Routledge's COVID-19 Pandemic series. This is for reviewing this book in draft form and for his insightful suggestions for improvements – many of which I have been happy to accommodate.

Unlike my *The Pandemic in Britain*, which was a straightforward work of politics and current affairs, focused obviously on the specificities and peculiarities of the UK crisis, this book draws much more on resources of critique in social theory in order to apprehend the crisis in world systems. These resources are chiefly (though not exclusively) those of:

- Critical Realism (CR) or critical realist social theory (CRT)– especially Margaret Archer's morphogenetic approach to analyzing the interface between structure and agency in social systems;
- Realist International Relations Theory (RIRT) – especially as developed by Robert Keohane, John Mearsheimer, Robert Gilpin, and others;
- Norbert Elias's theory of the civilizing dynamics of modernization processes;
- Alex Callinicos's work on the relationship between global political economy and contemporary imperialism, together with Chris Harman's work theorizing the interface between state and capitalism today – which allow for a Marxist reframing of the insights of RIRT;
- The critical "postmodern" sociology of modern individualism and consumerism developed especially by Zygmunt Bauman and Jean Baudrillard.

This book is therefore particularly conceptually indebted to the work of these scholars. If this all seems rather eclectic theoretically, I have no apologies to offer for it. However, these various conceptual elements are drawn together within a critical Marxist sociological framework that, hopefully, integrates them, more or less. These allow the COVID-19 pandemic to be contextualized (as it must be if it is to be sociologically comprehendible) in the socioeconomic and sociocultural orders of world systems – or such is my intention.

Introduction

This book is one of a pair whose purpose is to "sociologize" (culturally, politically, and economically) the global COVID-19 crisis, that is, to understand the pandemic as an event or connected series of events amenable to sociological inquiry, or which can be explained in part sociologically in the sense that certain of its aspects have socioeconomic and sociocultural dimensions, even drivers.[1] These sociological dimensions of the present crisis are not simply those that germinate new and dangerous diseases, and which allow them to globalize, but also those that, to a greater or lesser extent, impact negatively on the capacity of governments to protect their own peoples from the ill effects of pandemic events. Modern socioeconomic and sociocultural conditions not only make possible pandemics that have the potential to kill millions (if not tens or hundreds of millions) of people worldwide, but they also partially undermine the effectiveness of public health protection measures at the level of nation-states.

These conditions or drivers, as I will show, are not those that may be captured or grasped by the term "globalization". Nor do these conditions or drivers pertain to those lofty abstractions of "modernity" or "modernization" that are preferred by a depoliticized social science. Rather, these conditions or drivers are those generated by specific emergent social and cultural structures that are commonly associated with these ideas.[2] These ideas are especially those of corporate mega-capitalism, its neoliberal mode of political governance, its fundamental social inequalities and divisions (especially those of class but also those of "race" and ethnicity), and its cultural modes of "rights" individualism and technocratic instrumentalism. Some of these forms (neoliberalism, the multinational business enterprise, and individualism of certain kinds) have been the facilitators and drivers of processes of so-called globalization since the 1980s.

This book (*Modernity and the Pandemic*) and its companion volume (*Contagion Capitalism*) may be seen as a continuation and extension of my earlier *The Pandemic in Britain*. The latter book addresses the gross inadequacies of UK government policy with regard to COVID-19, in that this mounted a seriously compromised defence of public health and thereby caused tens of thousands of avoidable deaths. The basic cause of policy failure was a failure to prioritize people over profits. The British government's pandemic strategy failed, as I tried to demonstrate, because it was hemmed in by neoliberal ideology, the protection of corporate interests, and the peculiarities of a British model of capitalism that is more internationalized or

DOI: 10.4324/9781003437208-1

export-based than those of the other developed countries and which is focused especially on retail, hospitalities, tourism, and finance – with a substantial low-pay sector of the labour market characterized by precarity. Further constraints on effective anti-pandemic policy flowed from the politics of Brexit that dovetailed with the neoliberal fetish of open markets and open borders.

I described these failings as aspects of "British exceptionalism". This was not exceptionalism in the sense of uniqueness, however. On the contrary, British policy inadequacies (in terms of defending people's lives and protecting health-care services from bulging caseloads) were widely shared by other governments across the globe, and for the same reasons. Rather, the exceptionalism of British exceptionalism consists of the fact that the errors and inadequacies from a public health perspective that characterized to varying degrees governmental responses elsewhere were all found in a particularly concentrated form in the UK.

A purpose of the present volumes, therefore, is to consider the pandemic in its relation to state policymaking more generally, as this too has been constrained and facilitated (and hence undermined) by neoliberalism and by the international orders (world capitalist economy and international state system) that this helps sustain. This (the application of critique of the drivers of British exceptionalism more generally) is what perhaps renders these works a continuation of the earlier volume. However, these books also seek to situate the pandemic within the systems of global political economy and their attendant cultural modes in the sense that these not only place severe limitations on government health protection policies in response to pandemics but are also the facilitators or drivers of global pandemic risk. Critique, then, is twofold: firstly, of a type of society (ours) in which corporate-capitalist control of economy, of state, and of science, is institutionalized, and of the way in which this impacts perversely on the cause of public health policy everywhere; and secondly, of a type of economy and culture (ours) that is driving the ecological crisis of sustainability of which pandemic events such as COVID-19 are integral.

This volume will develop certain aspects of this critique, whereas *Contagion Capitalism* will develop the others. The division of labour is as follows. The latter will address COVID-19 and pandemic risk in the capitalist world economy and global ecological crisis. This will also explore critically the role of the clinical sciences – of pharmacology and industrial pharmaceutics, of the biomedical model upon which these are based, of mathematical epidemiology and virology, and of technocratic expertise – in addressing the pandemic and serving (or rather ill-serving) the cause of public health more generally owing to their absorption by corporate capitalism.

As for this volume, it is intended to accomplish two main objectives. The first of these is to explore the impact of processes of modernization characteristic of contemporary capitalism (especially of individualization, polarization, and marginalization – especially though not exclusively by class – which have been integral to capitalist development) in weakening or degrading community or societal protections from dangerous viruses such as COVID-19. These processes that once held sway mostly in parts of Europe and North America during the 150 years or so from the start of the Industrial Revolution have since World War Two begun to internationalize. The internationalization of modernization has accelerated since the 1980s. This aspect of the analysis sets out a thesis of *decivilization* as a pervasive feature of advanced commodity cultures. This is especially those in developed countries where consumerism extends into all corners of social life. However, this is also a growing tendency of the burgeoning urban middle classes of the developing countries of the Global South. Decivilization accounts for why lockdown policies and non-pharmacological interventions (NPIs) upon which the primary defence against COVID-19 depended during the pandemic's first, second, and third waves were only partially effective.

The concept of decivilization deployed here, as ought to be clear, is not intended to denote interruption or roll-back of those social processes that Norbert Elias famously identified as civilizing processes. Elias's theory of civilizing processes was, as Paddy Dolan points out, "developed…in the 1930s to describe and explain the generation of higher standards of various forms of conduct in the context of unplanned but structured changes in state formation and lengthening chains of social interdependencies".[3] The fundamental idea of the theory was that the emergence of the nation-state system allowed central-state control of powers of authorization (including the means of coercion and violence) so that violence and aggression were emptied from everyday civilian life. This occurred alongside socioeconomic processes (driven by industrialization and commercialization) that increased interdependencies among individuals and groups in a society so that competition was reduced and cooperation increased.[4] Now, Elias did not elaborate a theory of decivilization, though a concept of decivilization is discernible in his work. His positive reading of modernization precluded that. In this book, however, decivilization will be understood not as a reversal or regression of Elias's civilizing processes but as the "other face" of these same processes and as their negative consequences.

This "other face" includes the nurturing of cultural sensibilities in people that are corrosive of the social bond and which, by virtue of this, weaken a collective community response to pandemic events such as COVID-19. This is especially the impact of an egocentric rights-focused individualism driven to some degree by consumerism that licenses people to make self-centred cost-benefit decisions over whether to follow NPIs or to disregard them, or whether to get a vaccine or not to do so. Under modern citizenship, civic responsibilities are subordinated to civil rights. Rights pertain to individuals, not to communities, and this encourages the contemporary citizen to view these, first and foremost, as *my* rights, not those of *other* people.[5] What then gets rather lost sight of in liberalized "rights" cultures is that the individual is part of society so that "my" rights are always shared by others. "My" rights are *our* rights – and, if they were not, they would be privileges, not rights. Indeed "my" rights depend on others since, unless these are socially recognized, they have no efficacy. In short, *rights presuppose responsibilities.*[6]

But the consumer-mediated cultural way of life under contemporary capitalism ensures that rights are not simply interpreted as those of individuals, as our own private property, nor simply as entitlements to certain "public goods" (legal protections, welfare benefits, voter rights, etc.) but also as rights of consumption and indeed as user-pay entitlements to even life-sustaining goods (such as, for example, a vaccine). This is also consumption through the pursuit of libidinal experience so that hedonistic desires are interpreted as fundamental needs, the satisfaction of which is a matter of self-entitlement, integral to self-identity and social status. The consumer-mediated way of life is also a cultural force that renders people vulnerable to viewing other people instrumentally, as objects of exploitation, or as the means to acquire other objects of utility. This is as commodities to be bought and used (e.g. the hiring of labour power in an employment market or of sexualized bodies in the flesh industries) or as vehicles of consumption (e.g. people as passive "stomachs" or as various kinds of access points to consumer opportunities). These modes of individualism have allowed people to make decisions on whether or not to comply with NPIs on the basis mostly of judgements of self-risk, or of risk to intimates in their interpersonal circles, rather than on the basis of *societal* risk, that is, risk to the unacquainted multitude of a wider community.

These modes of individualism also license people to place their personal wants before social or community needs so that the temporary imposition of relatively trivial inconveniences (e.g. wearing a face mask in an enclosed indoor setting, or maintaining physical distancing, or avoiding physically socializing with friends as opposed to doing that virtually, or taking the trouble to get vaccinated) may be seen as a grievous assault on entitlements, injurious to self and personal wellbeing. Such egoistic rights-based individualism then licences – when this is thwarted by physical distancing restrictions – an epidemic of mental ill-health, or at least a moral panic over the expectation or prospect of one.[7] For those who suffered from lockdown-generated psychiatric distress, this was certainly a profoundly unpleasant and frightening experience. But this was, for many, a consequence less of physical distancing rules *per se* than of exposure to a culture that could only regard these as detrimental to the very foundations of self and wellbeing – and which would energetically impress this on the individual consciousness.[8] Interestingly, in the UK, the Health Foundation reported that the number of people in the country who reported experiencing feelings of loneliness during the first lockdown did not rise above the pre-pandemic levels.[9]

Research into the negative impacts of the pandemic on mental health has tended not to differentiate between those generated specifically by social isolation caused by lockdowns and by physical distancing and those generated by all of the other ill effects of COVID-19. Pandemic deficits then become translated especially or even exclusively as lockdown deficits.[10] This was because these were ideologically weaponized by opinion-formers and powerholders to legitimize fast-tracked re-openings. Those "other" effects include anxiety over the threat of becoming ill or of loved ones becoming ill; loss of income; loss of a job; loss of welfare benefits; and lack of access to mental health or wellbeing services (owing to general under-resourcing of healthcare that was exacerbated by the demands of the pandemic). Specific lockdown stressors also impacted largely low-income households. This was owing less to the inevitability of social isolation from physical distancing than from "cabin fever" generated specifically by poor quality and cramped housing lacking outdoor garden spaces plus lacking access to the internet that would allow virtual interactions with others.[11] In the latter case, then, factors of social-class disadvantage ensured that physical distancing became social and psychic distancing, with all of the mental wellbeing adversities that this brings.

A focus of this book is, accordingly, the negative impact of decivilization as driven by self-entitled individualism on public compliance with the pandemic NPIs and indeed on public compliance with pandemic pharmaceutical interventions (PIs), that is, vaccination. However, the COVID-19 crisis has thrown up plenty of other examples of people prioritizing self over society in a way that is detrimental to the cause of public safety, which I do not address. One of these particularly worthy of note is the phenomenon of vaccine queue-jumping, as discussed by Michael Ryan and Serena Nanda,[12] which the rich and well-connected have availed themselves of. This too fits the mould of decivilization. Such involved wealthy Westerners obtaining fast-tracked jabs from overseas as the commonfolk waited in line for their age cohort to get the call to the vaccination centres, and members of elites in poorer countries doing the same.[13] Moreover, "cutting the line", or getting ahead of others with a stronger need or entitlement for a vaccine, owing to status and money advantages, was also a practice of well-off citizens within their own countries and communities. Ryan and Nanda describe many such cases from rich and poor countries alike. In the West, for example:

> Italy is prioritizing vaccines for tourists going to the glamorous island of Capri, instead of more vulnerable categories of its population … Even Germany, with its high value on equality and government integrity, has experienced many cases of younger people attempting to get vaccinated by falsely claiming they are caretakers for their elderly relatives … And money talks: in New York City, some of the highest vaccination rates are in the wealthiest neighborhoods, like the Upper West Side and Upper East Side, where by late March 2021, approximately half the residents were vaccinated, while in the poor, immigrant neighborhood of Corona, Queens, where the virus was far deadlier, only 19% of the population had been vaccinated.

As for the rest, for example:

> Even in poorer nations, richer and politically connected people try to cut the line. Two ministers in Peru and one in Argentina have resigned for receiving or giving preferential access to scarce vaccines, and the doctor conducting Peru's first vaccine trial acknowledged giving vaccine priority to nearly 250 politicians, well-known political allies and their families, as well as university administrators. In Ecuador and Brazil, investigations are being held involving local politicians and their families trying to cut the line. And in early March 2021, in Palestine, even as Palestinians were clamoring for the vaccine that Israel has denied to their communities, their own leadership was accused of siphoning some of the few doses allotted to them to the senior ranks of the ruling party, allies in the media, and family members of top dignitaries.[14]

Decivilization as the "other face" of modernization also includes the reproduction of ever-deepening social divisions and inequalities (within countries and internationally).[15] This is under the auspices of intensifying international capitalist competition and a neoliberal governance of austerity and retrenchment of health and welfare services intended to boost corporate profits. The hardening of the injustice of inequality since the closing decades of the twentieth century has furnished the multitude of the working poor – included amongst which are the so-called precariat of low-income, low-status, (mostly) service sector, often zero-hours contracted employees – with compelling economic reasons to disregard those physical distancing norms that would undermine their ability to make ends meet or participate (albeit on the fringes) in consumerism.[16]

Not only that, but this also ferments in many of them resentments and antagonisms towards "wealthy achievers" (to borrow a term from the *British Crime Survey* of a few years ago) and towards a political establishment supportive or tolerant of a social order in which they are marginalized. Such further weakens, for millions of people, at least in potential, collective community responses to pandemic events such as COVID-19 – and especially for those who are members of oppressed minority groups or who are at the wrong end of the class divide – since basic trust in political authorities has been substantially undermined over several decades.[17] This is part of the explanation for why wild conspiracy stories citing the oppressive "hidden agendas" behind physical distancing rules and vaccination programmes go viral on social media.

The second purpose of this volume is to begin the task of analyzing global pandemics such as COVID-19 as products of "modern" social structures and relations rather than merely natural forces. To be clear, this is not a product of "globalization" but of particular modes of internationalization. These are the parallel though intersecting and mutually supportive orders of the capitalist world economy and international state system. Even though "globalization" (as I will argue in this book) is certainly partly mythical – so that the notion that capitalism today is trans-nationalized, a borderless utopia of free trade, is a neoliberal legitimation of untrammelled corporate domination of the world economy – capitalist internationalization as conveyed by a capitalism-affirming interstate system is certainly real nonetheless. And capitalist internationalism is fertile soil for new infectious diseases, the reinvigoration of older ones, and their rapid community and cross-border transmission.

These great engines of "globalization" (capitalist world economy and international state system) are radically asymmetrical in terms of the resources they divide and distribute worldwide, generating huge inequalities in the power of command or authorization and in the control of property and wealth. This renders them systems of domination and subordination: of non-owning classes by owning classes; of lesser states by greater states. This also ensures that both are systems of competition since domination can be secured only by competitive success in each of the systems. The world capitalist economy and the international state system are those in which the dominant actors (capitalist bosses and propertied elites in the economic sphere; state managers in the political sphere) seek to secure and extend their systemic advantages over their rivals (that is, other capitals and other states).

The relationship between the two systems is one of structural interdependence.[18] On the one hand, the international state system is the life-support system of the capitalist world economy since this, contrary to the myths of globalization theory, cannot function in a borderless or deterritorialized world. But, on the other hand, the interstate system can reproduce itself only inasmuch as state authorities in each and every country draw on the economic resources generated by local capitalist enterprises within their borders and from their overseas operations to sustain themselves. This relationship of structural interdependence of economy and polity in world systems ensures that the interests of powerholders in each are more or less congruent. This has rarely before been more transparent than it has become since the neoliberal era. This is because the neoliberal era has seen the dismantling of the postwar compromise between capital and labour (that is, the social-democratic state) that was once seen as necessary to preserve capitalism itself.

The focus of this volume is on the international state system in its relation to world capitalism, whereas the focus of *Contagion Capitalism* is on the world capitalist economy in its relation to neoliberal governance. This focus on the structural realities of the global political economy allows an explanation of the limits and failings of the COVID-19 international vaccination programme, as I will show. Much was promised for this programme, but (at the time of writing) much less was delivered. This ought to be baffling for those globalization theorists who have insisted that capitalist internationalization and the diffusion of liberal-democratic citizenship worldwide is ushering in a new era of global cooperation and cosmopolitan solidarity among nations and peoples (indeed even transforming people everywhere into "world citizens")[19] so that merely national interests can no longer hold sway. This is exposed for the nonsense it always was by the international political response to the pandemic, which has seen the wholly predictable prioritization of national interests over international ones as a matter of first and last resort.

Theory

The conceptual resources of critique that will inform the analysis contained in this volume include chiefly:

1. Theories and concepts illuminating modes of modern individualism developed by sociologists such as Emile Durkheim and Anthony Giddens. These allow the analyst to grasp the limits and potentials of social solidarity in contemporary times faced with pandemic events.
2. The critiques of contemporary consumer culture made by sociologists of postmodernity such as Zygmunt Bauman and Jean Baudrillard. This is in order to understand the decivilizing processes. Such usage does not imply any sort of endorsement on my part of the concept of postmodernity. Postmodernity is false, but the critiques of contemporary society offered by certain of its sociologists have considerable relevance to the task of making sense of aspects

of the modern, notably, of consumer capitalism in the corporate age. These may be incorporated into a critical Marxist theory of contemporary social (dis) order.[20]

3. My own critical realist theoretical reconstruction of Marx's socio-historical materialism, which draws heavily on Margaret Archer's morphogenetic social theory, and its application here to help make sense of global political economy today.

4. Concepts and insights drawn from the Realist School of International Relations Theory (RIRT). This is also in order to make sense of the interstate system and contemporary imperialism in relation to neoliberalism and world capitalism today. CRT and RIRT together support a critical understanding of the phenomena of "vaccine nationalism" and "vaccine imperialism", which account for the grave shortcomings of the international political response to COVID-19.

CRT and world systems

A few words on (2) are in order at this point, however. This is for the simple reason that analysis of global political economy constitutes the macroscopic framework that contextualizes and mediates not only the novel coronavirus pandemic but also the responses of nation-state actors to the crisis. Moreover, this also establishes the relevance and efficacy of the other resources of critique drawn upon in this enterprise, since these also require contextualization within a broader critical analysis of capitalist world economy and international relations as a systemic whole, which the authors of these critiques do not in most cases provide. Marx's critique of capitalist political economy – understood in my conception as a critical realist theory of societal dynamics – furnishes here, in this analysis, the conceptual toolkit for illuminating this macroscopic level of world systems.

Since global political economy (the interface between the international nation-state system and the capitalist world economy) is fundamental to making sense of the pandemic, one chapter of the present enterprise (Chapter 1) is therefore devoted to exploring the world system in its economic and political aspects, albeit with a particular focus on the political. In the companion volume, *Contagion Capitalism*, the analysis is also contextualized within these world systems but with the main focus on the economic. The philosophical case for an analysis of political economy informed by Critical Realism (CR) is as follows. This is that, as critical realist social theory (CRT) affirms, societies are dualistic systems. This means they are forged in the dynamic interface of social structure and human (social) agency, each of which is ontologically distinct from the other, and each of which is causally efficacious in the shaping and reshaping of system outcomes.[21]

Human agency is causal because it is animated by people who are the bearers of biologically based needs (albeit culturally prescribed and developed) that may be frustrated or satisfied by social relations so that they have real interests in either societal change or continuity. Human agency is causal also because only people are intentional systems, owing to the fact that they have properties of self or subjectivity, by which they may own motives in acting on their interests in societal change or continuity.[22] Social structure is causal because, as the ensemble of role positions and asymmetric resource distributions that people find "already made" from the moment they enter society, this impacts their capacities for thought and action. This is by immersing them within a framework of constraints and enablements that they experience differently depending on where they are positioned in relation to these role positions and distributions.[23]

Now, capital relations and state relations, like any other relations that make up a social system, have structural properties that are causally efficacious. These structural properties generate social practices that impact not only the social world (the reproduction and evolution of human relations) but also nature (the manipulation of physical laws and the harnessing of natural resources to service social goals). This means that the risks faced by humanity (whether these are those generated by group conflict or institutional dysfunctionality or by hazards of nature) tend to be socially constructed. It is no longer the case, or not so much the case, as arguably (though contentiously) it was in preindustrial times, that social and natural processes may be construed as distinct and independent sources of hazard.[24]

Rather, in the "global" age of universalized industrialism and technoscience, under the auspices of state relations and capitalist relations, the hazards are all sociologized,[25] and this includes the social production of disease. This is because the history of societal "modernization" is also a history of ever-deepening and ever-accelerating penetration of nature by forces of economic production and cultural knowledge (primarily the knowledge generated by technoscience) so that these are inextricably bound, for good and for ill. This invasiveness of the sociocultural in the natural (which resembles that of surgical interventions to reorder a living body) is aimed at extending and intensifying the utilization of its elements as exploitable resources of capitalism and dissolving their capacity to obstruct in the least their own subordination to servicing human and social needs. Human relations with nature under capitalist modernity have been anthropocentric to the core.

This also means that structural emergence sets the parameters (antecedent constraints and enablements) on and of social practices within which governmental and people's responses to socially produced hazards (such as pandemic events) are compelled to operate. CRT establishes that economic and political orders are not the immediate recursive artifice of collective human agency, the spontaneous outcome of our continual making and remaking of societal bonds and relations. There is, in short, more to society than the ongoing social practices that reproduce it. If this was not so, the orders and institutional patterns of society would not endure in the face of the flux of social intercourse. The "more" is what is emergent from previously materialized social interaction and human agency that we encounter as environment. These are the cultural and structural properties of society that every generation of human agents has to confront as a range of fetters, facilitators, impulses, and pressures that mediate its practices and motives for action.

These inherited structures of society are the essential starting point when analyzing social processes because, although history-making is the task of human agents alone, human agency is always rationally oriented to the material and cultural contexts in which it is situated and is comprehensible only by linking it to these action contexts.[26]

Social structures impart regularities and stabilities on processes of social interaction by virtue of which systems endure. Human interaction, if this was unbound by structures, would otherwise be free to deny these systems stability or dissolve them altogether. Historically this has been accomplished on the basis of hierarchy and asymmetry in the distribution of reward and command in society. Consequently, there is inequality in all of its forms – which, because this is antecedently given, is also injustice. Structural emergence accounts for the allocative and authoritative resources available for distribution among a population in any system of society.

This also determines how these resources are distributed socially,[27] thereby stratifying the members of a society into separate groups by virtue of their differing degrees of access to these resources and by fixing their relations with each other (as "owners" or "non-owners" or "greater owners" or "lesser owners") *vis-à-vis* these distributions.[28] The constraints and enablements that structures confront people with are thus experienced by them differently depending on where they are involuntarily placed within these structures in relation to role positions and resources so that some are more enabled and less constrained than others. This means that certain groups and role incumbents are granted the power to reimpose their own "orders" on others who are denied these resources and capacities so that the stabilization and ordering of social interaction are hardly consensual and may be threatened by inter-group conflicts between haves and have-nots.

By the same token, structures establish the situational logics that inform the strategic decision-making of those differently placed when they are seeking to maintain or improve their control of resources, individually or collectively. This is the case whether these be macro-actors such as governments, or micro-actors such as individual people. As Margaret Archer puts it: "It is the situations to which people respond that are mediatory because they condition (without determining) different courses of action for those differently placed, by supplying different reasons to them".[29]

Situational logics distribute different "vested interests to those differently placed". These are interests (individual and collective) of persons in pursuing different kinds of agency (political, economic, cultural) *vis-à-vis* other social groups that are aimed at preserving or extending their access to resources – typically at the expense of these other groups. Vested interests are "those appropriate modes of social agency that interactants have to engage in" – given their relationship to distributions of allocative and authoritative resources – "if they are to defend or enhance their life-chances against other interactants differently placed" in relation to these distributions.[30] Situational logics, as determined by "positions within relations", exert directional pressure on agents (individual and collective) to think and act in ways that do not undermine their vested interests. This is because structurally set situations in society

> attach specific opportunity costs to different modes of social agency. Forms of social agency which are out of phase with the vested interests of specific structurally situated collectives of interactants are likely to incur punishing sanctions.[31]

In summary, structures are causal owing to the fact that differential involuntary placement of people (or groups of people) *vis-à-vis* others distribute among them opposed vested interests (in social reform or transformation or reproduction) that are experienced as pressures they should, if they are being rational, act on. This is because human agents must face situational logics by virtue of their involuntary placement in structures whereby they would incur deficits or deductions from life chances (e.g. loss of income, status, or authority) if they acted in ways contrary to their vested interests.

The relevance of applying this CRT social ontology to the job of theorizing global political economy in the present work is as follows. The interstate system and the capitalist world economy confront human agents worldwide with emergent structures that situate them asymmetrically in relation to the main distributions of socially generated rewards (allocative or economic resources and authoritative or political resources) and which in doing so generate inequalities in power and reward and relations of domination and subordination between them. These economic and political structures, therefore, distribute for agents differently placed in them (as powerholders or non-powerholders, as beneficiaries or non-beneficiaries) vested interests in either their advancement or consolidation or in their abolition or transcendence.

In theory, at the level of concepts, the international nation-state system and the capitalist world economy could operate as rival systems that obstruct or counteract each other in the service of opposed vested interests. The possibility is afforded by the fact that these are governed by and sourced in different modes of social power – the power of authorization versus the power of allocation, or the power of command over people versus the power of control over property.[32] But, in practice, the development of modern society has more or less brought about a strategic alignment of polity and economy, of state and capital, of the power of ownership and the power of command – for reasons well theorized by Marx.[33]

This is because economic powerholders need political powerholders to guarantee their control of allocative resources, just as political powerholders require economic powerholders to bankroll the institutions by which they deploy their authoritative resources. Thus, for these reasons, global political economy is a force of *structural conditioning* that places definite and stringent constraints on the governance of crises that are invariably of its own making. These are economic and ecological crises generated by international capitalism, and political crises that stem from interstate rivalries that are linked to the capitalist mode. The only policy solutions to such crises that are allowable by powerholders are those that are compatible with the preservation of the systems that generate them. This, as I will show, is certainly true of the novel coronavirus pandemic.

This presents humanity with a fundamental, intractable problem. This is that the capitalist mode of production in the "global" age, as I argue in *Contagion Capitalism*, has become a force of economic ossification and zombification. The system has been characterized for 50 years by weak growth, stagnation, and recession so that its capacity to absorb major economic shocks (such as those that the present pandemic is delivering) is fatally compromised.[34] This is just as corporate capitalism's mode of relating humans to the physical world through production for its own sake is, by virtue of its international reach, generating conditions for new pandemics to arise.

Weberian sociologist David Lockwood's famous distinction between structural malintegration and social malintegration is relevant in this context.[35] The capitalist world economy today is *structurally* malintegrated owing to its inner institutional strains and antinomies – including the astronomical and widening gap between the incomes of rich and poor, its progressive tendency to subordinate human needs to capital growth, and the ecological havoc that it wreaks. The system is also *socially* malintegrated because from structural dissonance flows social disorder fanned by human discontent. This is why the "global" age has witnessed major convulsive upsurges of social conflict and the emergence of mass protest movements right across the world in response to the injustices and privations that the system imposes on billions of people worldwide.

Yet, in spite of this alignment of structural and social dissonance, corporate mega "zombie" capitalism perpetuates. It does so not owing to its own robustness but because the international nation-state system has been converted into its life-support system. This is due to the structural alignment of polity and economy that has been consolidated under neoliberal governance under the hegemony of the US and supported by the other "developed" countries.[36] To put it simply, wherever social conflicts and political protests and other forms of resistance happen to arise (and these are typically responses to economic pressures and assaults on entitlements – often originating outside national borders), and in response to whatever trigger events, these are more or less reined in by agents of state power. The universalization of social malintegration is countervailed by its splitting up or compartmentalization into "localisms" that are ring-fenced by national borders and policed by individual sovereign states.

The two great systems of global political economy – the economic order of zombified mega-capitalism and the political order of rival nation-states – are thus mutually reinforcing structures of domination. As long as their strategic alignment remains intact, these constitute radical obstacles to further progress in human development and in the global civilization process. A sustainable future for humanity – economically, ecologically, and socially – depends on transcending both systems or at least undermining the alliance of state power and capitalist power that is prolonging the demi-life of the latter.

Themes

This book, *Modernity and the Pandemic*, will draw on those resources of critique cited earlier to explore two main themes that seem to me necessary to a sociology of pandemics.

1. The impacts of cultures of individualism and consumerism, and of pervasive and deeply entrenched social inequalities (that is, *decivilization*), in weakening public compliance with NPIs and indeed with Pharmaceutical Interventions (PIs) – such as vaccination – that would protect us from pandemics such as COVID-19.
2. How interstate competition in world politics has undermined an effective international response to COVID-19. This is by subordinating worldwide human interests (and especially those of people in low-income countries) to national interests in the Global North and high-income countries more generally.

As for the companion volume, *Contagion Capitalism*, this draws on other resources of critique to explore new but related themes that also seem to me integral to pandemic sociology. These are:

1. How political mobilization of science and expertise as modes of legitimation for government policies compromised public health in the service of the interests of economic powerholders in the present pandemic.
2. How corporate mega-capitalism today – a system that mobilizes science and technology instrumentally, for the purpose of converting the natural world into mere resources of profit-driven industrial expansion, and which increasingly does this on an international scale – has rendered human populations the world over increasingly vulnerable to the threat of viral and other pandemics.
3. How the accelerated risk of global pandemics in our contemporary age is integral to the ecological crisis of unsustainability of the capitalist mode of production in the "global" corporate age. Thus, epidemiological rift is an aspect of planetary rift.
4. How the instrumental mode of biomedical technoscience under capitalism not only obscures a sociological understanding of the roots of global pandemics (thereby obstructing recognition of solutions that are possible only by recasting socioeconomic and sociopolitical orders) but also threatens public health and poses its own pandemic risks.

Structure

The book is set out in four chapters. Chapter 1 theorizes the emergent structures of contemporary global political economy, with a specific emphasis on the politics of the interstate system. Chapter 2 then situates the politics of pandemic management within these structures of global political economy. This is done by showing how pandemic politics were shaped (adversely) by the interface between the two intersecting orders of competition and domination – the world capitalist economy and the international state system – but with a specific emphasis on the role of interstate and imperial rivalries. Chapter 3 outlines the theory that decivilization is an integral aspect of capitalist modernization. Chapter 4 discusses the role of decivilizing processes in the COVID-19 pandemic. These processes are those which include diluting the effectiveness of NPIs as well as generating a degree of vaccine hesitancy, especially in poor and minority communities and social groups.

Terminology (a note on the efficacy of concepts)

Especially in the chapters of this book addressing global political economy (Chapter 1) and the pandemic in international relations (Chapter 2), I deploy the terms "developed", "developing", and on occasions, "semi-developed" and "underdeveloped", when referring to the economic status of countries within the international state system. This, as the editor of the Routledge Pandemic Series (Michael Ryan) observes, risks an "over-homogenized" representation of global divisions and inequalities as being set by national borders. Such terms, he opines,

> hold accurate for the vast majority of the time, but it is important to note that the elite in "developing" countries have often been able to avail themselves of the resources of the "developed" world to a far greater degree than even many of those living in that world ... It is important to distinguish between resources available within a given country and resources available to given individuals (from whatever country).[37]

Ryan provides the example of global vaccine inequities (which I address in Chapter 2) to demonstrate his point. On my account, the chief explanation of these inequities is precisely the division of the world into clusters of countries (developed, developing, and underdeveloped) that have a greater or lesser command of allocative and authoritative resources. But, as the series editor points out, and as he shows in his own work,[38] there is also the international social-class dimension that has shaped vaccine injustice.

Elites in developing or underdeveloped countries, as I noted earlier, have been able to sidestep local vaccine shortages that are generated by unequal vaccine competition between nation-states and fast-track their own protections by travelling to the high-income countries (where supplies are plentiful) to get their jabs. For example, "wealthy tourists from Latin America are traveling to the United States, where many hesitant citizens of that country are not getting vaccinated; they are finding vaccines easily available in tourist spots like Las Vegas and Miami".[39] This is just as elites in the developed world have been able to jump ahead or "cut the line" in the vaccination queues by paying for their doses overseas in certain developing countries. Ryan and Nanda cite "vaccine tours" for better-off Britons in the United Arab Emirates (UAE) and for wealthy Americans in the Caribbean as examples of this.[40] These benefits for the rich (of "globalization"), he suggests, may somewhat counteract or qualify my arguments that "states still matter"[41] in the global political economy (Chapter 1) and that these have been the crucial players in determining vaccine advantages and disadvantages worldwide (Chapter 2).

Now, Michael Ryan is right that focusing on inequalities at the level of international relations does risk losing sight of the inequalities generated by global class divisions, including those of vaccine allocation. However, I think this is a consequence that flows unavoidably from any focus on the interstate system, such as is the focus in this book, which I have shown is indispensable for apprehending global inequalities. Thus, it is a fact that vaccines were largely monopolized by governments of high-income countries – and this was on behalf of *whole* national citizenries rather than on behalf of *particular* citizenship groups. That is, of course, a different matter to elites everywhere looking after themselves by means of border-hopping queue-jumping. Yes, elites in developed and developing countries doubtless got ahead in the race to inoculate as "ordinary folk" were left further behind. Nonetheless, ordinary folk in high-income countries benefited from fast-tracked vaccine rollouts, whereas those in the low-income countries did not. This was and still is, for the latter, the consequence of being "ordinary" in a *developing* or *underdeveloped* country, where governments can less afford mass vaccine procurements and are reliant on the "charitable" donations of the wealthier nations.

The concepts of "developed", "developing", and "underdeveloped", as applied to making sense of the economic status of countries in the hierarchized international state system, thus have crucial explanatory relevance in accounting for pandemic-related inequities, including and especially those of vaccine distribution and supply. Consequently, the reality of cross-border vaccine exploitation by footloose elites, as ordinary feet-of-clay people were compelled to wait in line within national borders for their doses, hardly undermines my argument that states matter (and indeed matter a lot) in shaping world affairs, including those affairs of the pandemic. It is commonplace that some states have a much greater command of powers of authorization and allocation than others. This is what explains how everyone in developed countries within 12 months was offered an opportunity to have a COVID-19 jab and why this was not the situation elsewhere in developing countries. As I show in this book, the main issue for high-income countries is now vaccine hesitancy (a demand-side problem), not vaccine inaccessibility (a supply-side problem), whereas the reverse is true of the low-income countries.

Sean Creaven

3 July 2021 (updated May 2022 and May 2023)

Notes

1 Bringing the insights and tools of social science to bear on the pandemic is the purpose of the Routledge COVID-19 series, of which my books are a part. See especially these collections: Gammel, I. and Wang, J. (Eds.) (2022). *Creative Resilience and COVID-19: Figuring the everyday in a pandemic.* London and New York: Routledge; Ryan, J.M. (Ed.) (2023). *COVID-19: Individual rights and community responsibilities.* London and New York: Routledge; Ryan. J.M. (Ed.) (2023). *COVID-19: Surviving a pandemic.*

London and New York: Routledge; Ryan, J.M. (Ed.) (2021). *COVID-19: Global pandemic, societal responses, ideological solutions.* London and New York: Routledge.

2 By structure or structures I mean the antecedent structural properties of social systems that are ontologically distinct from human agency and social practices by virtue of their emergence from social interaction, which operate causally in the reproduction of social systems. This is elaborated later in this introduction.

3 Dolan, P. (2011). *Civilizing Processes.* Centre for Consumption and Leisure Studies: Technological University Dublin.

4 Elias, N. (2000). *The Civilizing Process: Sociogenetic and Psychogenetic Investigations.* (Revised edition). [1939]. Oxford: Blackwell.

5 See also: Nanda, S. and Ryan, J.M. (2022). 'The Importance of Culture in Understanding the COVID-19 Pandemic'. J.M. Ryan (Ed.) *COVID-19: Cultural Changes and Institutional Adaptations.* London and New York: Routledge.

6 Yet, as Michael Ryan (p. 18) observes, "the word 'responsibility' appears nowhere in the UN Universal Declaration of Human Rights, or in the Constitution of the USA". See: Ryan, J.M. (2023). 'Individual Rights, and Community Responsibilities'. J.M. Ryan (Ed.) *Individual Rights.*

7 Campbell, D. (2021). 'Extent of mental health crisis in England at "terrifying" level'. *Guardian* (9 April). This is of course driven by opponents of lockdowns rather than champions of the mental wellbeing of young people. This was especially strident in the campaign to reopen schools as the pandemic raged. See: Trick, S. (2022). '"A classic moral panic": A psychiatrist on school and kids' mental health during COVID-19'. *TVO Today* (online). (17 February).

8 This is especially so for the young who, although low risk for COVID-19 physical illness, are socially constructed (by the media, parents, and assorted experts) as particularly vulnerable to "lockdown" mental illness owing to their supposed lesser "resilience" compared to older people. Naturally, the young then respond in the expected ways when questioned by researchers, not least because they do not enjoy lockdowns. See: Catling, J.C. *et al.* (2022). 'Effects of the COVID-19 lockdown on mental health in a UK student sample'. *BMC Psychology*, 10 (110), pp. 1–7. This study imagined, bizarrely, that mental distress in undergraduates could be gleaned from their increased rates of "smartphone usage". Such, it was surmised, was indicative of "smartphone addiction". Yet increased smartphone usage would be a way of ensuring that physical distancing did not become increased social distancing. More credibly, perhaps, the study found that rates of self-reported depression among young people increased from 30 percent to 44 percent during the pandemic and that rates of anxiety increased from 22 percent to 27 percent. This author has never been convinced that "anxiety" as such is a mental health indicator. Anxiety is a natural response to a global pandemic, especially given the failure of governments to prioritize public health over money-making.

9 Marshall, L., Bibby, J., and Abbs, I. (2020). *Emerging evidence on COVID-19's impact on mental health and health inequalities.* Health Foundation (online). (18 June).

10 Catling *et al.* (2022); Karantzas, G. (2022). 'Lockdowns doubled your risk of mental health symptoms'. *Conversation* (12 April). This was the author's remarkable conclusion from his review of 33 published papers, even though, he claims, many of these were lacking in research quality.

11 Gillard, S. (2021). 'Experiences of living with mental health problems during the COVID-19 pandemic in the UK: a coproduced, participatory qualitative interview study'. *Social Psychiatry and Psychiatric Epidemiology*, 56, pp. 1447–50; Marshall *et al.* (2020); Mind (2021). *What has the impact of coronavirus been on mental health?* (online). (June).

12 Ryan, J.M. and Nanda, S. (2023). 'Vaccines – are we really in this together?' J.M. Ryan (Ed.). *Surviving a pandemic.*

13 Ryan and Nanda (2023), p. 84.

14 Ryan and Nanda (2023), p. 85.

15 This is explored in Ch.2.

16 As I argue in Ch.3.

17 See Ch.3.

18 Harman, C. (1991). 'The state and capitalism today'. *International Socialism*, 2 (51), pp. 3–54.

19 See especially: Jacobson, D. (1997). *Rights Across Borders: Immigration and the Decline of Citizenship*. Baltimore: Johns Hopkins University Press.

20 My theory selection may appear rather eclectic – this drawing together of "postmodern-ist" and "modernist" concepts and theorists. However, sometimes "filing cabinets" are not useful. My interest in the "two B's" (Baudrillard and Bauman) is not their supposed "postmodernism" but the power of the substantive critiques they offer of our society, which are quite compatible with a materialist-oriented critical theory of capitalism, unlike the bulk of stuff produced under the auspices of radical social constructionism and anti-humanism. Bauman certainly does not fit the definition of theoretical "anti-humanist", for example.

    The Baudrillard upon whom I draw is the one who saw his work as updating Marx, as complementing Marx, by addressing the mode of consumption which the capitalist mode of production generated as this shifted to Fordism. I do not read these critiques as especially or definitively postmodern. Indeed, this would not have been a descrip-tion of his work that Baudrillard at that stage of his intellectual journey would have accepted.

    The same point applies to the Bauman upon whom I draw. Bauman's work on con-sumerism is really after he has ditched the postmodernism in favour of notions of hyper-modernization as "liquid" and "light". But, even if Bauman may be considered "postmodern", his radical critique of consumer culture is perfectly compatible with a humanistic critical theory such as Marxism offers. Indeed, he is sometimes accused of "Marxism" by critics.

    My reason for utilizing the critiques of these two is thus simply that I find them powerful and persuasive. They are far more useful to a *critical* theory of contemporary society than those offered by "modernists" such as Giddens and Beck (though even these have their uses, as I will show). This is because the cultural developments they explore are recognized as profoundly alienating (or, as I would put it, *decivilizing*). Moreover, in my view, the cultural developments they relay cannot be grasped outside the structures of corporate capitalism today, which is something that they themselves rather lose sight of.

21 Archer, M.S. (1995). *Realist Social Theory: The Morphogenetic Approach*. Cambridge: Cambridge University Press.

22 Creaven, S. (2000). *Marxism and Realism: A materialistic application of realism in the social sciences*. London and New York: Routledge. See esp. Ch.2 and Ch.3.

23 Creaven (2000), Ch. 4.

24 Beck, U. (1992). *Risk Society: Towards A New Modernity*. London: Sage.

25 Beck, U. (1999). *World Risk Society*. Cambridge: Polity Press.

26 Creaven, S. (2007). *Emergentist Marxism: Dialectical Philosophy and Social Theory*. London and New York: Routledge, p. 177.

27 Archer (1995), p. 201.

28 Creaven (2000), Ch. 4; Creaven (2007), pp. 142–43.

29 Archer (1995), p. 201.

30 Creaven (2007), p. 177.

31 Creaven (2007), p. 178.

32 Mann, M. (1986). *The Sources of Social Power: A History of Power from the Beginning to AD 1760*. Vol. 1. Cambridge: Cambridge University Press.

33 As elaborated in his theory of socio-historical materialism. See: Marx, K. and Engels, F. (1970). *The German Ideology*. [1845]. London: Lawrence and Wishart; Marx, K. and Engels, F. (1967). *The Communist Manifesto*. [1848]. Harmondsworth: Penguin;

Marx, K. (1970). *A Contribution to the Critique of Political Economy*. [1859]. London: Lawrence and Wishart; Marx, K. (1978). *The Poverty of Philosophy*. [1847]. Peking: Foreign Languages Press; Marx, K. (1934). *The Eighteenth Brumaire of Louis Bonaparte*. [1852]. Moscow: Progress Publishers. For excellent introductions see: Callinicos, A. (1995). *The Revolutionary Ideas of Karl Marx*. 2nd edition. London: Bookmarks; Collier, A. (2004). *Marx*. Oxford: One World. For useful reconstructive defences see: Callinicos, A. (1987). *Making History: Agency, Structure and Change in Social Theory*. Cambridge: Polity Press; Cohen, G.A. (1978). *Karl Marx's Theory of History: A Defence*. Oxford: Oxford University Press; Creaven (2000, 2007); Levine, A. (1984). *Arguing For Socialism: Theoretical Considerations*. London: Routledge and Kegan Paul.

34 Brenner, R. (2006). *The Economics of Global Turbulence: The Advanced Capitalist Economies from Long Boom to Long Downturn, 1945–2005*. London: Verso.
35 Lockwood, D. (1964). 'Social Integration and System Integration'. G.K. Zolschan and H.W. Hirsch (Eds.) *Explorations in Social Change*. Boston: Houghton Mifflin.
36 This is the interstate system grasped as *imperialism* as explored in Ch.1.
37 Ryan, J.M. (2023). *Personal Communication*. (27 February).
38 Ryan and Nanda (2023).
39 Ryan and Nanda (2023), p. 184.
40 Ryan (27 February, 2023); Ryan and Nanda (2023), p. 184.
41 Ryan (27 February, 2023).

1 Neoliberalism, capitalism, and imperialism

In my book *Contagion Capitalism*, I addressed one good explanation of how the asymmetries or imbalances in the world economy are reproduced. This was that these are the necessary effects of the unfettered markets that neoliberal governance has imposed internationally.[1] But this is only part of the explanation. A second answer to this "how" question – which actually dovetails with the first – is simply *imperialism*. Imperialism in this book is to be understood as generated by the dynamic interface of two kinds of competition – economic (inter-capitalist) and geopolitical (interstate) – in their evolving forms and connections, in the pre-neoliberal and post-neoliberal epochs, which together constitute the global political economy. This chapter is intended to grasp the relationship between neoliberal capitalist economics and neo-imperial geopolitics in reproducing the structures of advantage and disadvantage, domination and subordination, of global political economy today.

Mega-capitalism and global disorder

A world economy that is structured by (for the most part) unregulated inter-capitalist competition is inherently unbalanced, and hence potentially dangerous and unstable politically, as well as ideologically volatile. Such an economy must generate, owing to the operation of its own structurally based generative mechanisms, vast and growing asymmetries between social classes within countries and across the world – and along with these a hardening of class grievances and antagonisms domestically and across borders. Thus, a capitalist world economy based on free trade is structurally incapable of eliminating world poverty and delivering economic or social justice for the majority of the world's population.

Such an economic system, if left to its own structurally generated "laws of motion", must also reproduce widening development and income gaps between high-income countries and those "Third World" countries locked into underdevelopment and dependency in the system's periphery. This means that conflicts over the distribution of allocative resources are not simply those between possessing and non-possessing classes or between privileged minorities and underprivileged majorities. Rather, these conflicts are also between various other constituencies of "haves" and "have nots" or those between "greater haves" and "lesser haves" on the international canvas – that is, between rival states, rival imperialisms, and

DOI: 10.4324/9781003437208-2

sub-imperialisms, and between the US-hegemon-led developed world and the rest. These conflicts are integral or internal and necessary to mega-capitalism because this mode is constituted by an international state system dominated by great powers that are committed to preserving an economic status quo that serves their national advantages in the global pecking order.

This means that the contemporary world order is socially malintegrated because it is structurally malintegrated at the levels of polity and economy. The real-world phenomenal or empirical effects of this are manifold. These include Huntington's "clash of civilizations" (especially between the Christian West and the Islamist East);[2] international "blow-back terrorism" (the weapon of economically marginal-ized and politically disenfranchised non-state actors from usually poor countries against oppressor governments or states and their supposed civilian "accom-plices");[3] civil wars and border wars in the economic wastelands of the periphery; and inter-communal or ethnic group antagonisms everywhere (usually motivated by asymmetries of allocative or authoritative resources between minorities and majori-ties).[4] However, the social malintegration that world capitalism and its life-support system of interstate political governance generates is also more or less, and for the most part, politically contained for reasons that will be discussed in this chapter.

Not only is mega-capitalism integrally or structurally dissonant, but it has become ever more so in the era of neoliberalism, owing in part to the multiple fail-ures of the neoliberal project. As I will argue,[5] the neoliberal age has witnessed, as might be predicted given its global architecture, a hardening of wealth and income inequalities between rich and poor in most places. This is despite record levels of people in waged employment worldwide and the decline of those in subsistence farming – the traditional bastion of rural poverty. The world economy today is rooted in mostly urban-based wage labour.

In 1800, just three percent of the world's population lived in towns and cit-ies. Today, 54 percent of the world's population does.[6] By 1980, the share of the world's economically active population employed in the industrial and service sectors surpassed for the first time that employed in the primary sector (mining, agriculture, fishing, and forestry).[7] At the time of writing, just one-third of the world's economically active population still derive their primary livelihood from the land, from subsistence farming, though the absolute number of peasants, petty farmers, and landless rural workers is higher than ever before.[8] This represents a massive expansion of the world's working class. By the start of the twenty-first century, Marx's proletariat – those propertyless economic actors who derive the main part of their income from the commodification of their own labour power – was poised to become the majority social class of global humanity.[9]

Such radical socioeconomic disequilibria may be offset by other system-wide benefits, however. These are exactly those that were promised by neoliberal cham-pions of boundless capitalism. Two are especially worthy of note – upon which the legitimacy of neoliberal politics arguably hinges. One of these is simply the gradual elimination of the most extreme forms of poverty as the world's poor are pulled away from subsistence agriculture into paid employment, reducing the old peasantry to a residual or rump class, in effect proletarianizing the global workforce. The other is the supposed "trickle down" impacts of faster growth and bigger profits, which it was promised would flow from unleashing the "dynamism of the market" (that is, maximizing capital freedoms).

Now, worldwide proletarianization has indeed substantially reduced "extreme" poverty (on the World Bank's definition). But the global rise of the world's working class, driven by capitalist internationalization and by post-colonial modernizations in the Global South, precedes the neoliberal age. This, indeed, had its biggest push during the postwar boom. Moreover, under neoliberalism, the reduction in the proportion of the world's population who are among the "very poorest" (based on the World Bank's definition) has been accompanied by a dramatic increase in the number of "working poor".[10] This is the global multitude whose number often hovers precariously (by the odd dollar or two) above the World Bank's arbitrary and pitiless poverty threshold. Finally, as also discussed in my *Contagion Capitalism*, neoliberalism simply has not delivered on its promise to restore dynamism to the world economy in the long period since the collapse of the postwar boom. Even if trickle-down economics was not ideological, the opportunities for it are curtailed by conditions of weak GDP growth, stagnant foreign direct investment (FDI), and fragile profits, which characterize our present times.

Neoliberalism and globalization theory

But, as I have argued elsewhere,[11] neoliberalism sets itself against a divergence theory of world economy based on the ideas of neo-classical economist Robert Solow. Instead, for neoliberalism, the unfettered operation of world markets is reckoned to usher in an era of global economic convergence. Now, the ideology of convergence sits at the heart of a particular strain of globalization theory that regards the world economy as becoming increasingly integrated owing to capitalist transnationalism. "Globalization", of course, has become all the rage in business studies and the social sciences since the 1990s, at least at the level of economic processes. According to this, since the 1980s, capitalism has essentially globalized. This means that world trade, investment, and production have become or are becoming *de-territorialized*. Hence *trans-state capitalism* is, according to globalization theory, either an established fact or one that is at least on the horizon.[12]

This "globalization", it is said, is driven primarily by technological change and innovation. This is especially by the "communications revolution" (hence virtually mediated stock exchanges and finance markets that instantaneously shift capital to the four corners of the earth) and "weightless" production (carried by the technologies of computerization, automation, cybernetics, and the worldwide web). But it is also carried by the "new capitalism", consumerist and corporate, of global leisure and tourism and of "footloose" (that is, totally mobile) mega-corporations. As such, this globalization is said to have drawn each corner of the globe into a fully *integrated* global marketplace – or to be well along the road to doing so. This, on some accounts, has generated a world economy where production and exchange are driven by global consumerism and "sign-value" (that is, the purchasing decisions of a burgeoning urban-based global citizenry for reasons of identity- and status-affirmation).[13]

For virtually all globalization theorists, however, the ascendancy of the world market and global economic integration has completely or at least substantially subordinated the nation-state to a capitalism that is supposedly *trans*national. This is because "global enterprises" – or "stateless corporations" (as *Business Week* dubbed them)[14] – have emancipated themselves from reliance on any state in particular, it is claimed. This allows them to curtail or even undermine the capacity of governments to implement policies that would place any kind of limits on commodification, consumer-driven growth, and corporate profits.[15]

Most hyperglobalists regard globalization as a good thing because the subordination or disciplining of nation-states by the market ensures that the citizen-as-consumer is empowered. Collective state actors, owing to trans-nationalization, cannot impinge on individual market-actors. These supportive hyperglobalists are thus champions of free-market *capitalism*, hence of neoliberalism. Globalization is, for them, exactly trade liberalization, privatization, and financial deregulation writ large on a world scale – and these developments will (if supported by a politics that disposes of the interventionist social-democratic or socialist state) guarantee worldwide economic growth and prosperity, expand consumer opportunity, and substantially abolish world poverty.[16]

As arch-neoliberal then UK Prime Minister Tony Blair put it when patronizing the Seattle anti-capitalism protestors in 2000: "World trade is good for people's jobs and people's living standards. These protests are a complete outrage".[17] Yet a minority of hyperglobalists regard globalization as disastrous by virtue of exactly those same economic processes and policies lauded by neoliberals (that is, trade liberalization, unrestrained cross-border capital flows, deregulated labour markets, and subordination of state to market). These, they hold, trap the world's poor in poverty, empower the corporate elite at the expense of the workers, strengthen the dominance of the developed countries over the others, and widen wealth and income disparities worldwide.[18]

But globalization theory is false because globalization is partly mythical. As Emmanuel Todd rightly says: "The debate about 'globalization' … is in part disconnected from reality because we too often accept the orthodox representation of commercial and financial exchanges as being symmetrical and homogeneous".[19] This, after all, is the meaning of global economic *integration* that globalization is reputedly all about. This can be empirically substantiated by examining patterns or trends in the main cross-border exchanges (that is, in trade, investment, and production) since World War Two. These are some distance from being "symmetrical" and "homogeneous". Nor are these "borderless" or trans-nationalized. These are not generating or sustaining an economically integrated world in any straightforward kind of way.

International trade

Starting with international trade, globalization theorists are right that the period has witnessed an enormous expansion in the volume of world trade. Indeed, this has been especially the case since the 1990s, when so-called globalization really accelerated. World trade doubled between 1960 and 1990.[20] But, more suggestive still of globalization, this increased 27 times between 1950 and 2008 – a rate three-times faster than world output growth.[21] Consequently, the trade-to-GDP ratio rose from 25 percent to 60 percent over this period.[22] Yet, despite this, by 1990, 80 percent of world output was still for domestic or national markets rather than for export.[23] And today, a further 25 years down the line, approximately 30 percent of the value of world GDP (WGP) is traded internationally, whereas 70 percent is still bought and sold within national borders.[24]

Now, the share of world trade of the developed countries (especially of North America, Japan, and the European Union) was 72 percent of the total in 1990 – so that the rest of the world had only 28 percent.[25] By 2012, however, the developed world's share of world trade had diminished to around 56 percent,[26] whereas by 2017, NATFA, the EU, and the AFTA accounted for 58 percent of the total.[27] This was because, according to the World Trade Organization (WTO), the share of world trade going to developing countries increased from 26 percent in 1995 to 39 percent in 2014.[28] This, they suggest, demonstrates globalization at work – which is a force for the growing global *integration* of trade.

Further progress in equalizing world trade has stalled since 2012, however. In 2020, the developing world's proportion of it was 44 percent, the same as eight years earlier.[29] Of much greater importance, the apparent globalization of trade was almost entirely owing to just a select few countries joining the club of NICs and BRICs over the past 20 or so years (China, India, Argentina, Brazil, and so on). In fact, the rise of India, but especially of China, has been responsible for nearly all world trade growth outside the developed world over this period. China increased its share of world trade from just one percent in 1980 to 13 percent by 2011, as the WTO itself acknowledges.[30] This means that 85 percent of world trade today is circulated in very specific places – North America, the European Union, developed Oceania, Southeast Asia, China (or rather specific coastal regions of China), India, and one or two other BRICs – rather than being globally diffused. By contrast, the share of world trade of that part of the Global South that cannot be counted as among its handful of economic success-stories (that is, the so-called *under*developed world) was just 16 percent at the start of the 1990s. Yet, in the early 1960s, these "Third World" countries enjoyed a 24 percent share.[31]

Today, just 20 countries monopolize almost three-quarters of export trade in goods or merchandise. These are all either the developed countries or NICs and BRICs – namely, the US, Canada, China, Hong Kong, Japan, Russia, Mexico, Brazil, India, Singapore, Taiwan, South Korea, the UK, plus seven of the EU nations (Germany, France, Belgium, Spain, Italy, the Netherlands, and Switzerland).[32] This pattern of divergence rather than convergence is even more marked for export trade in IP services and in services generally – the so-called cutting edge of "post-industrial" capitalism. This is most asymmetric in IP, with 92 percent of world trade in these services circulating within and dominated by developed countries. As the WTO reports: "39% of exports are from EU, 34% from US, 11% from Japan and 8% from other developed countries".[33]

Trade in services generally is also dominated by the developed world (with a 70 percent share), whereas the share of all but six percent of the remainder circulates to the newly emergent South Asian economies (especially China, India, and the other NICs of the Pacific Rim).

In 2019, developing economies' share of world services exports (US\$6.1 trillion) was 30 per cent (US\$1.83 trillion). The highest share of world services exports was recorded by developing Asia at more than 24 per cent. The top three services exporters are China (4.6 per cent), India (3.4 per cent) and Singapore (3.5 per cent). They account for more than 40 per cent of developing economies' services exports.[34]

Even though the "contribution of developing economies to trade in services grew by more than ten percentage points between 2005 and 2017", this was "mainly concentrated in five economies. The share of least developed countries remains small".[35] Ever the masters of credulity and understatement when it comes to admitting the development failures of world capitalism, the WTO observes that the "participation of developing countries in services trade is *not yet* [my emphasis] inclusive".

A close look reveals that trade is very concentrated, with the same five economies ranking both as leading services exporters and importers, although in a different order. In 2017, China was the leading services trader, followed by Hong Kong (China), the Republic of Korea, Singapore and India. These five Asian economies accounted for 56.7 per cent of developing economies' exports and 58.1 per cent of imports.[36]

Not *yet* indeed – or rather simply not so. The share of trade in services of 125 other developing countries was just 10.7 per cent for exports and 16.1 percent for imports in 2018. But, not in the least bit deflated by the fact that this "not yet" has so far taken more than 70 years to materialize since the end of the colonial period, or by the lack of any sign that this happy state of affairs is on the way, or by the fact that the development failures outnumber the successes by 25:1, the WTO instead heroically assumes that global inclusivity is merely deferred. This is just as it lauds the five's "impressive trade performance…From R&D and IP-related services to ICT services, professional services and finance". Yet even the successful five, the WTO admits, "make up only 14.2% of exports and 17.3% of imports" in the global marketplace.[37]

The pattern of world trade thus does not look terribly global. These statistics do not support the idea that global integration of trade *has* happened. This is contrary to the claims of the hyperglobalists or globalization boosters. Nor indeed do these statistics support the lesser notion that global integration of trade *is* happening or is *in the making*. Rather, the pattern revealed is triadic, evidencing more a regionalization rather than a globalization of world export trade, as flows of goods and services are chased by "price signals" to those places where consumer markets are

most profitable. Regionalization of trade is most marked in the developed economies of North America and Europe. Trade within the EU accounts for 63 percent
of its exports, whereas trade within the North American Trade Area (NAFTA)
accounts for half of its exports.[38] Most of the rest of EU export trade flows, firstly,
to NATFA, and secondly, to the Association of Southeast Asian Nations (ASEAN).
Most of the rest of NATFA export trade flows, firstly, to the EU, and secondly, to
the ASEAN. Trade within the ASEAN, by contrast, accounts for 24 percent of its
exports, with the bulk of the rest flowing to either NATFA or the EU or China.[39]
This patterning is contrary to the claims not only of hyperglobalists but arguably
also of moderate globalists or self-styled transformationalists.

International production

But enough has now been said about international trade. I will now focus on world
goods production. Is there *here* evidence of global integration, either as fact or as
process? The following statistics may shed some light on this issue. Between 1990
and 2005, the level of manufacturing taking place in developing countries rose from
19 percent to 30 percent of the world's output.[40] So, on the face of it, this is a sign of
a growing global diffusion of industrial production from the wealthier Global North
to the poorer Global South. Now, this is not indicative of "globalization" in the
sense of accomplished fact, since, after all, 71 percent of manufacturing output was
still in the advanced economies by the mid-2000s. Indeed, three-quarters of it was
in 2004 concentrated in just 21 countries.[41] But at least this might be indicative of a
globalizing dynamic at work – and one that is leading towards economic globalism.

   However, even the lesser argument of moderate or cautious globalists does not
really fit the facts. This is because only five countries – China and certain other
Southeast Asian "tigers" – accounted for 62 percent of the increase in industrial
goods production in the whole of the developing world between 1980 and 2005.
Most of the rest was accounted for by the other BRICs in Asia and Latin America.
Elsewhere, across the Global South, there was little evidence of industrial growth.[42]
Again, as was the case for international trade, this indicates that the pattern of
industrialization in the developing world does not, as this first appeared, provide
evidence in favour of economic globalization. Not only that, since "production" is
not simply of goods, of course, but also of services, a decline of control over the
former by the high-income countries is not necessarily indicative of the erosion
of their primacy in the world economy generally. Far from it. The Global North's
dominance of international trade in services is in fact indicative of its control of
output from services.

   In any case, since the mid-2000s, the manufacturing industry worldwide has
become if anything more concentrated in fewer industrial centres than before, even
though the most recent pattern does at least reveal erosion of the dominance of
the developed countries in world goods production. Just ten countries accounted
for around 72.2 percent of WGP from manufacturing in 2017.[43] Despite the "post-
industrial" shift of the developed countries away from goods-production industries and towards service industries, six of the top ten manufacturing countries

nonetheless remained in the Global North, whereas the others were either NICs or newly emergent BRICs. This further centralization and concentration of industrialization (rather than its globalization), which also finally broke the primacy of the advanced or developed countries in manufacturing, was almost wholly driven by China's continued breakneck economic expansion and the US's and Japan's relative decline as "factory" economies. In 2000, China accounted for 6.5 percent of the world's industrial goods production, whereas the US accounted for 26.3 percent and Japan 18.3 percent of it. By 2017, China was responsible for 27.5 percent of global factory output, whereas the US's share has fallen to 17 percent and Japan's to 7.6 percent.[44]

Today, 70 percent of world trade and 25 percent of world production is carried out by MNCs or MNEs), and their sales account for 50 percent of WGP.[45] As Lesley Sklair points out, the majority of these MNCs are Western companies, hailing from the Global North. Hence their predominance in the world economy is also the predominance of the West or of the Global North.[46] A total of 24 of the world's largest MNCs are US corporations, whereas 72 of the world's biggest 100 MNCs hail from a handful of developed countries: the US, Japan, the UK, Germany, and France.[47] This is not evidence of a global diffusion of corporate power. Nonetheless, as Alan Rugman has shown, the West by no means monopolizes corporate power. By the start of the twenty-first century, although a large majority of the biggest MNCs were US or European, a significant number of South Asian companies had joined this elite capitalist club. "Of the fifty largest MNEs in manufacturing, twenty-five have their home region in North America, fifteen in Europe, and ten in the Asia-Pacific".[48]

The investments and sales of these mega-corporations are also heavily concentrated in their home regions. Thus, a triadic regionalization of corporate-capitalist power has been consolidated in recent decades, not its globalization. This is where the bulk of production, sales, and assets of the MNCs are situated in their home regions within the triad. By contrast: "Extremely few MNEs operate globally; nearly all are regionally based".[49] Much is made by globalists of the results revealed by the trans-nationalization index. This measures the proportion of sales, investments, and assets of the biggest corporations that are located outside their home countries. These results, it is claimed, establish the transnational status of corporate capitalism today.

But the trans-nationalization index tells us nothing about the proportion of corporate business activity that is situated within a home region or within the triad as a whole; the focus is narrowly nationalistic. Yet, even according to this data, 35 percent of the business of the top 100 MNCs today is conducted in their home countries,[50] whereas by the early 2000s, more than half of the business of the world's 50 biggest MNCs was situated in their home countries.[51] Even the most "global" companies make the bulk of their sales within the triad (spreading these across North America, the European Union, and Southeast Asia) rather than outside. According to statistics gathered at the close of the 1990s, 85 percent of the output of these corporations (whether from goods or services) is produced in their home countries and home regions and just 15 percent by their overseas subsidiaries.[52]

International investment

These statistics too appear to challenge the views of both hyperglobalists and moderate globalists. Neither production nor sales have been globalized – and the present trends do not, as far as can reasonably be supposed, support the view of a definite move in that direction. Rather, these indicate less a global pattern and more a regional one. But what about cross-border money flows? Is world investment globalized or becoming global? Does this differ significantly from the patterns for trade and production? There has certainly been a massive increase in cross-border investment in the postwar period – and this has been especially pronounced since the 1990s.

> Foreign direct investment shot up: flows of it rising from $37 billion in 1982 to $1,200 billion in 2006; the cumulative stock of FDI rose from 4 percent of world gross domestic product in 1950 ... to 36 percent in 2007.[53]

For the Organization for Economic Co-operation and Development (OECD), the stock of incoming FDI as a proportion of GDP increased from 28.8 percent in 2009 ($12.32 billion) to 44.3 percent ($22.12 billion) in 2017. The OECD's stock of outgoing FDI increased from 36.6 percent ($15.66 billion) to 50.5 percent ($25.22 billion) over the same period.[54] Nonetheless, the global imbalances in the distribution of FDI are striking.

In 2015, the developing world – which has 83 percent of the global population – received around 45 percent of FDI, according to the UN. Therefore, the developed countries, including North America, Japan, and the EU – which have almost 17 percent of the world population – obviously received the larger share of 55 percent.[55] In 2016, the developed countries did even better, increasing their share of global FDI to 59 percent of the total, meaning the share of the rest of the world shrank to 41 percent.[56] This certainly looks remarkably asymmetric. Per head of population investment in the developed world is more than seven times higher than in the developing world. Yet there has been a longer-run tendency since 2007 for the global distribution of FDI to shift away from the Global North and towards the Global South – or at least certain parts of the Global South. From 1986 through to 2007, the proportion of FDI going to developed countries averaged 68.5 percent per annum.[57] Since 2008, though, this has been reduced to an average of 48.5 percent per annum.[58] These statistics do support, on the face of it, a globalizing dynamic at work, at least in terms of FDI, though this tendency towards apparent redistribution of investment funds from the developed to the developing world also shows signs of partial reversal over the past few years.[59]

However, the initial phase of capitalist internationalization under the spur of neoliberal policies in the 1980s and 1990s led to a massive increase in inequality of world investment to the advantage of the developed countries. At the start of the 1960s, the developing countries (which, of course, includes those that are not developing) received half of world FDI.[60] By contrast, with the consolidation of the neoliberal "globalization" era, from 1986 to 1990, the proportion of world FDI going to the developed countries reached an all-time high of 82 percent per year on average, and this was running at 69.2 percent over the course of the 1990s.[61]

Thus, in 1960, there was an "even split" between the developed world and the rest in the distribution of world FDI (though investment per head of population was five times higher in the former), whereas in 2018 the share going to developing and transitional economies was 55 percent.[62] From a longer historical view, then, the levelling gains of supposed globalization look much less impressive. Between 2015 and 2018, the developed world absorbed an average of 52.5 percent of total world FDI.[63] This was marginally more than was the case six decades earlier.

But, indeed, if one considers *all* cross-border capital flows (not simply FDI), the asymmetry between the Global North and the Global South widens still further. In 2018, for example, developed countries received 70 percent of all capital inflows. Not only that, the imbalance within the developing world itself over who gets what is even more marked in terms of total capital investment funds than in terms of FDI inflows. "Developing Asia" received 39.4 percent of the FDI that went to all developing countries in 2018, for example, yet that same year received three-quarters of total capital investments bound for the developing world.[64]

These FDI statistics, which seemingly indicate a tendency since the mid-2000s for a more even global pattern of foreign investment, may in fact disguise a growing *inequality* of world FDI allocation. This is because almost two-thirds of FDI that goes to the developing world is received by just a few countries. These are, of course, the NICs and BRICs, which the World Bank in recent years has dubbed the newly emerging markets (NEMs). These select few countries received, in 2015 for example, almost two-thirds of the total that went to the developing world. Now, one can finger-count these countries: China and Hong Kong (which alone had 18 percent that year), Singapore, Taiwan, Korea, India, Brazil, and Mexico.[65] By 2018, of the top 20 countries receiving incoming FDI, ten were developed, whereas the others were mostly NEMs. The US was by far the biggest recipient, with around 21.5 percent of the total, followed by China (12 percent) and Hong Kong (ten percent). Of the top ten countries for receiving FDI in 2018, half were developed, whereas the other half were made up of NICs and BRICs. Together, these received approximately 79.3 percent of the total.[66]

These statistics reveal also major intra-regional imbalances. In recent years, by far the biggest recipient of FDI in the developing world has been the cluster of NICs referred to by the World Bank as "developing Asia". In 2012, these received 27.5 percent of it, but by 2018, their portion of it had grown to 39.4 percent. But even here – the most dynamic part of the developing world – the asymmetries in resource allocation are radical. Almost three-quarters (73 percent) of FDI received by "developing Asia" in 2018 went to just four countries: China, Hong Kong, India, and Singapore.[67] The same pattern is true of Latin America and the Caribbean. These regions received 11.3 percent of world FDI in 2018. But 71 percent of this went to just three countries: Brazil, Mexico, and Argentina.[68]

There is also another problem with these statistics. This is that they disguise the fact that quite a lot of so-called FDI is actually a form of economic imperialism. This is basically in two ways. Firstly, this is because the subsidiaries of (mostly Western) MNCs operating in poor countries actually raise a lot of capital for investment in the host countries themselves.[69] But this is then counted as FDI being brought into the poor host country by the MNC. As the UN's 2019 *World Investment Report* observes: "A significant part of investment between developing countries (South–South FDI) is ultimately owned by developed-country MNEs".[70] Thereafter, the profits made by the MNC are then exported or repatriated to the MNC's home country or home region, which partly explains why the poorer countries are net exporters of capital.[71]

Secondly, a lot of FDI is also used to buy up or buy out existing enterprises rather than generating new ones, which amounts to the foreign appropriation of "resources for development" rather than the generation of additional investment in them. This may be called neoliberal imperialism. This amounts to a transfer of ownership – from local ownership to ownership by a foreign MNC. This is so-called "brownfield" or "merger-and-acquisition" (M&A) FDI, which may be preferred by foreign MNCs and other investors to "greenfield" FDI owing to the lower financial risks and higher profits. This has often involved the privatization of formerly publicly owned industries, often infrastructural (power, water, communications, and so on), but often other sectors such as media and banking.

> In developing countries, the share of cross-border mergers and acquisitions in FDI was about 10% in the mid-1980s and increased to more than a third at the beginning of the 2000s. The lion's share of the increase in cross-border M&A is explained by the privatization of state enterprises that took place during the 1990s in many developing countries. The share of cross-border M&A in FDI also increased markedly in industrial countries.[72]

Neoliberal-driven capitalist internationalization has thus also driven a worldwide merger-and-acquisitions boom, the majority of which in the developing world have been acquisitions. In the 1980s, virtually all FDI going to the developing world was greenfield. But, since the 1990s, FDI from M&A began to increase. Between 1991 and 1998 it rose from an average per country of just $40 million compared to $260 million for greenfield (approximately 14 percent of total FDI) to $700 million compared to $1,300 million for greenfield (around 54 percent of total FDI). By 2006, M&A FDI going to the developing world was approximately $1,110 million on average per country compared to $2,600 million for greenfield (around 43 percent of the total).[73]

A body of research has found that brownfield FDI is much less advantageous for the recipient economies than greenfield FDI. Compared to greenfield investment, it tends to have lower benefits; indeed, it may have negligible benefits or even negative impacts on the host country's economic development.[74] This is for reasons that ought to be obvious:

> Foreign entrants may exploit the superior position in the global marketplace, on which their internationalization is based, to crowd out domestic entrepreneurs. Associated product market power will also result in higher entry barriers for domestic entrepreneurs. Moreover foreign entrants may also absorb a disproportionate share of domestic factor endowments (e.g.,

finance, managerial and skilled labor), raising the costs of entrepreneurial entry.[75]

In any case, ignoring the problem of how much FDI is genuine and adding value to the local economies into which it is exported, if we exclude the NICs and BRICs, so that our focus is on the so-called Third World, what we find is that the share of world investment received by this part of the world has been *falling* for decades. For example, it fell from 50 percent in 1960 to 25 percent by 1974, and then to just 17 percent by 1988.[76] This has meant that, by 1995, more than 80 percent of total foreign investment ended up in just 12 countries – in North America, Western Europe, and the Pacific Rim – and this pattern has changed since then only inasmuch as China has gate-crashed the development party. By contrast, by the close of the 1990s, the 48 least developed countries attracted just half a percent of total world investment.[77] Since then, more than 25 years later, the basic situation remains incorrigible. From 2010 until now FDI flows to the least developed countries (LCDs) still make up less than two percent of total world investment. The LCDs, which are home to 14 percent of the world's people, had just 1.8 percent of global inward FDI in 2018 – and this has been static since 2010. The average incoming FDI to the LCDs from 2000 to 2018 was just 1.3 percent.[78]

The hardest-hit continent has, of course, been Africa, home to almost 17 percent of the world's population. In 2016, while the whole of the developing world (excluding the NICs) received just 15 percent of total world investment, Africa was especially marginalized, since it got just 3.1 percent.[79] Africa today receives 3.5 percent of global FDI inflows compared to 3.9 percent in 2012 and has received on average 3.8 percent of the total since 2012.[80] Indeed, the continent's share of world FDI has scarcely shifted in 20 years, fluctuating between a low of 2.6 percent in 2007 to a high of 4.6 percent in 2009 and averaging just 3.4 percent up to and including 2019.[81]

Africa has also suffered a devastating 42 percent fall in incoming FDI since 2014.[82] But Latin America and the Caribbean's developmental woes since the 2000s have also continued. In the mid-2000s, these regions (home to almost 8.5 percent of the world's population) had between them an 8.6 percent share of global FDI, which was actually a lower level than ten years earlier.[83] Fuelled by a primary commodities boom, however, they increased their share of world FDI to 20.1 percent by 2013, eliciting much talk by the WTO and World Bank of newly emerging markets and another economic miracle.[84] But, with the inevitable collapse of the boom, their share of global FDI had plummeted to 8.1 percent by 2017.[85] Not only that, they experienced a calamitous 27 percent drop in inward FDI between 2014 and 2018.[86]

These statistics indicate that *global* investment does not exist. More seriously, they do not even demonstrate that a trend *towards* genuinely global investment exists. Rather, the data appear to indicate reinforcement of the pattern of regionalization or triadization of world economy that is also suggested by other indicators. Owing to asymmetrical capital flows, nearly two-thirds of the globe is virtually bypassed by overseas (mostly Western) FDI and capital flows generally.[87] The problem for the globalization theorists, therefore – whether these be hyper or moderate globalists – is that much of the world and its population is simply superfluous to the profit-driven needs of the capitalist world economy. And so they are just not included. These become impoverished backwaters populated by "non-peoples" or "unpeoples".[88]

Asymmetrical patterns of FDI confirm that "globalization" is a myth. But other empirical data demonstrate that even the trend for world FDI to expand has stalled in recent times – so that what is taken as globalization has hit the buffers. This was apparent even before the Great Financial Crisis of 2007/09 and the austerity decade that ensued. This was due to the impact of low profit rates and weak GDP growth (discussed in my *Contagion Capitalism*) in retarding cross-border capital flows. Global net inflows and outflows of FDI as a proportion of WGP were lower in 1985 than they were in 1970. Thereafter, though, the secular trend was upwards, despite ebbs and flows, reaching a peak of 10.81 percent of world output in 2007 – more than 13 times higher than in 1985.

This trajectory was far from a smooth ride, however. In response to the crises of the early 2000s, from 2000 to 2003, the value of world FDI fell by almost 57 percent. Thus, it was not until 2006 that its value surpassed the pre-crisis thresholds.[89] Moreover, since the 2007 peak, net FDI inflows and outflows as a proportion of world output have entered a long period of decline. The rate was lower in 2018 than it was in 1994, whereas the rate in 2019 scarcely surpassed that of 1998 and was almost three-and-half-times lower than in 2007 (Table 1.1).

The great financial crash triggered a drop of 53 percent in the volume of global FDI (16 percent in 2008 and 37 percent in 2009).[90] The recovery from these crisis years was painfully slow and undermined with setbacks. Modest upswings in 2010, 2011, and 2013 were undone by bigger downswings in 2012 and 2014.[91] Only by 2015 were FDI global flows restored to the (low) levels of the crisis years (2008 and 2009), and this required an unexpected 38 percent increase from the year before. But these cross-border transfers were still much below the 2007 level. And no sooner were the investment losses recovered than they were reversed owing to the ongoing "fragility" (as the UN's *World Investment* Reports regularly put it) of the world economy.

Table 1.1 Average FDI (net inflows and outflows) as % of world GDP 1970–2019[a]

1970–1979	0.9877
1980–1989	1.2988
1990–1999	3.0717
2000–2010	6.4409
2011–2019	4.9939

[a] World Bank (2021). *Foreign direct investment, net outflows (% of GDP)* (online); World Bank (2021). *Foreign direct investment, net inflows (% of GDP)* (online).

For three consecutive years (2016 to 2018) levels of global FDI registered declines, indeed often sharp contractions. Worldwide it fell by two percent in 2016, by 23 percent in 2017, and by 13 percent in 2018.[92] In 2019 there was only a very modest recovery, of just three percent, which was below the average of the previous decade and some 25 percent below the 2015 level.[93] Global FDI flows then plummeted in 2020, by 42 percent, so that it was at its lowest level since the 1990s and more than 30 percent beneath the "investment trough that followed the…financial crisis".[94]

During this same period, FDI flows to the developing world registered an overall drop of 14 percent, whereas those to the LCDs fell by 16 percent.[95] 2020 then saw further falls of 12 percent for the developing countries (37 percent in Latin America and the Caribbean and 18 percent in Africa) and a calamitous 77 percent for the "transitional economies".[96] Yet the biggest casualties of the decline of world investment over the past five years have been the developed countries. Here FDI inflows dropped by 54 percent between 2016 and 2019 and then by a further precipitous 69 percent in 2020.[97] This has led to a sharp (if likely temporary) swing in the balance of FDI in favour of the developing world, albeit from a drastically shrinking pot of investment funds.[98] World capitalism has never before been in direr straits than it is today.

Global inequality and the interstate system

Owing to the asymmetries of "globalization" (by trade, by production, by investment), the neoliberal era has reinforced longstanding trends of world economic development for the income gap between most developed countries (mostly in the Global North) and least developed countries (mostly in the Global South) to grow. This is somewhat obscured by certain statistics. "In 1980, the mean incomes in developing countries were 12.6 percent of those of the industrialized world; in 2000, these relative incomes had increased to 14 percent".[99] Such may be claimed as a triumph for globalization's capacity to reduce the gap between low-income and high-income countries, albeit an exceedingly modest one. But even this would be illusory.

Such raw figures are misleading because this apparent minor improvement in the fortunes of the developing countries has been, as I have pointed out, driven by a handful of NICs and BRICs, chief among which has been China – none of which has achieved these results by strict adherence to neoliberal free-market nostrums. GDP growth in the developing world from 1980 to 2000, if India and China are taken out of the picture, reduces from a yearly average of 2.4 percent to just 0.7 percent. Moreover, even though the developing world increased per capita income by 53 percent over this same period, the corresponding gains in poverty reduction in the Global South were much more modest. From 1987 to 1999, for example, the World Bank estimated a reduction of absolute poverty globally of just five to six percent.[100] This data is inconsistent with the ideology of growth-driven convergence.

Rather, the pattern has been mostly divergence – or convergence for a few alongside divergence for many others. Only a select number of countries have since World War Two managed to significantly close the income gap between the most developed ones and the rest. Even China, the big economic success story of the past few decades, had (by 2014) achieved a per capita income that was only one-seventh of the US's. And this was despite spectacular rates of growth – averaging over ten percent, seven percent per annum higher than the US economy managed to achieve – over the past 35 years.[101]

The majority of countries have remained stuck either in the so-called "middle-income trap" (with per capita incomes three to five times lower than in the US) or in a "poverty trap" (with per capita incomes 10–50 times lower than in the US). The industrialized countries had a level of daily per capita income that was 6.2 times higher than non-industrialized countries in 1960, which was a reduction from 6.5 times higher in 1950. However, by 1980, the gap had increased back up to 6.5 times, and by 2000 this was 6.7 times higher.[102] Latin America and Africa have fared particularly badly since the 1980s. "After almost doubling per capita income from 1960 to 1980, Latin American economies barely maintained their 1980s levels, and that also over a 20-year period. Africa did worse, as its per capita incomes declined by 12 percent" over this stretch.[103]

There are other indicators of divergence. "In 1980, median income in the richest 10 per cent of countries was 77 times greater than in the poorest 10 per cent; by 1999, that gap had grown to 122 times".[104] The average earner in the US (the archetypal high-income country) had during the 1950s and 1960s an income 50 times bigger than that of average earners in the world's poorest country. By 2000, this was 70 times larger. But, if the average income of US earners is compared with that of earners in the tenth-poorest country, the divergence is even more radical. In 1960, the average American earned 23 times more than the average earner in the world's tenth-poorest country; by 2000, this was 45 times more.

Comparing and contrasting the world's 20 richest and 20 poorest countries yields the same result. While the richest ones were 23 times wealthier than the poorest ones in 1960, by 2000 they were 36 times wealthier.[105] Similarly, as was reported by the UN's *Human Development Report of 1999* and the World Bank's *World Development Report of 2000/2001*:

> The income gap between the fifth of the world's population living in the richest countries and the fifth in the poorest countries was 74 to 1 in 1997, up from 60 to 1 in 1990 and 30 to 1 in 1960 … The average incomes in the richest 20 countries is 37 times the average in the 20 poorest countries – a gap that has doubled over the past 40 years.[106]

These trends have continued unabated in the new century. Income differentials between the richer and poorer countries have continued to climb.[107] Today, the world's least developed countries (LCDs), 47 in number, contain within their borders 14 percent of the world's population but more than half of the world's poorest people. These are those people who live on $1.90 a day or less. These LCDs account for just 1.3 percent of world gross product (WGP). They have "been diverging over a long time from other (non-LCD) developing countries", let alone the developed ones.

In 1990, the gross national income (GNI) per capita of other developing countries was three times higher than that of LCDs. Nowadays, it is almost six times higher. While in the early 1990s the labour productivity of these LCDs corresponded to 25% of that of other developing countries, at present it amounts to just 18%.[108]

But, of course, neoliberalism itself as a political project fully understands that trade and financial liberalization is not a force of convergence. Its purpose is exactly to confirm and reproduce the international market-power asymmetries and to deepen or extend these as far as possible. This is because neoliberalism is the politics of mega-capitalism that dominates the world economy and also of the state managers of the developed countries whose function is to serve this mega-capitalism (especially their "own" MNCs in the world market).

The state managers of the high-income countries (and hence political governance in the Global North) have formed a strategic alliance with corporate-capitalist power for mutual advantage. This is both internationally (against rival competitors in the Global South) and locally (against working classes and labour unions or other popular forces that would disrupt optimal competitiveness). Neoliberalization driven by the state managers obviously defends and extends the interests of their own national MNCs internationally and attracts inward investments from the MNCs of other developed countries. This protects the prosperity and advantaged position of these countries (and their locally based industries) in the international state system *vis-à-vis* the others and hence stabilizes the rule and privileges of their state elites.

This accounts for the radical disconnect between neoliberalism as *politics*, on the one hand, and neoliberalism as *ideology*, on the other. Neoliberalism as utopian ideology legitimizes this political project by representing it as something other than it is. This is as a politics that is about undermining world poverty, encouraging worldwide democratization (which is represented as a natural consequence of the export of trade liberalization), and levelling income and wealth disparities everywhere – all of which are supposedly bounties flowing inevitably from the "dynamism of the market".

Mega-capitalism and the interstate system

However, the globalists perceive a different relationship between neoliberalism and world capitalism. As we have seen, a fundamental claim of globalization theory is that the new mega-capitalism has escaped dependence on the state system and therefore undermines the capacity of national governments to adopt policies that obstruct or constrain corporate profit-making. This, it is claimed, is largely the consequence of two developments. The first is the unprecedented mobility across national borders of money capital (where billions or even trillions can pass through national turnstiles at the touch of the "send" button on a computer keyboard). The second is the structural power of the "nationless" MNCs in the world economy owing to the fact that they control the bulk of the world's resources and have the capacity to pick and choose which countries they will invest in and set up operations in.

Since the MNCs and finance capital are mobile or "footloose", say the globalists, they can set up in or transfer funds to countries that better serve their interests in high profits and low costs and exit those countries that serve these interests less well. Nation-states are forced to compete to attract inward investment from the MNCs and state managers have to keep international speculators and financial markets onside. They cannot therefore afford to levy high taxes in order to fund expansive welfare programmes.[109] Nor can they do this by increasing government borrowing. Nor can they afford to lower interest rates to stimulate demand-led growth.[110] They cannot even afford to introduce a decent minimum wage.

If states attempt to "buck the market" in these ways, their creditworthiness rating will suffer so that interest charges on debts increase and loans are harder to acquire. Moreover, "global capitalists" will simply take their resources to where governments offer low interest rates and low taxes and can guarantee a highly skilled but "affordable" workforce. This means, it is argued by globalists of all hues, that national governments are no longer in charge economically of what happens to or within the countries they administer. The economic stability or prosperity of the territories they rule is determined not by themselves but by the market and by international capitalism. Governments in practice are forced to share sovereignty over national affairs with the mega-capitals. If they want economic stability and prosperity (which after all will also stabilize the state) they must work with international capitalism and market forces rather than against them. This means that the role of government is to outcompete or outbid rival states in ensuring that the "supply side" of things (labour skills, wage rates, taxation policy, employment law, infrastructure, etc.) is as attractive to corporate investment as possible.[111]

For these reasons, it is claimed, national governments are forced to define their role as serving above and beyond all else the interests of the MNCs and global financiers.[112] If they are to attract (as they must) the trade custom, R&D, expertise, investment revenues, and employment opportunities afforded by mega-capital, they are compelled to adopt exactly the kinds of economic policies that the big corporations would like to see. Thus, in the words of Peter Gourevitch: "Whatever the difference in partisan outcomes, all governments have been pressed in the same direction ... [that is, to] curtail state spending and interventions".[113]

In practice, this means ensuring that the price of labour power is "competitive" (hence legal restrictions on the labour unions) and lowering the cost of the "social wage" (hence abandoning policies of progressive taxation, welfarism, nationalization, and full employment). As Geoffrey Garrett and Peter Lange explain: "The new international economic environment has undercut the partisan strategies of the left and right based respectively on broadly 'Keynesian' and 'monetarist' fiscal and monetary policies".[114] Or, as aspirant UK Prime Minister Tony Blair put it shortly before winning his first electoral stint in 1997, since "the determining context of economic policy is the new global market ... the room for manoeuvre of any government in Britain is already heavily circumscribed".[115]

Such policies demanded by the MNCs and by the "footloose" financiers are then exactly the neoliberal ones: low rates of taxation on business and wealth; labour market deregulation – that is, flexible working, temporary contracts, and so on; privatization of profitable state assets; dismantling of controls on the free movement of capital and goods; downsizing of the welfare state; and legal restrictions on the rights of trade unions to cause economic "disruption" through excessive industrial action. Neoliberal ascendancy is thus, according to the globalists, the inevitable consequence of "global" capitalism's dominance of the state system; it reflects the disempowered state, which is converted into a mere means of serving the imperatives of the marketplace.

This renders neoliberalism passive – the creature of mega-capital – according to its apologists and some of its left-wing critics. Neoliberalism expresses the crisis of competence of the nation-state that results from its drastically reduced autonomy in the sphere of economic policymaking. This in turn erodes its legitimacy and authority in the eyes of the citizenry who can perceive its weakness and lack of independence of action from market forces.[116] This may indeed (as it arguably has done) generate widespread popular disillusionment with politics and government. These are the pessimistic claims of the left globalists in particular.

Now, as powerful as the thesis of the "declinist" or even "disempowered" state appears,[117] faced with the pressures of globalization, it is far from being convincing. Indeed, it has been subject to damaging criticism, which in my view is decisive in dispelling it. As the sceptics point out, the state system is integral to the capitalist world economy, for two main reasons. Firstly, this is owing to the fact that states retain their monopoly on the means of destruction (military power) and of judicial authority. This renders them indispensable to the maintenance of social order and hence of economic order.

Secondly, this is because the national state remains in possession of sufficient authoritative and allocative resources to exercise a measure of control over economic processes and relations with its own borders, despite the contrary claims of the globalists. Indeed, in recent decades, it could even be said that the capacities of the state to intervene in the marketplace to secure economic or other goals have been enhanced rather than diminished. This is because since World War Two states have sought to re-empower themselves (or rather re-embed or re-consolidate their powers) by means of alliance-building, international cooperation, and the formation of multilateral partnerships and associations in various supranational political organizations that are all about global "governance" of the world economy.

Recent decades have seen a dramatic increase in the capacity of states to control the global environment by cooperating with each other. The postwar creation of a range of international governmental organizations (IGOs) or interstate supranational organizations (such as GATT, the IMF, the World Bank, the UN, NAFTA, AFTA, the EU, the ASEAN, etc.) does not necessarily evidence that the autonomy and competence of the nation-state is declining. Rather, this may more plausibly be indicative that nation-states (or rather some of them) are becoming more competent at asserting their own national interests on the international stage.[118]

This shows that different states have reached an understanding that they have common interests that are best served through multilateral agencies. This also shows that they have found ways to pursue their particular interests through collaboration rather than through unilateral action. So, for example, international coordination of currency exchange rates can enhance state autonomy rather than diminish it by imposing a measure of order or stability on cross-border exchanges. In particular, the growth of the IGOs is evidence that a particular group of states – the US and its high-income allies – have constructed international regimes that help preserve a particular geometry of global power relations. So, for example, the UN, the IMF, the World Bank, and the WTO are not simply neutral international bodies concerned with the welfare of all nations. Rather, they are US- and Global-North-dominated institutions that allow the more powerful states to assert both common interests and particular interests against weaker, more dependent states.[119]

So, to suggest that globalization necessarily undermines state autonomy is to lose sight of the ways in which states empower themselves against the vagaries of global forces (including the world market) through collective action. International relations theorists of the Realist School have pointed out that the world capitalist economy depends on the maintenance of law and order worldwide.[120] In short, the economic order of global markets is contained or embedded within the political order of states.

States have a monopoly on the means of violence and the legal right to exercise it. They are, as participants in a system of states, collectively invested (to varying degrees) in maintaining some kind of global order through power-balancing. Moreover, states provide police and legal protections for the wealth and property of those MNCs that are situated within their borders from rival states and rival firms and from alienated labour and the propertyless.[121] States also secure the social and normative conditions and relations of commodity exchange more generally, including by the judicial administration and policing of contracts. Unless this is done, what is called economic globalization (in reality worldwide competition between capitals and class conflict between capital and labour) could degenerate into violence, banditry, and war.

The military and political capacities of states also provide their citizens with relative security. Such is made necessary in a world made dangerous by national rivalries without which even a semblance of economic stability would not be possible.[122] Only states can provide citizens with security, internally and externally, whether by means of the dispensing of legal entitlements, the provision of social welfare rights, or the protections afforded by police and military forces. Capitalist markets and business firms obviously cannot provide these securities, since their function is simply the business of economic exchange between private actors in pursuit of individual gain, not the provision of public goods to service collective goals.

The absence of military conflicts between the leading states since World War Two is explained by globalists as resulting from global economic integration that disassociates economic interests from national politics.[123] This is illusory because the disassociation of the two is much less than globalists think. The military functions of states may *seem* less significant in the postwar world compared to before because these are exercised less often than previously. But this is arguably a measure of the relative effectiveness of the international relations of state actors since World War Two in maintaining a balancing of powers that has secured world order in its political and economic aspects.[124]

As Kenneth Waltz puts it: "Possession of power should not be identified with the use of force, and the usefulness of force should not be confused with its usability…Power maintains an order; the use of force signals its breakdown".[125] Where state actors withdraw from international relations so that state powers no longer are deployed to "balance" or "stabilize" interstate competition, as occurred in the 1914–45 period, the system dissolves into anarchy and violence. This 1914–45 period that was characterized by depression and war among the great powers was in fact preceded by the first wave of so-called globalization. During this period (from the mid-nineteenth century up until the outbreak of the Great War) world trade grew by 900 percent, whereas by the 1890s half of the total investments of the UK (still the world's biggest economy) were exported overseas.[126] Yet this period of growing international economic "interconnectedness" or "integration" through foreign trade and overseas investments did nothing to arrest the world's plunge into war driven by the intersection of inter-imperial and inter-capitalist rivalries.

The interstate system also continues to play a key role in regulating and stabilizing the world market, whereas particular states prop up the largest of their "own" corporations when they run into difficulties. Since the 1970s, as noted by David Gordon, in response to economic liberalization, and in order to head off or ameliorate recessionary pressures in the world economy, "the role of the state has grown substantially". Moreover, "state policies have become increasingly decisive on the international front, not more futile…And…everyone including transnational corporations has become increasingly dependent upon coordinated state intervention for restructuring and resolution of the underlying dynamics of crisis".[127]

In response to the East Asian crisis that broke out in 1997, and its spread to Latin America and Russia in 1998, massive bailouts organized by the IMF totalling more than $179 billion (and by Japan totalling $30 billion) eventually stabilized these economies.[128] At the same time coordinated state intervention in the financial markets by governments of the high-income countries led by the US prevented (albeit narrowly) these meltdowns from dragging the developed world into crisis.[129] Trillion-dollar bailouts of the corporate banks in the developed world prevented a collapse of the financial sector and a far more severe global depression than perhaps would otherwise have been the case in the aftermath of 2007/08.[130] Trillion-dollar state and central bank subsidization of a wide swathe of big corporations is presently being rolled out to head off a potentially even bigger global economic slump than ten years ago provoked by the COVID-19 pandemic.[131]

Here a number of observations are pertinent. (1) Even the lone or stand-alone nation-state can still actively buck the world market and oppose the forces of international capitalism when it has to. The case of Malaysia provides a not-too-distant example of what is possible in the "global" age. Hardly a central player in the world economy, Malaysia was nonetheless able to weather the Asian economic crisis of 1997–98 rather better than most of the neighbouring states by resorting to counter-market measures. Basically, there was here an abrupt turn towards protectionism – imposing controls on the movement of capital into and out of the country – in express disregard of the free-market mantras of the Washington Consensus neoliberals.[132]

Another recent example of "market-bucking" state action is provided by Argentina. In this case, in response to the economic crisis, the government defaulted on its debts.[133] This, according to neoliberalism, is the cardinal sin, tantamount to committing economic suicide. Yet, although the defaults helped trigger sharp contractions in GDP, the withdrawal of foreign investments and currency devaluation, economic calamity did not come to pass. These were relatively fleeting ill-effects under the impress not simply of the defaults but the economic crisis that motivated them. Foreign investments were soon restored.[134] Inflation soon dropped back.[135] GDP growth was quickly restored.[136] Argentina has since continued to be regarded as a profitable site by international financiers and MNCs, despite still carrying major debts and debt default status. Argentina's default status was not lifted until 2016.[137]

(2) By the end of the 1980s, as Ruigrock and van Tulder have pointed out, at "least 20 companies in the 1993 *Fortune* 100 would not have survived as independent companies if they had not been saved by their respective governments in the last decade and a half".[138] Such rescues (whether by means of subsidy, non-market loans, or temporary nationalizations) characterized the economic crises of the 1970s and 1980s. Even though more bankruptcies were tolerated by governments in the 1990s and 2000s, there were still major bailouts,[139] and these have as we have seen mushroomed in response to the financial meltdown of 2007–09 and the present coronavirus crisis. In the teeth and claw of the current crisis, hundreds of billions have been thrown at the corporate sector, much of which has found its way into the pockets of shareholders and executives. The reason for this "bailout culture" of neoliberal governance of contemporary mega-capitalism is clear enough. Rescues of the corporate sector have been indispensable tools for blunting the impact of recessionary crises, preventing these from spiralling into global depressions, just as state-coordinated financial stimulus measures have boosted lending by the banks to kickstart corporate investments and consumer spending.

(3) Whenever MNCs set themselves up in any specific country, they are dependent on the patronage of the host nation-state, just as they are dependent on the support of their "own" state in their home markets. Nation-states provide corporations with access to the resources and safeguards they need: infrastructure (energy sources, water supplies, transport, communications); stable currencies and exchange rates; skilled labour power; secure labour markets and acquiescent workers; access to supply chains; tax concessions; legal protections of their property; and an effective police force to ensure industrial peace and armed forces to safeguard national security, etc.[140]

Not every state can guarantee these conditions. Indeed, it is quite often only those of the high-income countries that can. This explains why the MNCs largely confine the bulk of their business activities to their home countries and home regions – hence the regionalization or triadization (not globalization) of corporate power already discussed.[141] Moreover, MNCs also rely on their own home nation-states to help them gain access to foreign markets and to bat for their interests in negotiations with foreign states within which they have set up operations or in which they wish to set these up. So-called globalization is not a process that generates "stateless corporations" (or *trans*national or *trans*-state capitalism). Rather, this is a process whereby MNCs seek to dominate overseas markets by establishing partnerships with foreign states that bind these to supporting their goals.[142]

This means, as Stopford and Strange observe, that very "few firms can operate in a genuinely borderless world". Rather, they must operate within an international state system in which governments, "both host and home...continue to play a crucial and, perhaps paradoxically... increasing role".[143] This role is in securing and extending their interests in competition and sometimes cooperation with the rival firms of rival states. This establishes the relations between states and capitals as one of "structural interdependence" rather than one of the utter dependence of the former on the latter.[144] Such gives governments, especially of the advanced or developed countries, considerable leverage to influence the decisions of the international corporate elite. This leverage exists also because MNCs cannot simply "up stumps" whenever they encounter government policies of which they disapprove or other unexpected obstacles to profit maximization. MNCs establish themselves in local national economies by placing themselves at the centre of complexes of enterprises that are cultivated as suppliers, distributors, retailers, etc.).[145] "Neither individual firms nor states but *industrial complexes* constitute the centre of gravity of the international restructuring race".[146]

Therefore, for an MNC to exit a particular country where its operations are heavily consolidated would involve major liabilities. These would include writing off considerable investments (premises, plant, machinery, etc.); abandoning networks of partners and clients; eschewing local sources of financing and labour skills that are particularly weaned to its needs; and turning its back on a range of other benefits and concessions underwritten by the local state.[147] There are also the costs of establishing these complexes and negotiating these benefits from scratch somewhere else. This is not an undertaking that can be taken lightly or oft-repeated. This, again, is exactly the reason why there are very few genuinely transnational corporations operating in the world economy today. This is why corporate enterprise tends to cluster within specific regional zones and national borders. MNCs simply cannot be as "footloose" as globalization theory asserts.

Globalization theory represents money as especially borderless and footloose, however. This is on the grounds that this has an immateriality or virtuality that industrial capital lacks. The notion of the deterritorialization of capital (that is, of its independence from the state system) gains its strongest empirical case owing to the growing internationalization of finance.[148] Billions, it is said, may be shifted from one part of the world to another, at the flick of a switch, in the restless search for higher returns on investment, so that states and governments are at the mercy of financial speculators and must optimize local conditions for profit-making in order to attract the funds or deter their flight. Yet even in the case of finance capital the mobility in question is hugely exaggerated. This is because, as Susan de Brunhoff reminds us, "a global single market of capital does not exist". There is "no single world rate of interest" any more than there are "single world prices for produced goods".[149]

Nor is there a global currency. Rather, there are different national (or sometimes regional) currencies that do not convert into each other as equivalents – which largely reflects the varying strengths of the different *national* economies. This explains why finance capital does not circulate freely across the globe (instead concentrating especially in the developed world and a handful of developing countries) despite the opportunity allowed for total mobility by the "telecommunications revolution". What the technology allows the economics refuses. This demonstrates, as Dick Bryan points out, "the centrality of nationality within global accumulation":[150]

> International finance ... maintains national characteristics. It does not move systematically so as to equalise savings and investment ... A global financial system comprised of nationally designated currencies signals that globalisation cannot be devoid of a national dimension.[151]

(4) Nor is it the case that nation-states have been forced into the service of international capitalism in their promotion of trade liberalization. The thesis that these everywhere have been compelled to submit to identical neoliberal policies under the pressure of "globalization" encounters an empirical difficulty. This is simply that, despite the constraints on state action imposed by international capitalism and neoliberal IGOs, important variations in government economic and social policies remain. As I have noted elsewhere,[152] the export-oriented NICs and Japan built their competitive success by means of high levels of state support, investment, and direction in their economies. Even more so, China's ascendancy to the world's second-largest economy is built on state-capitalist methods of national economic planning and management.[153]

As for the developed countries, many of these have not travelled as far down the neoliberal path as the UK and the US. All have travelled some way down it (since reducing budget deficits and maintaining low inflation is almost a universal goal of state managers), but national differences remain significant. The marketization of public services is much less advanced in France and Germany than in the pioneers of the Washington Consensus, for example. The trade unions in these countries are also far more robust than they are in the UK or US. Welfare and health spending as a proportion of GDP and general taxation to support public services are also significantly higher in Germany and France (and also in the Scandinavian countries) than they have been in the US and UK in recent decades. The former also maintain higher levels of tax on capital and wealth and corporations and more regulated labour markets than is the case in the Anglo-American world.[154] In short, these countries retain significant aspects of social-democratic policies alongside neoliberal ones. Yet none of these countries are being outperformed economically by the purer liberal market "competition states". This is despite the fact that these are all oriented to import-export trade, and are hence open to "globalization". Indeed, Germany is one of the world's biggest exporter economies.

A second problem with the notion that the irresistible power of world capitalism has forced states into adopting neoliberal policies (hence the thesis of the "declinist" or "powerless" state) pertains to the question of intentionality or agency. This is simply that so-called economic globalization was pioneered by some of the most powerful state actors, just as it has since been promulgated worldwide by US- and Western-dominated multilateral state organizations (IMF, World Bank, WTO, G7, etc.). In short, the internationalization of mega-capitalism was made possible by the intentional *policy goals* of government actors. Central to this agency was building the three pillars of neoliberalism – deregulation, trade liberalization, and privatization. These "created the foundations for globalization" so that, as Manuel Castells rightly says, "the global economy was politically constituted".[155]

A fundamental problem with the globalist perspective, therefore, is that this tends to regard politics as the passive mirror of economics. Aside from the philosophical objections that can be made to economic determinism generally, this lets neoliberalism off the hook rather too easily. Indeed, the myth of the powerless state functions as ideological legitimation for neoliberal policies, since these are represented as matters of economic necessity rather than as matters of political choice, albeit constrained choice in response to capitalist crises. Rather than neoliberalism representing a browbeaten accommodation or adjustment of state politics to a resurgent internationalizing capitalism, this was instead a major driver of capitalist internationalization. "Globalization was actively sponsored and promoted by powerful western governments, including and especially those of Reagan in the US and Thatcher in Britain".[156]

Since deliberate state action was indispensable to unleashing the "runaway world" of free-market capitalism, it follows that deliberate resolute state action ought to be capable of bringing this world back under a measure of control that would restore limits to capital in the popular interest. For example, there seems no reason why the leading states administering the high-income countries could not seek to secure international agreement to rein in markets by imposing taxation on financial speculation (hence discouraging the destabilization of national currencies for financial gain), or de-penalizing protectionism for weaker economies, or re-instituting higher taxes on wealth in order to reduce inequalities. But the obstacle to this is simply that the dominant powers of the interstate system lack the *will* to contain capitalism – or, rather, they simply *do not wish* to confront capitalism. This is not because they are rendered powerless by "globalization", but because they positively identify with the agenda of corporate empowerment that "globalization" serves. It was, after all, this politics of preference – of commitment to untrammelled corporate exploitation of the world – that unleashed worldwide hyper-commodification in the first place.

(5) Finally, theorists of the "powerless state" exaggerate the *unique* nature of the pressures and constraints exerted by so-called economic globalization on national

governments today. After all, capitalism has been afflicted by crises which have had an international impact since its birth. There have been plenty of major ones (1880s, 1930s, and 1970s) before the neoliberal age. This means that it is problematic to attribute the failure of the state to confront capitalism simply to the forces of "globalization". Capitalists have always resorted to economic sabotage – that is, withdrawing or withholding their money from a country – in order to get their way when faced with the challenge posed by left-leaning reformist governments. Capital flight and investment strikes are longstanding weapons of big business to try and deter or deflect such governments from pursuing even modest welfarist or redistributionist agendas.

Unfortunately, social-democratic governments have historically demonstrated very little willingness to confront or resist these tactics of economic destabilization, just as neoliberal governments have shown no inclination to do anything to provoke them in the first place. Rather, they have backed away from confrontation (and hence from social-democratic reforms), because fundamentally they are compromised by their reformism, which commits them primarily to capitalism and only secondarily to reforming capitalism.[157] In Britain, for example, this was the pattern of every Labour government elected into office during periods of economic turbulence: the MacDonald governments of 1924 and 1929; Attlee's 1947 government; and the Wilson governments of 1967 and 1974.[158]

This history demonstrates that the main barrier to state autonomy (though hardly an insuperable one) is simply *capitalism* rather than capitalist "globalization". But, again, if this is the case, there seems no good reason to suppose that corporate power has rendered states incapable of reintroducing the kinds of constraints on capitalism that existed in most of the developed countries right up to the start of the 1980s. Regulated labour markets, rent controls and social housing, restrictions on cross-border capital flows, progressive taxation of wealth and property and corporations, welfare inclusivity, public ownership of key utilities, de-commodification of public goods and services, etc. – none of this is beyond the power of *collective* government agency under the leadership of the US and the other leading state actors.

International relations under US hegemony

The great insight of the theorists of the Realist School of International Relations (or RIRT) is their sober assessment of world politics as a system of interstate rivalries under the hegemony of the US state in which international cooperation is typically used by rival states as a means of securing national rather supranational goals. The concept of "hegemony" warrants particular attention given its centrality to RIRT. As Robert Keohane argues, "hegemonic powers must have control over raw materials, control over sources of capital, control over markets, and competitive advantages in the production of highly valued goods".[159] The US state possesses such controls in abundance, owing to structural emergence (that is, the "inheritance of advantage" from prior competitive success in previously materialized social interaction), as the Realist scholars correctly diagnose.

A hegemonic state is one, says John Mearsheimer, "that is so powerful that it dominates all of the other states in the system". This would be a state against which "no other state has the military wherewithal to put up a serious fight".[160] Hegemony, therefore, is obviously not merely a question of the capacities of a specific state, but of how those capacities are exercised in international relations. In other words, a hegemonic state operates in a hegemonic *system*, whereas a hegemonic system is one where, as Robert Gilpin points out, "a single powerful state controls or dominates the lesser states in the system". This " type of system", Gilpin instructs, "has, in fact, been most prevalent, at least in modern times, and scholars of international relations have detected a propensity for every international system to evolve in the direction of a universal empire".[161]

The US's GDP is (at $20.89 trillion in 2020) larger than all of the EU states combined and four times larger than Japan's (the world's third-biggest economy).[162] The US's economic power bankrolls its military power. US arms spending (at $766.58 billion in 2020) is almost four times higher than the EU's (at $198 billion), and this dwarfs the military resources of each and every other developed country.[163] This, according to the Realist School, allows the US to perform the role of "stabilizer" of a world order that would otherwise be in danger of being pulled apart by the dynamics of competition. As Charles P. Kindleberger, the founder of a particular version of RIRT, that is, Hegemonic Stability Theory (HST), succinctly summarized the argument: "for the world economy to be stabilized, there has to be a stabilizer, one stabilizer".[164]

Since, ultimately (as Marx as much as Hobbes understood), *might* is the basis of *right*, a particular state can act as a stabilizer power in world systems, according to Realists, only if that state is in possession of such an overwhelming preponderance of material (economic and military) resources that challenging the orders that it maintains is so fraught with hazard that this is almost ruled out. For Barry Posen, the US's "command of the commons" – that is, of the airways, oceanways, and landways – grants it the basis of military hegemony, since US military power can be deployed worldwide in all of these "commons".[165] But hegemony is also a matter of ambition and of will. As Christopher Layne points out, a powerful state makes itself a hegemon by acting "self-interestedly to create a stable international order that will safeguard its security and its economic and ideological interests". Moreover, a state with the "hard" military and economic power to make itself a hegemon can do so only by self-consciously deploying "that power to impose order on the international system".[166] Again, there is little doubt that the US state is a hegemon, under these definitions.

Now, the world capitalist economy *and* international state system require a single dominant state power to incentivize enough cooperation and deter enough conflict among rivals to secure normative order. This is necessary, as Gilpin affirms, to generate and maintain "an open and liberal world economy",[167] just as, in Keohane's words, it is necessary "to maintain the essential rules governing interstate relations".[168] On the one hand, according to HST, "a particular type of international economic order, a liberal one, could not flourish and reach its full development other than in the presence of such a hegemonic power".[169] On the other hand, "hegemonic structures of power, dominated by a particular country, are most conducive to the development of strong international regimes whose rules are relatively precise and well obeyed".[170] Hegemonic state power is thus fundamental to world order in the context of a capitalist world economy so that geopolitical and market competition between rival state-capital actors does not degenerate into a Hobbesian war of all against all that undermines the basic functionality of the two systems.[171]

According to HST, the US alone has been capable of performing the stabilizer role in the postwar world. And the US has taken on the role because the preservation of the international status quo serves the specific interests of its power elite of state managers and corporate bosses.[172] Competitor states (including and especially those of the Global North) allied to the US have acquiesced to US hegemony in world politics for three reasons. First, this is because they have lacked the economic and hence military clout to challenge it. Second, this is because their own self-interest is better served by the US's stabilizer (of the world market and international relations) role than by the absence of a stabilizer. As Robert Gilpin puts it: "There can be no liberal international economy unless there is a leader that uses its resources and influence to establish and manage an international economy based on free trade, monetary stability, and freedom of capital movement".[173] Since that is what US hegemony provides, those states that are relatively invested in the world market and derive major benefits from their investments in it will tend to accept the legitimacy of US leadership in world affairs.

Finally, this is because the US state has extended to them a share of the spoils derived from economic imperialism (the inherited advantages of structural emergence) that reproduces asymmetric competition and unequal exchange in order to maintain them as a cluster of relatively friendly states that act as a bulwark against any others which may undermine US hegemony. A major function of any hegemon state is to be ready and willing to deploy authoritative resources (rules, economic sanctions, and force of arms) to preserve the emergent structures of the world capitalist economy from which an array of other state actors (primarily those that run developed countries) may also prosper.[174] US political hegemony is thus earned by the military and normative protections it provides for the militarily weaker states of the Global North and Japan. These protections allow others to partake in the lesser but substantial benefits that the US's securitization of the capitalist world market for the primary benefit of its own MNCs provides. These protections also legitimize the hegemon's right to exercise global hegemony in their eyes.[175]

Thus, as Keohane's important distinction between what he describes as Kindleberger's "basic force model" and his own "force activation model" of world politics makes clear, the US state's hegemony in world systems is not simply a question of the material forces at its command or of hegemonic ambition or will. Rather, this is also based on its willingness to take on political and ideological *leadership* in world affairs. Hegemony is achieved where "one state is powerful enough to maintain the essential rules governing interstate relations" and is also "willing to do so".[176] This allows hegemony to operate through domination as consensus-building by means of the exercise of leadership. As Keohane elaborates, the hegemon plays a distinctive role, providing partners with leadership in return for deference; but unlike an imperial power, it cannot make and enforce rules without a certain degree of consent from other states.[177]

This means, says Keohane, that the stability of hegemony also relies on the hegemon being prepared to act "in a collectively beneficial manner", albeit ultimately in the service of its own national self-interest.[178] Benefits must be distributed beyond the hegemon in order to facilitate cooperation with the world orders that this hegemony defends and acceptance of the hegemon's right to exercise hegemony. This also involves the construction of "regimes" under the auspices or guidance of the hegemon – that is, "sets of implicit or explicit principles, norms, rules, and decision-making procedures around which actors' expectations converge in a given area of international relations"[179] – including by means of which "public goods" are distributed to other states. Public goods include military protection, shared access to markets, maintenance of international commercial law, transfer of foreign aid and other credits through supranational organizations, and so on. This also means that hegemony through consensus-building "is related in complex ways to ... institutions such as international regimes".[180]

This pattern of hegemony manifestly corresponds to the US model. Indeed, Keohane's general theory appears almost written to make sense of it specifically. But Keohane's own analysis of US hegemony considerably underplays imperialism. This is because he imagines that the US's hegemonic leadership is for the betterment of "the system" and that consensus-building divests from its hegemony the power of coercive domination of other states. As he puts it, the "hegemon plays a distinctive role, providing partners with leadership in return for deference; but unlike an imperial power...[i]t cannot make and enforce rules without a certain degree of consent from other states".[181]

Perhaps Keohane has in mind here that imperialism is only *really* imperialism if it is always direct colonization. But, in any case, the problem with this is twofold. First, since consensus-building, on Keohane's own account, can be built only by the US, and only because the US excels in terms of its capacity for "hard" power, this would suggest that consensus is not separate from domination. Second, claiming "system benefits" for the US hegemony rather loses sight of the fact that "the system" is shaped by virtue of the "inheritance of advantage" to serve US interests (economic and geopolitical) in particular – or rather those of America's elites. The capitalist world economy is, as we shall see, radically structurally asymmetric so that "system benefits" do not actually correspond to human or social benefits – or not to those of most people, and not anywhere in the world – and especially not to the multitude of the Global South. Finally, as critical realists would rightly point out, the notion of "system benefits" is in any case a reified or fetishized one. The "system" of global political economy is made not of people in their interactions with other people but of positions and attendant powers in structures that are given by positions. Purposive interest-governed agency is a property of people not of the structures they inhabit.

In the real world, of course, states and capitals of the Global South remain subordinate to those of the Global North and especially subordinate to the developed world's leading power, the US, as I will show. This also renders the poorer countries (and the working classes within them) vulnerable to super-exploitation at the hands of the big corporations. Such is owing to lesser command of resources (economic and military) in the two systems, notwithstanding the exception of Japan and the new ascendancy of China. Yet, as many RIR theorists argue, the relative decline of the US's economic power faced by the rise of new capitalisms, especially of China's, is beginning to pose a challenge to the US's dominance of world commerce, though the US's economy remains a tad bigger on most estimates and certainly much stronger than China's on qualitative indicators.[182]

But, if this challenge continues to grow, China may also be able to challenge the US for hegemony outside the developed world.[183] Equally, with the US's relative economic decline, if this should continue, its legitimacy as the guarantor of normative order worldwide and as leader of the developed world may falter. Nonetheless, presently, the US's political hegemony over the interstate system remains intact. This is due to the fact that currently as much as before the US alone commands superpower status since it is the only nation-state that combines the most advanced economic capacities with a level of military investments that is more than three times higher than the world's next biggest arms spender, China.[184]

Imperialism and the interstate system

The preceding analysis of the relationship between state and capital in the "global" age brings us to a second good answer to the questions of *how* the economic imbalances between and within countries exist and *why* they have these radicalizing since the 1980s. This is because some account is needed of how the spectacularly economically unbalanced world (which even though this is, to be sure, one that is reproducible by the market mechanism alone at the level of economy) has not been rendered politically untenable by virtue of massive social dissonance and popular resistance. That is, how revolt of the impoverished masses of the Global South against the rule of the US hegemon and the Global North in world affairs and against their own rulers who acquiesce with a world radically hostile to their interests has been avoided. This is the question of how a world of massive and growing economic injustice can be politically stabilized. Since social malintegration is definitely real and unavoidable (given the magnitude of the structural antinomies that the capitalist mode confronts global humanity with), why has this not given rise to the kind or intensity of social malintegration that would undermine the current world order?

As I stated at the start of this chapter, the good answer to this question is exactly that which some Realists deny, *imperialism*. This imperialism is made in the interface of economic (inter-capitalist) and geopolitical (interstate) competition under conditions where the protagonists have radically asymmetric access to authoritative and allocative resources by virtue of structural emergence. It is important to recognize in this context that the well-documented pattern of US political interventions and interferences in the sovereign affairs of a vast swathe of countries of the Global South in the postwar period was never motivated simply by Cold War geopolitical and ideological rivalries. Such interventions and interferences are the paraphernalia of trade embargoes, economic blockades, strategies of political destabilization aimed at non-compliant governments, and overt and covert support for repression of oppositionists by compliant governments and aspirant governments. The latter includes arming and training insurgents, supporting military coups, hostile encirclements with military installations, supporting international terrorist networks that have abducted and murdered opponents or dissidents across the world, military and financial and intelligence assistance for "friendly" regimes, and even direct military interventions.[185]

This was only partly motivated by fears over Soviet expansionism (though anti-Soviet paranoia played a part). In short, this was no mere artifice of what Alex Callinicos has dubbed "superpower imperialism", though this is how its excesses were typically rationalized or legitimized.[186] On the contrary, this was motivated as much by a politics committed to ruthlessly binding the countries of the Global South to the capitalist world market – a world market dominated especially by American MNCs and trade.[187] But this was also one in which the other developed capitalisms would benefit owing to the logic of comparative advantage in a system of free competition where they were sheltered from political disruptions of the economic mechanism by the global projection of American political and military power. Breaking free of the Cold War, with the decline of Soviet "communism" towards the end of the 1980s, the role of US military power in securing the "developing" world for the imperialism of unequal exchange and the rule of US-led free trade could assume centre-stage.

As President George Bush Senior's 1990 *National Security Strategy of the United States* review put it:

> In a new era, we foresee that our military power will remain an essential underpinning of the global balance, but less prominently and in different ways. We see that the more likely demands for the use of our military forces may not involve the Soviet Union and may be in the Third World, where new capabilities and approaches may be required ... Since World War II, the threat posed by the Soviet Union has dominated much of our planning for the Third World. But we have ... long identified specific interests independent of a Soviet factor. In the future, we expect that non-Soviet threats to these interests will command ever greater attention ... Third World conflicts may no longer take place against the backdrop of superpower competition. Yet many will, for a variety of reasons, continue to threaten U.S. interests ... and place serious demands on our forces.[188]

The US's war on the Global South in the Cold War era was aimed not simply at national movements and governments that were formally (or informally) aligned with the USSR or committed to building Stalinist-type command economies. Rather, this was just as much aimed at governments and movements – populist, nationalist, social-democratic, socialist – that were merely left-of-centre (that is, those committed to a policy spectrum including land reform in favour of the rural poor, increasing taxes on wealth and property, limiting foreign ownership, placing controls on the export of capital, and so on). Sometimes it was aimed simply at governments or movements that were set on liberal-democratic reforms (that is, free elections). This was because a preference of US foreign policy – especially though not exclusively in the Cold War era – was for regional "strongman" states (that is, right-wing dictatorships) absolutely committed to private property and capitalist enterprise *without limits*, and hence resolutely set against the trade unions and pro-worker or pro-peasant reforms.[189]

This was on the grounds that these would insure against the rule of the "wrong" kind of government (that is, "weak" government that would bend to popular pressures) and would better protect US corporate property, investments and profits in "emerging" markets. As US State Department lead policy strategist George Kennan observed in 1949, "it is better to have a strong regime in power than a liberal government if it is indulgent and relaxed and penetrated by communists".[190]

In Latin America, regarded by Washington as its own captive marketplace, this allowed foreign policy to be projected and translated as equivalent to US internal security policy from the Kennedy presidency onward. This meant that any socialist, social-democratic, or nationalist movement or government in the subcontinent was viewed as "communist" or "ultranationalist" by default, hence opposed to US interests and bent on undermining US national security. This, as Lars Schoultz has argued, enabled the permanent undermining of "a perceived threat to the existing structure of socioeconomic privilege by eliminating the political participation of the numerical majority...the popular classes".[191] This same point could be made with equal force with regard to US foreign policy in the Middle East, which has also been read by its artificers through the "internal securitization" lens, and with the same purpose in mind.

So, at work in the state system were two distinct but intersecting forms of imperialism – the bipolar imperialism of interstate competition between the US-led alliance and the USSR and its allies, and the US-led imperialism of the developed countries that was imposed on the Global South. Thus, although superpower imperialism has gone with the demise of the USSR and its allies, the other axis of imperialism (the Global North's domination of the Global South) remains as entrenched as ever. This is why the post-Cold War (and neoliberal) world is one that has seen the continuation of US-led imperial power politics, indeed their extension into previously uncharted territories that were reined in at least in part by Cold War partitions.

But, since imperialism is, as Callinicos says, "constituted by the intersection of two forms of competition, namely economic and geopolitical",[192] the demise of bipolar superpower rivalries has led to a transformation of the system of imperialist competition since the 1990s. And so imperialism in the neoliberal world is reconstituted as a triadic political system based on three great power centres: those of the US (the lone superpower), the EU, and Southeast Asia (Japan and China – the latter being a regional power that has perhaps global superpower ambitions and which if so is likely to increasingly challenge worldwide US political hegemony).[193] This triadic pattern is the correspondence of power of authorization (political domina-tion) to power of allocation (economic exploitation) – the latter of which is also, as we have seen, triadic.

This re-ordered international state system is the power container of the new mega-capitalism and of its neoliberal governance. Its architecture is asymmetric in the sense of polycentric, with the US leading the other developed countries by virtue of: (1) its greater economic strength (a GDP almost as big as Japan's and the EU's combined);[194] (2) its strategic control over access to the bulk of the world's energy supplies in the Middle East (by virtue of its military protection of the petrol monarchies) upon which all of the other advanced capitalisms are dependent;[195] (3) its global policing role (primarily for the protection of the interests of its own MNCs in the world market – but which entails safeguarding international free markets from which its "partners" also benefit);[196] (4) its much bigger contribu-tion than its North Atlantic Treaty Organization (NATO) partners to overall world military spending and to funding NATO that is integral to this policing of world order role;[197] and (5) its political domination of the various multilateral institutions of global governance (UN, G7, OECD, GATT, APEC, World Bank, IMF, and most recently WTO) that ensures that Washington Consensus (neoliberal) policies are internationally endorsed and are ideologized as multilateral and consensual.[198]

In this hierarchical trilateral structure, the developed countries (those of the EU bloc and Japan) can be viewed as sub-imperial states, under the leadership of the US. This is inasmuch as they are participants (as junior partners) under US hegem-ony in the "imperialism of free trade"[199] that reproduces their mutual advantages and the disadvantages of others in the world economy. Yet free trade (neoliberal-ism) as global policy is supported by the US and the high-income countries only to the extent that it extends or defends the interests of their MNCs in the world economy and does not compromise their national economic competitiveness.

As was the case in the Cold War era, free trade is something to be imposed as far as possible on the developing and underdeveloped worlds rather than fully embraced by the developed countries themselves. Consequently, the US and EU both heavily subsidize their agriculture sectors, R&D in the public and private sectors, as well as certain core enterprises of strategic importance (telecommunica-tions, computers, pharmaceuticals, aeronautics, automobiles, fossil-fuel industries, etc.), in effect defending these against foreign competition. The US and EU also maintain trade barriers (tariff and non-tariff) on imports from overseas.[200] As Noam Chomsky rightly says:

> Free market doctrine comes in two varieties. The first is the official doctrine imposed on the defenceless. The second is what we might call "really exist-ing free market doctrine": market discipline is good for you, but not for me.[201]

The developed countries may also be viewed as junior partners of US imperialism in a different way. This is inasmuch as they may be mobilized through multi-lateral though US-dominated international organizations to endorse and support the sanctioning of weaker states for maintaining barriers on foreign imports or to approve US economic or military measures intended to discipline or undermine "outlier" states.[202] However, these sub-imperialisms have their own national interests, meaning that tensions and conflicts are also integral to the interstate system, though these are containable so long as the US hegemon can maintain its economic and military power and hence political authority over the developed world. This cannot be guaranteed in the long *durée*, however, owing to the continuing relative decline of US economic power in a centrifugal world order of sovereign nation-states and resurgent NEMs[203] and the growing dependence of its relatively weakened economy on capital and commodities from overseas (hence bourgeoning trade deficits).[204]

Neo-Weberian sociologist Michael Mann diagnoses four major sources or modes of social power – economic, political, ideological and military.[205] Hegemonic power over society, Mann argues, is achieved by securing control or dominance of the four sources or modes. But, as Marx understood it, economic power constitutes the basis of the social power centres, since capacities of authorization are resourced by capacities of allocation. Therefore, the US's relative economic decline threatens its control of ideological capacities (exercised through the global corporate media) and political resources (exercised through supranational bodies of international governance) and its ability to maintain military capabilities far in excess of its competitors.[206] Faced with relentless inter-capitalist competition, the capacity of the US to solidarize its hegemony in the strategic theatres of global geography (the EU, Southeast Asia, and the Middle East and Southcentral Asia – where the bulk of the world's oil resources are to be found) will come under increasing strain.[207]

This may be part of the explanation for the US's resort to unilateral military interventions under the Bill Clinton and George Bush Junior presidencies in order to rein in outlier states – for example: in the Balkans in 1999; in Afghanistan in 2002; and in Iraq in 2003 – rather than the preferred and more typical "consensus-building" method of enticing or bribing or coercing multilateral support for military interventions through the agency of the UN and under the cloak of international law.[208] A greater willingness of the US to deploy military force unilaterally outside its own regional theatre of influence in the Americas could be symptomatic of a declining capacity to project political power by virtue of economic ascendancy. This is as the decline of American economic power weakens its political and ideological dominance of the Western Alliance, making it harder to build multilateral support for acts of military or economic coercion against outlier states in regional hotspots.

There is certainly evidence that US hegemony in the sphere of political ideology and in matters of general culture are facing increasing contestation, despite the virtual monopolization of global media and communications by US media corporations. The 2007 *Global Attitudes* Survey, for example, revealed considerable popular scepticism towards the US's claim to uphold human rights, democratic freedoms, economic justice, and the rule of law internationally. A majority of people in 20 out of 47 countries included in the survey viewed the US negatively overall under various criteria, whereas in 43 of the surveyed countries, a majority of people thought that the US's support for democracy overseas was merely equivocal and strategic, governed by its own national self-interest.[209]

However, the supposed discontinuity of US imperial policy during this period with what went before (and what has come since) – that is, the shift from instrumentally multilateral to instrumentally unilateral military interventions in the sovereign affairs of other countries – is perhaps overstated. After all, Washington's *National Security Strategy* review of 1990 sanctioned the US "to act either in concert with our allies or, if necessary, unilaterally, where our vital interests are threatened",[210] just as its predecessors did. If US imperialism had been able to win UN backing for the second Gulf War against Iraq in 2003, as it did for the first one in 1991, for example, the latter would also have been an exercise of instrumental multilateralism rather than instrumental unilateralism.

Notably, the Obama presidency that followed those of Clinton and Bush Junior eschewed new unilateral military interventions, indeed multilateral ones as well, in favour of waging proxy wars. As Luke Martell points out, despite relative economic decline, the US retains the world's largest economy, both absolutely and in terms of per capita income.[211] This still makes it the dominant global player politically and ideologically (hence the worldwide appeal of "American values" of individual freedom, consumerism, market liberalism, etc.), even though this dominance is eroded. Certainly, the US's military ascendancy has not yet been seriously contested.

Now, the key aspect of the US's de-territorialized power network is the dispersal of military bases across the globe, especially in theatres of strategic importance to the US. With the Cold War world 30 years past, the US still maintains almost 800 overseas military bases worldwide at a cost of between $80–100 billion.[212] At the end of World War Two, by comparison, the number was 400,[213] whereas Britain, France, and Russia today have 30 foreign military installations between them.[214] This leaves little room to doubt that the US is the world's dominant imperial power, and the only one with global reach.

The locales of US military installations include Europe, in order during Cold War times to contain the threat of the former Soviet bloc, but latterly of post-Soviet Russia. They include as well Southeast Asia and Indochina, in order to contain the threat of China and other "communist" countries such as North Korea, as well as other potential sub-imperialisms, and to maintain regional watchdog states. They also include Latin America, in order to police the US's client and vassal states, buttressing allies and deterring enemies, and on occasions engaging in covert operations against popular left-wing insurgency, or in support of right-wing insurgency. Finally, they include the Middle East, Persian Gulf, and Central Asia regions. This is to buttress the oil monarchies and securitize oil fields and supply lines upon which US capitalism and its chief rivals – Russia, the EU, Japan, and China – depend. This is also to rein in "rogue" states (that is, those that pose a threat to US control of these resources). Such "rogues" include or have included Islamicist Iran, Ba'ath Iraq, and other secular nationalist regimes (such as Nasser's Egypt in the 1950s) that were committed to versions of "state socialism" and to building regional alliances based on ideologies of pan-African/pan-Arab unity.[215]

Imperialism and NATO

Most recently, with the collapse of the Soviet bloc, the global reach of US militarism and imperialism has been extended to the far-flung fringes of Eastern Europe and the Balkans, and towards Southern and Central Asia adjoining the Caspian Sea.[216] Especially since the Yugoslav civil war, US and NATO military bases have been implanted in former Soviet territories and satellites that have been pulled into the US camp by the lure of American money, ring-fencing the Russian Federation on its western and southern frontiers. The expansion of NATO deep into Eastern Europe that started under the Clinton presidency (drawing initially the Czech Republic, Hungary, and Poland into the Western Alliance) has been one aspect of this strategy of containment and encirclement of a state (Russia) with the potential to become a regional hegemon.[217]

Alarmingly, recent decades have seen this strategy of containment being accelerated, especially under the presidencies of George W. Bush and Barack Obama. This is with the incorporation into NATO of Bulgaria, Romania, and the Baltic Republics.[218]

In November 2002, Bush backed NATO's invitation to seven nations – including former Soviet republics Estonia, Latvia and Lithuania – to begin talks to join the Western alliance. In 2004, with Bush as a driving force, the seven Eastern European nations joined NATO.[219]

Shortly afterwards, the US courted longstanding Russian allies Georgia and Ukraine by making them recipients of generous Western aid.[220] This was just as Bush Junior's government tore up the Anti-Ballistic Missile Treaty as the prelude to setting up new surveillance installations and anti-ballistic missile bases in several NATO-aligned countries in Eastern Europe.[221] The US- and EU-supported "pro-democracy" insurgency orchestrated by right-wing nationalist groups in Ukraine that chased out the democratically elected president Viktor Yanukovych in 2014 for courting closer economic ties with Russia rather than the EU is the latest dangerous escalation of this strategy.

Before then, NATO expansion had reduced Russia's security buffer with the West to just two states, Belarus and Ukraine. Consequently, for Moscow, the preservation of friendly relations with the Kyiv regime was geo-strategically vital. Now, Ukraine is a country divided between an anti-Russian and pro-EU West and a Russia-leaning East. Such renders it inherently unstable and ripe for a tug-of-war between, on the one side, the US and EU, and on the other side, the Russian Federation. The "Orange Revolution" of 2014 motivated Russia's retaliatory strategic annexation of Crimea. Looking ahead, these events risk all-out war between Russia and Ukraine This is owing to the latter's pursuit of NATO membership, which the US state has done nothing to deter, and for which it has declared its support, along with support for Georgia's membership) since 2008.[222] Indeed, drawing Ukraine into NATO would be entirely consistent with the US's established strategy of hostile encirclement and neutralization of a potentially dangerous regional hegemon.

But this is a hazardous game because keeping Ukraine "neutral" is for Russia an absolute red-line national security issue, irrespective of who happens to lead the government in Moscow.[223] It is even possible that the US's refusal to concede Moscow's demands for a "neutral" Ukraine, or to rule out granting the country NATO membership, is intended to goad Russia's president Vladimir Putin into making war on his neighbour. After all, faced with a similar situation (that is, hostile encroachment from a foreign power in its own "backyard" or regional sphere of influence), US governments would behave in exactly the same way as Putin's regime in Russia is threatening to behave. This is sanctioned by the so-called "Monroe Doctrine", according to which the US reserves the right to take military action in Latin America or in the Caribbean in defence of its national security interests.[224] As such, Washington would understand, based on the US's own imperial precedents, that Russian military action in Ukraine in response to NATO expansion into the country would be a reasonable case scenario.

If conflict provocation is the goal of US planners, there are signs that this is yielding results. Since the spring of 2021, there has been an upscaling of Ukrainian military action against pro-Russian separatists in the Donbas region and of "retaliatory" Russian troop mobilizations close to the border, accelerating in October.[225] Military action would be attractive to Putin because this could force Ukraine's nationalist government to abandon allying itself with the West or, failing that, allow a more Russian-friendly regime to be installed in Kyiv. But the advantage to the US of such a war would be that it would allow a radical upscaling of sanctions against Russia, setting back its economy for decades. Not only that, it would offer the opportunity to seriously degrade the Russian military since this would legitimize NATO member states in providing Ukraine with massive amounts of advanced weapons aid, which could draw Russia (and Ukraine) into a prolonged and costly conflict.

But, if provoking Russia to wage war in Ukraine is indeed the US's intention, the risks this would pose to political security and economic stability worldwide, if the strategy succeeds, would be astronomical. Military aid for Kyiv from the West in the context of an all-out war between Russia and Ukraine would risk military escalation and cross-border conflict-widening from Moscow. US-led economic sanctions against Russia may bolster nationalist support at home for Putin. They would inevitably beget Russian retaliatory action – including the suspension of energy supplies to Europe and beyond. This would accelerate those recessionary pressures on world capitalism that stemmed immediately from the COVID-19 pandemic but that also reflect decades of weak growth culminating in the Great Financial Crisis of 2007/09 and the long periods of economic stagnancy that followed.

The US's and EU's efforts to draw Ukraine away from closer ties with Russia and into their own economic, political, and military camp have been accompanied by US attempts at alliance-building with the new Central-Asian states on Russia's southern borders. This is intended to thwart Russia's own geopolitical goals which are energetically being pursued by Putin in Central Asia – to extend its regional influence, build new allies, or restore old ones. This is also to obtain control of the bountiful oil and gas reserves of the Caspian Basin on Russia's southern rim and its supply lines westwards (towards and through the Balkans) and southbound (through Turkey) to international waters, and so by the same token to restrict or deny independent access of rival states to these resources– not only opposed or "othered" states such as Russia and Iran, but also competitor states such as China and those of the EU.[226]

US hegemony and subordinate allies

Of these strategic alliances, Japan's with the US for mutual advancement appears most secure. Japan has been bound to US hegemony by its strategic decision to ally itself with the world's biggest economic and military power in exchange for its protection. The advantage for Japan is that this has virtually eliminated expenditure on self-defence that would slow down investments in the country's civilian economy (assisting Japan's ascendancy to the world's second-largest economy by the mid-1980s), whereas the advantage to the US has been twofold. First, this pre-empts any strategic alignment of Japan with China, indeed placing Japan at the centre of a network of states encircling China that are cultivated as allies by the US. Second, this allows Washington the technological means to sustain its military machine, since this is dependent on the import of a range of high-tech Japanese products and parts.[227]

With the rise of China as a regional great power, overtaking Japan as the biggest capital investor in Southeast Asia, this alliance is more likely to be strengthened rather than diminished, as tensions with China grow. This has generated political pressures in Japan for re-militarization, the renouncing of the pacifism clause in the constitution and even the acquisition of nuclear weapons. The US–Japan strategic alignment also contributes to growing tensions with other Southeast Asian states that remain suspicious of Japanese intentions owing to Japan's colonial record and the refusal of its leaders to officially acknowledge the country's culpability for its colonial exploits. Yet there are also growing tensions between Japan and the US fuelled by Japan's economic doldrums since the 1990s that have caused GDP growth to fall far behind the US's just as national debt piles up. This too has helped reinvigorate Japanese nationalism, which, owing to Japan's subordinate status in the US–Japan alliance, contains a strand of anti-Americanism. This has led to calls by Liberals for the return of the US Yokota military base to Japanese control, for example.[228]

The US's hegemony over Europe looks less secure though hardly endangered at present. The EU and its predecessor the EEC, after all, were forged not only to rein in the kind of destructive interstate rivalries that had led to two world wars[229] but in order to act as a counterweight to US and Soviet power, by unifying the constituent states in a relatively protected (from the greater economic power wielded by the two superpowers) single market zone.[230] Greater European alliance-building also served the US, however, because this would – by modernizing and stabilizing the continent economically – help fuel the expansion of the capitalist world market and better repel the threat of Soviet "communism" in Europe. A further benefit, from the US standpoint, was that this would allow the economic resurgence of Germany without the risk of reinvigorating German nationalism, German political domination of Europe, or the re-establishing of Germany as a great power that could challenge the US.[231] But a major source of Washington's hegemony over Europe was the military protection it offered against the USSR, which considerably waned with the end of the Cold War.

Imperialism and the Global South

Beyond the great regional hubs (US, China, Japan, and the EU), the rest of humanity is dispersed in mostly vassal and client nation-states developed or underdeveloped, to varying degrees, to service the needs of the high-income countries of the North. These are the multitude of semi-developed (or "developing" or "emerging" as the World Bank would have it) countries, mostly in the Global South, which are turned into open markets for North American, European, and Japanese commodities, suppliers of key energy resources, and net exporters of capital especially to the US but also the other developed countries.

The maintenance of this asymmetric geopolitical international structure of subordination (of the Global South to the US-led Global North) crucially depends on the worldwide "projection" of US military capabilities (hence the vast global network of US military bases), as those who do the projecting admit:

> The underdeveloped world's growing dissatisfaction over the gap between rich and poor nations will create a fertile breeding ground for insurgencies. These ... have the potential to jeopardize regional stability and our access to vital economic and military resources. The situation will become more crucial as our Nation and allies, as well as potential adversaries, become more and more dependent on these strategic resources. If we are to have stability in these regions, maintain access to these resources, protect our citizens abroad, defend our vital installations, and deter conflict, we must maintain within our active force structure a credible military power projection capability with the flexibility to respond to conflict across the spectrum of violence throughout the globe.[232]

Many if not developing countries are poor, minimally industrialized to varying degrees, over-reliant on the limited export earnings to be made from a limited range of primary and unsophisticated products, and locked into a subordinate and dependent market position *vis-à-vis* the developed countries whereby they are heavily dependent on imports of manufactured goods to function as even minimally industrial economies.[233] Even the economically successful countries of the Global South – such as the East Asian tigers, Brazil, Argentina, Mexico, India, and China – are unbalanced and not fully industrialized. This is inasmuch as these are unevenly developed (with advanced industrial enclaves alongside stagnating regions) and wage rates that are a fraction of those in the developed world – which is a major source of their attractiveness for investors.[234] This is also because these have huge proportions of workers in the informal sector, in casualized employ-ment,[235] and with large rural populations in at best semi-modernized agricultural sectors.[236]

These NICs and BRICs are also heavily reliant on the foreign earnings to be made from the exports of a limited number of usually high-tech companies (mostly to the developed world) which have been favoured by state support to render them internationally competitive. These countries thus produce much more for foreign high-income consumer markets than for their domestic ones since the latter are deficient in the purchasing power (given the suppression of wages to render exports inexpensive) required to sustain growth.[237] Outside the favoured capital-intensive companies driving export-driven growth, the rest of the economy remains rela-tively neglected, with labour productivity much lower than in the US, Europe, and Japan.[238] These countries too are net exporters of capital to the developed countries, especially the US.[239]

Included in the NICs of course is China, which has emerged as the biggest economy in Southeast Asia, with a GDP second only to the US,[240] but which shares the economic imbalances and vulnerabilities of the others. China is too large and powerful economically to be considered as less than a fully fledged imperial power in the making with aspirations for regional dominance and with the potential to challenge US world leadership. Indeed, that China is prepared to pursue its own national interests in geopolitics, without kowtowing to the US, is revealed by its willingness to loan money to poorer countries in the Global South (disregarding the IMF and its neoliberal conditionalities on capital transfers), its drive to add mili-tary strength to economic strength (expanding and modernizing its armed forces), and its intention to reclaim full sovereignty over Taiwan.[241] Add to that China's alliance-building with North Korea, Cuba, Iran, and Russia (all of which are "off-message" states from the perspective of the Washington Consensus, outside the US coalition – and one of which, Russia, is a sub-imperial state with regional ambi-tions, engaged in geopolitical competition with the US for control of the Caspian region, and with vast natural resources at its disposal as well as a vast stash of nuclear weapons) – and the potential for growing imperial conflict is clear.[242]

"Rogue" states and "failed" states

The large group of countries of the Global South that is home to the majority of the world's population includes those countries vulnerable to US-enacted or US-orchestrated or US-led neo-imperial sanctions – denial of foreign credit, trade embargoes, political destabilizations (e.g. funding or arming oppositionists or involvement in military coups), and direct military interventions, albeit usually as a weapon of last resort – if they fail to tread the free-trade path or if they disrupt the established geopolitical order of things.[243] The poorer or weaker of these countries are especially vulnerable to political instabilities in their own right.

Thus: "The most protracted and deadly ethnopolitical conflicts are likely to occur in poor, weak, heterogenous states like those of Africa".[244] This is owing to the pre-carity of their economic situation, the consequential incapacity of governments to dispense basic social functions or accommodate the minimal aspirations of many, and the acute internal conflicts this generates over access to resources. Such conflicts may then often be expressed in ethnic or tribal antagonisms, and where these are most acute dissolve the authority or legitimacy of the state altogether so that people must fend for themselves. In short, in such cases, class conflicts over allocative rights may be experienced as ethnic tensions and antagonisms between groups, which when state authority fails may even degenerate into banditry and civil war.[245] Somalia, the Democratic Republic of Congo, the Central African Republic, and Rwanda are recent cases.[246]

These precarities or vulnerabilities of the poorer countries are radicalized owing to the intensification of interstate economic competition under the whip-hand of neoliberal politics and the pressures this places on local states to retrench public services and redraw and draw in the distribution of social or community entitlements. And so,

> ethnic and sectarian violence is ironically linked to the apparent triumph of economic globalization and institutional transformation – the opening of new markets for goods, services, capital, and people; the construction of new democracies; and the implementation of "state-shrinking" ideologies that have swept the globe ... And transition to the market and the pressures of globalization – increased demands for industrial competitiveness and rising external debt that weakens the state's capability and willingness to allocate resources – are associated with high levels of conflict and even violence ... [C]ultural violence erupts most vociferously where secular economic decline, neoliberal economic reforms, and institutional transformation have broken old "social contracts" – that is, where they have broken the rules and norms by which access to political and economic resources was once granted. Globalization and liberalization are thus "triggers" for cultural conflict.[247]

Indeed, where membership of a particular ethnicity confers market advantages over non-members, ethnic antagonisms fuse with class antagonisms or, in the experience or perceptions of those encountering these injustices, replace them so that these become the main political drivers of conflict – or so it is argued.[248] These pressures or strains (resource stress, economic precarity – and intensifying struggles between groups over the distribution of entitlements) may even be motives for vulnerable states to wage war for territorial or economic advantage on other of their weak, underdeveloped neighbours – hence acting as minor sub-imperialisms in their own right. These border wars can be a way of alleviating the inner tensions and conflicts or deflecting these onto an external foe.

Such sub-imperial wars were also a legacy of the colonial period where antagonisms between clans and tribes were engineered by imperial authorities for purposes of divide and rule and where the clans or tribes were cut off from each other by colonial border-drawing. This has certainly been the case for interstate conflict in Africa, where border wars are sometimes fought to "liberate" and reunite wider ethnic or tribal groups. Again, Somalia is a classic example.[249] Other economically stronger, but nonetheless dependent or underdeveloped states, may aspire to exploit the freedom afforded by not being under the exclusive control of a specific imperial state (as was the case in the colonial era). This allows them the latitude to manoeuvre between the great powers (and between different MNCs from the rival great powers seeking investment opportunities within their borders),[250] in order to try and make of themselves regional sub-imperialisms – as, for example, Iran has tried to accomplish in the Middle East and Central Asia in recent decades, since the Islamic Revolution.

Watchdog states

Scattered among the vassal states, dependencies and protectorates under the new de-territorialized imperialism are what may be termed "watchdog" or "surveillance" states. These are nation-states situated in areas of the globe that are of particular or vital economic or strategic value to US corporate-capitalist interests and which are sanctioned to act as bulwarks against local forces (countries or movements) that may threaten these interests in exchange for economic patronage and military aid. These are thereby elevated to regional sub-imperialisms by their strategic role in policing or neutralizing their neighbours.

Suharto's brutal military dictatorship in Indonesia responsible for between 500,000 and a million deaths in internal pogroms and up to 300,000 deaths during its invasion and occupation of East Timor was one such case. Suharto secured power through a US- and British-assisted coup that unseated Sukarno's popular democratic government on the trumped-up pretext that the Marxists of the KPI were themselves planning one. Thereafter, Suharto enjoyed US (and British) patronage for "stabilizing" Indochina in the Cold War era and after, firstly as a bulwark against "communism", then latterly as a key ally against China, for which the regime was rewarded not simply with lavish military aid but by a blind eye being turned to its purging of dissidents and its war crimes in East Timor.[251]

The Middle East and watchdogs

The Middle East, owing to its vast concentration of energy resources, has been the region where US governments have perhaps sought most energetically to maintain such watchdogs. Almost 80 percent of the world's total oil reserves are in Organization of Petrol Exporting Countries (OPEC), with more than two-thirds of that in those countries which are situated in the Middle East.[252] Historically, the US economy has relied, to greater or lesser degrees, on oil exports from the Middle East, though some degree of reliance has been the norm since the late 1960s.

By the start of the 1970s, a third of US oil consumption needs were met by imports from the region.[253] By the close of the 1990s, 52 percent of the US's energy needs were being catered for by imported oil.[254] In the early 2000s, around 60 percent of US oil consumption was from imports, with around 21 percent of this coming from the Middle East.[255] The Bush Junior administration's *National Energy Plan* of 2001 predicted that US oil consumption would rise by 33 percent by 2020, which would require oil imports to increase by 30 percent. This, the report said, would create "increased dependency on foreign powers who do not always have America's interests at heart" so that the Middle East "would remain central to world oil security" and the "primary focus of US international energy policy".[256] By 2015, however, US imports from the region were reduced to 19 percent, owing to upscaling of domestic shale oil production, which greatly downsized the country's total foreign imports.[257]

Nonetheless, for most of the period, including most recently, these have been major volumes and hence real dependencies, which provide US governments with pressing interests in securitizing these energy sources for reason simply of economic national self-interest. Yet, in recent times, US foreign energy dependency has been in decline (owing to the shale oil boom), and this is projected to continue so that the US economy will soon achieve energy self-sufficiency.[258] In fact, energy self-sufficiency has been a longstanding goal of US policy exactly in order to help preserve its international hegemony.[259] And, if the US can produce major volumes of oil beyond its domestic needs (and the US is a major oil exporter), this creates the potential to render economic and geopolitical rivals more dependent on the US for their energy requirements.

Notwithstanding these observations, US imperialism's interests in securitizing the Middle Eastern oilfields and controlling the regional supply chains remain firmly intact, for two main reasons. Firstly, this is to prevent disruption of the international energy marketplace and hence ensure the stability of world prices. "The oil market is still global, which means the price Americans pay for fuel is still set by global oil prices and is vulnerable to supply disruptions, wherever they occur".[260] Secondly, this is also because competitor capitalisms (such as those of the EU bloc and Japan) and international rivals (most notably, China) are very much energy-dependent on the Middle East, whereas potential enemy states (such as Russia) which are much less so would become much more powerful rivals to the US if they could secure greater control of these resources at Washington's expense.[261]

US control of Middle Eastern oil (and indeed attempts to control it elsewhere – especially in the Caspian) is primarily for geopolitical rather than economic reasons. Oil, as Simon Bromley rightly says, is for the US a "strategic commodity".[262] From the US perspective, controlling access to the world's biggest oil reserves is a powerful lever for ensuring that it continues to get what it wants in world politics. This is by virtue of the capacity this bestows for economically disciplining existing competitors and rivals and for obstructing the ability of new rivals or opponents to challenge the US economically and hence politically. Indeed, this has the further advantage of permitting the US to cripple economically any "outlier" state in the Middle East that may be tempted to disrupt the security of oil supply or the stability of oil prices or the established balance of interstate power relations in the region in pursuit of its own national interests.

Up until the 1970s, US control of the Middle East's oil was secured by virtue of the direct corporate ownership or possession of much of the oil extraction and refining business across the region by its energy MNCs. Consequently, the patrimonial petrol monarchs or oil sheikhs of the Persian Gulf were tied to US imperialism by virtue of minority share ownership in as well as executive board membership of the "Seven Sisters" (mostly US-owned or US-majority controlled oil companies that possessed refining and processing and extraction facilities and which owned drilling rights right across the region). They were, in effect, "coupon-clipper kings".

Other rewards included receipt of tax revenues from the oil operations of these companies (which instead of being repatriated to their home governments were diverted into the coffers of the local kingdom-state) and, of course, military aid to prop up these deeply unpopular autocracies.[263] Since then, however, direct foreign ownership or control of oil by Western (mostly American) energy companies has been largely replaced by state ownership in the various regional oil-exporting nations, though the Western oil corporations do still largely control sales and refining.[264] By the end of the 1970s, unfettered access of international energy companies to oil supplies worldwide was reduced from 85 percent in the 1960s to just seven percent.[265]

Nonetheless, US domination of the Middle East's oil has since persisted by means of a system of control through *indirect* influence, pressure and patronage. The key US watchdog state of the region is of course Israel. Israel, since it was founded under US patronage and UN mandate in 1948,[266] has been the beneficiary of astronomical amounts of US economic and especially military aid. This accounted for a third of Washington's total foreign economic assistance budget from 1948 to 2000,[267] which bankrolled Israel's transition from a low-income to a high-income country. As for military aid, Israel has been the single biggest recipient from the US since it was carved out of Palestinian land.[268] "By 1999 the accumulated total was over $90 billion".[269] This shows no sign of slowing down after 70 years. In 2021, Israel remained

> the largest recipient of U.S. Foreign Military Financing. For FY2021, the President's request for Israel would encompass approximately 59% of total requested FMF funding worldwide.[270]

Such bounties and privileges have been bestowed on this apartheid-colonial state in return for policing its Arab neighbours in the interests of regional "stability". As was noted by the US National Security Council in 1958, containing the threat of radical Arab nationalism to US control of energy supplies in the Middle East necessitated continuing "to support Israel as the only strong pro-West power left in the Near East".[271] Nor, obviously, was this lost on Israeli leaders. As was reported by the Jewish *Ha'avetz* newspaper in 1951: "Strengthening Israel helps the Western powers maintain equilibrium" in the region.[272] Consequently, US arms and money have also bankrolled the Israeli state's regional imperialism, that is, its wars of territorial expansion that started with the swallowing up of the Palestinian state (and expulsion of much of its population) that was established alongside Israel in 1948[273] and that culminated in the annexation of the West Bank and Gaza Strip in the 1960s and 1970s.[274]

For a while, Saddam Hussein's Ba'athist regime in Iraq was also courted by Washington, by means of the usual economic and military inducements. This was in order to pull the oil-rich state beyond Soviet influence at the tail end of the Cold War and to weaponize it against Islamist Iran in an attempt to destabilize the regime in Tehran.[275] This particular watchdog got ideas above its station, however, by attempting to annex Kuwait, or at least to grab some disputed Kuwaiti oilfields, and so was neutralized. The regime was subject to two US-led military assaults that targeted (and destroyed) civilian and industrial infrastructure as well as military targets. This was on either side of a brutal economic embargo that killed up to, on some estimates, a million people, including 500,000 children.[276] (More conservative estimates of sanctions-related child mortality during this period put this at a minimum of 107,000 and a "more likely" 227,000).[277] This was owing to malnutrition and disease caused by the chronic state of disrepair of electricity, water and sewage infrastructure, degradation of healthcare, lack of basic medical supplies,[278] and exposure to warzone contaminants such as white phosphorus and depleted uranium (DU) shell fragments.[279]

The first of the Gulf Wars (which secured UN approval and hence was sanctioned under international law) was waged to expel the Iraqi army from Kuwait and to restore the Kuwaiti royalists to power. Such was the war's official rationale. But this was also to encourage leadership change in Baghdad. This was its unacknowledged objective (which was not sanctioned by those UN resolutions that approved military action).[280] The first Gulf War killed on US estimates between 50,000 and 100,000 Iraqi combatants (on Israeli estimates between 150,000 and 200,000),[281] plus unaccounted numbers of civilians.[282] This also made 1.8 million Iraqis homeless as well as sowing the seeds "for famines and epidemics".[283] The second Gulf War (which did not win UN backing and so was contrary to international law) was waged to occupy Iraq and destroy its ruling party altogether.[284] Estimated civilian deaths from the start of the second war in 2003, including the long period of insurgency against the Anglo-American occupation up until 2011, and also the prolonged political instability and civil violence that followed the Anglo-American withdrawal, ranging from 175,792 to 196,572.[285]

As for the petrol monarchies (Saudi Arabia, Bahrain, the UAE, Oman, Qatar, and Kuwait), these are in effect US vassal states by virtue of receiving copious US military aid and the security bulwark that the distribution of US military forces across the region provides them with against their own peoples and against local state rivals.[286] The US spends "$81 billion annually to protect oil supplies, mostly in the Gulf".[287] Such patronage and the pressure to cultivate it is necessary because the rulers of the oil kingdoms command little support outside elite and middle-class circles in the countries they rule because they are oligarchs, heading family-run absolutist states. They are opponents of any semblance of popular democracy, repressing all opposition to their rights of sovereignty, usually under the guise of extinguishing the threat of radical Islam and combating "terrorism".

These states are almost wholly dependent on guest workers devoid of those entitlements of citizenship (economic, political, legal) beyond the cash nexus. "In the UAE, Qatar, Bahrain and Kuwait, migrants substantially outnumber the overall national population, while Saudi Arabia has most foreign workers overall with 12 million, compared with its national population of 20 million".[288] The cheap labour power of these migrant workers supports the fabulous wealth of the elite and the high living standards and negligible taxes of the local middle classes.

The oil monarchies are also rentier states because of the tax income they accrue from granting permissions for overseas companies to do business within their borders and the export dividends they receive by means of their monopoly of natural resources – in this case, of course, crude oil.[289] These regimes are themselves bulwarks against those popular or democratic movements that pose a threat to US access to oil in return for US protection (especially against secular nationalist or socialist movements – since historically these are recognized by the US as posing the greatest threat to the political and economic status quo).

But the oil states are also rivals, competing with and intriguing against each other for regional influence, including by supporting rival insurgency or counter-insurgency movements or organizations in neighbouring countries (most recently, for example, in Libya, Syria, Tunisia, and Yemen).[290] Of these absolutist states, Saudi Arabia, which straddles the biggest oil reserves in the Middle East, has been especially feted and rewarded for the watchdog role it performs in maintaining regional "stability", and has been a virtual US protectorate since 1947.[291] This is despite the regime's covert support in recent times for Salafist Jihadist groups (which the US has itself classified as terrorists) that operate to undermine or obstruct its regional rivals.[292]

For these reasons, popular or "street" opinion in the Arab world has traditionally been anti-American and anti-Western. US governments throughout the period have been fully aware of this negative gaze from the "Arab street" focused on their regional role (and on the role of the Arab elites in the US's vassal states). Not only that, they have also tacitly conceded the validity of the reasons informing the negative judgement. In 1958, US President Dwight D. Eisenhower made the observation that hostility towards the US came not from Arab governments but from "the people" who supported the goals of Arab nationalism or Arab socialism. As the US National Security Council explained in the same year:

> In the eyes of the majority of Arabs the United States appears to be opposed to the goals of Arab nationalism. They believe that the United States is seeking to protect its interests in Near East oil by supporting the status quo and opposing political or economic progress.

This perception exists, as the USNSC put it, because

> our economic and cultural interests in the area have led not unnaturally to close US relations with elements in the Arab world whose primary interest lies in the maintenance of relations with the West and the status quo in their countries.[293]

Indeed, quite so.

****

This concludes my analysis of imperialism and international relations in their connection to neoliberalism and mega-capitalism. This dovetails with my analysis of the relationship between neoliberalism and corporate mega-capitalism in the ("global") age contained in my *Contagion Capitalism*. Neoliberalism is a form of politics that supports and promotes the freedoms of capital and the market internationally and that represents this ideologically as serving classless interests. Radical marketization was thought by neoliberals to be the solution to the tendencies towards stagnation, recession, and declining profits that had been characterizing world capitalism since the collapse of the postwar boom. However, neoliberal solutions have not solved these problems of capitalism. Indeed, they have exacerbated them. The economic system has become more rather than less structurally malintegrated in the neoliberal age.[294] At the same time, since neoliberal policies are strongly implicated with the resurgence of hardening or radicalizing class inequalities within and across borders, structural dissonance threatens to fuel social dissonance and conflict everywhere.

This chapter has sought to analyze the relationship between neoliberalism, imperialism, and the international state system. To restate my earlier formulation, imperialism, as I have sought to demonstrate, is made in the interface of economic (inter-capitalist) and geopolitical (interstate) competition under conditions where the protagonists have radically asymmetric access to authoritative and allocative resources. Imperialism is a force that operates to stabilize the world political order of nation-states under the umbrella of a hegemon, the US state. This is not only so that the high-income countries of the developed world under US leadership can reproduce their economic and other advantages over the others in the interstate system but also so that the interstate system can contain the social dissonance that is inevitably generated by fallout from the structural malintegration of the capitalist world economy in the corporate age. This means that neoliberalism is not simply a force of capitalist economics but is also a force of imperial politics.

The COVID-19 pandemic and the response of governments to it have to be understood as embedded in this political-economy context. This is the world in which the pandemic was made. And this is a world that made rather a hash of managing it to the detriment of people's lives, public health, wellbeing, and livelihoods across the face of the planet. Situating the pandemic in global political economy is the task of the next chapter, which focuses on nationalism and imperialism in relation to particular aspects of pandemic management in international relations.

19 April 2021 (updated November 2021)

Notes

1 Creaven, S. (2024). *Contagion Capitalism: Pandemics in the Corporate Age*: London and New York: Routledge, Ch.1. (Forthcoming).
2 Huntingdon, S. P. (1996). *The Clash of Civilizations and the Remaking of World Order*. London: Simon and Schuster.

3 Johnson, C. (2004). *Blowback: The Costs and Consequences of the American Empire*, 2nd edition. London and New York: Henry Holt and Co; Johnson, C. (2002). 'American Militarism and Blowback: The Costs of Letting the Pentagon Dominate Foreign Policy'. *New Political Science*, 24 (1), pp. 21–38; Briant, E. (2015). *Propaganda and Counterterrorism: Strategies for Global Change*. Manchester: Manchester University Press.

4 Chua, A. (2003). *World on Fire: How Exporting Free-Market Democracy Breeds Ethnic Hatred and Global Instability*. London: Willian Heinemann.

5 See Ch. 3.

6 UN (2014). *World Urbanization Prospects*. New York: UN.

7 Satterthwaite, D., McGranahan, G. and Tacoli, C. (2010), 'Urbanization and its implications for food and farming', *Philosophical Transactions of the Royal Society B*, 365, pp. 2809–20.

8 Douwe Van der Ploeg. J. (2008). *The New Peasantries: Struggles for Autonomy and Sustainability in an Era of Empire and Globalization*. London: Earthscan, p. xiv.

9 Harman, C. (2002). 'Workers of the world'. *International Socialism*, 2 (96), pp. 3–46. See especially pp. 6–8

10 See Ch. 3.

11 Creaven (2024), Ch.1.

12 Those who subscribe to this point of view may be distinguished between hyperglobalists and moderate globalists. The hyperglobalists are those who claim that global economic integration (that is, the trans-nationalization of the world market) is either here or approaching in the manner of world-historical inevitability. The moderate globalists (who describe themselves as "transformationalists") are those who perceive in postwar economic trends a definite and growing trend or dynamic towards global economic integration, though this globalization is not yet an accomplished reality worldwide and may not any time soon owing to the imbalances and divisions that capitalist internationalization also generates. These perspectives do not clearly divide by Left and Right on the political spectrum, despite Anthony Giddens' dismissal of the globalization sceptics as "Old Left". See: Giddens, A. (2002). *Runaway World: How Globalisation is Shaping our Lives*. London: Profile Books, p. 9. Globalists (whether hyper or moderate) may be broadly supportive or even enthusiasts of the process or its opponents and critics – though the "boosters" (as Callinicos calls them) predominate. See: Callinicos, A. (2001). *Against the Third Way*. Cambridge: Polity Press, p. 19.

Supportive hyperglobalists include Albrow, M. (1996). *The Global Age*. Cambridge: Polity Press; Crouch, C. (2004). *Post-Democracy*. Cambridge: Polity Press; Fitzgerald, N. (1997). 'Harnessing the potential of globalisation for the consumer and citizen'. *International Affairs*, 73 (4), pp. 731–43; Friedman, T. (1999). *The Lexus and the Olive Tree: Understanding Globalization*. New York: Farrar, Straus and Giroux; Giddens, A. (2002). *Runaway World: How Globalisation is Shaping our Lives*. London: Profile Books; Jakšic, M. (1997). 'Globalizacija i makroekonomska politika. Ekonomska politika stabilizacije'. *Ekonomiski fakultet*: Beograd; McMichael, P. (2000). *Development and Social Change: A Global Perspective*. CA Thousand Oaks: Pine Forge Press; Ohmae, K. (1990). *The Borderless World: Power and Strategy in the Interlinked World*. New York: Harper Business; Ohmae, K. (1995). *The End of the Nation-State*. New York: Free Press; Reich, R. (1991). *The Work of Nations: Preparing Ourselves for 21st Century Capitalism*. London: Simon and Schuster; Waters, M. (1995). *Globalization*. London and New York: Routledge; Wolf, M. (2004). *Why Globalization Works: The Case for the Global Market Economy*. New Haven: Yale University Press.

Critical hyperglobalists include Bauman, Z. (1998). *Globalization: The Human Consequences*. Cambridge: Polity Press; Forrester, V. (1999). *The Economic Horror*. Cambridge: Polity Press; Gray, J. (1998). *False Dawn: The Delusions of Global*

Capitalism. London: Granta; Holloway, J. (1995). 'Global Capital and the Nation State'. W. Bonefeld and J. Holloway (Eds.) *Global Capital, National State and the Politics of Money*. London: St Martin's Press; Klein, N. (2000). *No Logo*. London: Flamingo; Marshall, A. and Horsman, M. (1997). *After the Nation State: Citizens, Tribalism and the New World Disorder*. London: Harper-Collins; Sklair, L. (1995). *The Sociology of the Global System*. Harvester Wheatsheaf: Hemel Hempstead; Sklair, L. (2002). *Globalization, Capitalism and Its Alternatives*. Oxford: Oxford University Press.

13 Bauman, Z. (1998). *Work, Consumerism, and the New Poor*. Cambridge: Polity Press; Waters (1995). These sorts of ideas are clearly influenced by Jean Baudrillard's pre-globalization "postmodern" theory. See: Baudrillard, J. (1973). *The Mirror of Production*, St Louis: Telos Press; Baudrillard, J. (1981). *For a Critique of the Political Economy of the Sign* [1972]. London: Telos Press; Baudrillard, J. (1983). *In the Shadow of the Silent Majorities* [1978]. New York: Semiotexte.

14 Cited by: Harman, C. (2009). *Zombie Capitalism: Global Crisis and the Relevance of Marx*. London: Bookmarks, p. 257.

15 The notion that world capitalism has emancipated itself from dependence on the nation-state and by so doing has emasculated any national politics that would run counter to corporate interests is shared by right-wing or "Third Way" globalization enthusiasts and by left-wing critics of globalization (Bauman, Klein, etc.).

16 Friedman (1999); Ohmae (1990, 1005); Wolf (2004).

17 Blair quoted in: Pallast, G. (2003). *The Best Democracy Money Can Buy*. London: Constable and Robinson, p. 142.

18 Bauman (1998); Gray (1998); Marshall and Horsman (1997); Sklair (1995, 2002).

19 Todd, E. (2004). *After the Empire: The Breakdown of the American Order*. London: Constable, p. 15.

20 Hirst, P. and Thompson, P. (1999). *Globalization in Question: The International Economy and the Possibilities of Governance*. 2nd edition. Cambridge: Polity Press.

21 Giddens (2002), for example, dismisses the arguments of the sceptics owing simply to the unprecedented growth in the volume and dollar value of international commerce of recent decades. This is despite the fact that empirical measures of cross-border trade volumes tell us nothing about the international distribution of trade or the proportion of world trade to output.

22 Hoekman, B. (2015). *Trade growth – end of an era?* Centre for Economic Policy Research (online). (24 June).

23 Hirst and Thompson (1999).

24 WTO (2015), *International Trade Statistics 2015*. Online Report, p. 19.

25 Marfleet, P. (1998), 'Globalisation and the Third World', *International Socialism*, 2 (81), pp. 91–130.

26 WTO (2015), p. 26.

27 WTO (2018). *World Trade Statistical Review 2017* (online), p. 50.

28 WTO (2015), p. 24.

29 SDG Pulse (2020). *International trade in developing economies* (online); UNCTAD (2020). *Handbook of Statistics 2020* (online).

30 WTO (2013), *World Trade Report 2013*. Online Report. See pp. 57–58.

31 Marfleet (1998).

32 International Trade Centre (2019). *Trade Map: Trade Statistics for International Business Development – 2018* (online); UNCTAD (2020). *International trade in developing economies* (online).

33 WTO (2020). *World Trade Report 2019: The Future of Services Trade* (online), p. 30.

34 SDG Pulse (2020).

35 WTO (2020), p. 6.

36 WTO (2020), p .32.

37 WTO (2020), p. 33.

38 NAFTA (established by the North America Free Trade Agreement–also NAFTA) was superseded by the US-Mexico-Canada Agreement (USMCA) in July 2020.
39 WTO (2020), p. 12.
40 Dunn, C. (2009). 'Myths of globalisation and the new economy'. *International Socialism* (online), 121 (Winter).
41 Dunn (2009).
42 Dunn (2009).
43 Perry, M. (2019). *World's Top 10 Countries by Share of World Factory Output, 1970–2017*. Flourish: Data Visualisation and Story Telling (online). (5 July 2019).
44 Perry (2019).
45 Stefanovic, Z. (2008). 'Globalization: Theoretical Perspectives, Impacts and Institutional Response of the Economy', *Economics and Organization*, 5 (3), pp. 263–72. See pp. 267–68.
46 Sklair (2002).
47 Kuzel, M. (2016). *Global Activity of the World's Largest Transnationals: A New Dimension of International Business*. Faculty of Economic Sciences and Management: Nicolaus Copernicus University.
48 Rugman, A. (2005). 'Globalization and Regional International Production'. J. Ravenhill (Ed.) *Global Political Economy*. Oxford: Oxford University Press, p. 269.
49 Rugman (2005), p. 270.
50 Kuzel (2016).
51 UNCTAD (2007). *The Universe of the Largest Transnational Corporations*. New York and Geneva: UN, p. 13.
52 Wood, E.M. (1998). 'Modernity, Postmodernity, or Capitalism?' R.W. McChesney, E.M. Wood, and J.B. Foster (Eds.) *Capitalism and the Information Age*. New York: Monthly Review Press.
53 Harman (2009), p. 255.
54 OECD (2019). *OECD International Direct Investment Statistics, 2009–2018* (online), pp. 18–19.
55 UNCTAD (2016). *The World Investment Report 2016: Investor Nationality – Policy Challenges* (online), p. 4.
56 UNCTAD (2017). *The World Investment Report 2017: Investment and the Digital Economy* (online), p. x.
57 UNCTAD (2002). *The World Investment Report 2002: Transnational Corporations and Export Competitiveness* (online), p. 7.
58 This calculation is distilled from the UNCTAD *World Investment Reports* from 2003 to 2014.
59 See also: UNCTAD (2015). *The World Investment Report 2015: Reforming International Investment Governance* (online); UNCTAD (2018). *The World Investment Report 2018: Investment and New Industrial Policies* (online); UNTAD (2019). *The World Investment Report 2019: Special Economic Zones* (online). See also: UNCTAD (2016, 2017).
60 Hoogvelt, A. (2001). *Globalization and the Post-Colonial World: The New Political Economy of Development*, 2nd edition, London: Palgrave, p. 77.
61 UNTACD (2002), p. 7.
62 UNTACD (2019), p. xiii.
63 UNTACD (2016, 2017, 2018, 2019).
64 UNTACD (2019), p. 12.
65 UNTACD (2016), pp. 4–5.
66 UNTACD (2019), p. 4.
67 UNTACD (2019), pp. 40–41.
68 UNTACD (2019), p. 49.
69 Hayter, T. (1990). *The Creation of World Poverty*, 2nd edition. London: Pluto Press, pp 77–79; Barnet, R.J. and Muller, R.E. (1974). *Global Reach: The Power of the Multinational Corporations*. New York: Simon and Schuster.
70 UNCTAD (2019), p. xi.

71 Hayter (1990), pp 77–79; Barnet and Muller (1974).
72 Calderon, C. and Loayza, N. (2004). *Greenfield foreign direct investment and mergers and acquisitions: feedback and macroeconomic effects*. World Bank (online), pp. 15–16.
73 Harms, P. and Meon, P-G. (2011). 'An FDI is an FDI is an FDI? The growth effects of greenfield investment and mergers and acquisitions in developing countries'. Working Paper no. 11. *EconStore* (online), p. 27.
74 Danakol, S.H., Estrin, S., Reynolds, P.D., and Weitzel, U. (2017). 'Foreign direct investment via M&A and domestic entrepreneurship: blessing or curse?' *Small Business Economics*, 48 (3), pp. 1–30; Neto, P., Brandao, A., and Cirqueira, A. (2008). *The Impact of FDI, Cross Border Mergers and Acquisitions and Greenfield Investments on Economic Growth*. (October 2008). Research Gate (online).
75 Danakol *et al.* (2017), p. 3.
76 Hoogvelt, A. (1997). *Globalisation and the Post-Colonial World: The New Political Economy of Development*. London: Palgrave.
77 Pilger, J. (1999). *Hidden Agendas*. London: Vintage, p. 75.
78 UNTACD (2019), pp. 66, 67.
79 UNTACD (2016), p. 4.
80 UNTACD (2019), pp. 34, 35.
81 UNTACD (2014, p. 37; 2020, p. 28; 2019, p. 28; 2018, p. 34; 2017, p. 44; 2016, p. 38; 2015, p. 32).
82 UNTACD (2019, p. 28; 2018, p. 34; 2017, p. 44; 2016, p. 38; 2015, p. 32).
83 UNTACD (2014, p. 61; 2020, p. 46; 2019, p. 48; 2018, p. 50; 2017, p. 57; 2016, p. 51; 2015, p. 58).
84 UNTACD (2014), p. 61.
85 UNTACD (2018), p. 50.
86 UNTACD (2019, p. 48; 2018, p. 50; 2017, p. 57; 2016, p. 51; 2015, p. 58).
87 Harman, C. (1996). 'Globalisation – a critique of a new orthodoxy'. *International Socialism*, 2 (73), pp. 3–33.
88 These are, respectively, Noam Chomsky's and Mark Curtis's terms for the anonymous victims-at-a-distance beyond-our-borders of American and Western economic and political domination.
89 UNCTAD (2010). *World Investment Report: Investing in a Low Carbon Economy* (online), p. 3.
90 UNCTAD (2010), p. 3.
91 UNCTAD (2011, p. x; 2012, p. xi; 2013, p. ix; 2014, p. ix; 2015, p. x; 2016, p. x).
92 UNCTAD (2017, p. x; 2018, p. 2; 2019, p. x).
93 UNCTAD (2020). *World Investment Report 2020: International Production Beyond the Pandemic* (online), p.11.
94 UNCTAD (2021). 'Global FDI Flows Down 42% in 2020'. *Investments Trends Monitor* (online), 38. (January).
95 UNCTAD (2017, p. x; 2018, p. 2; 2019, p. x).
96 UNCTAD (2021).
97 UNCTAD (2017, p. x; 2018, p. 2; 2019, p. x; 2021).
98 UNCTAD (2020, p. 8) predicts that the greater negative economic impacts of the COVID-19 crisis looking ahead will likely be the developing countries. "Developing economies as a group are expected to see a larger decrease in the range of 30 per cent to 45" of FDI in 2021.
99 Institute for International Economics (2002). *The Pattern of Economic Growth, 1950–2000* (online), p. 17
100 IIE (2002), p. 23.
101 Maria, A. and Wen, Yi. (2015). 'Trapped: Few Developing Countries Can Climb the Economic Ladder or Stay There'. Federal Reserve Bank of St Louis (online). (7 October).

102 IIE (2002), p. 18.

103 IIE (2002), p. 21.

104 Weller, C.E. and Hersh, A. (2004). 'The long and short of it: Global liberalization and the incomes of the poor'. *Journal of Post-Keynesian Economics*, 26 (3), pp. 471–505. See p. 471.

105 IIE (2002), p. 24.

106 UNDP (1999). *Human Development Report 1999: Human Development in this Age of Globalization*. New York: UNDP, p. 3; Kanbur, R. *et al.* (2001). *World Development Report 2000/2001: Attacking Poverty*. New York: World Bank, p. 3.

107 OECD (2011). *Divided We Stand: Why Inequality Keeps Growing*. New York: OECD.

108 UNCTAD (2020). *The least developed countries report 2020:productive capacities for the new decade* (online). (3 December).

109 Giddens, A. (1994). *Beyond Left and Right: The Future of Radical Politics*. Cambridge: Cambridge University Press.

110 Held, D. (1991a). 'Democracy and Globalization'. *Alternatives*, 16 (2), pp. 201–08; Held, D. (1991b). 'Democracy, the nation-state and the global system'. *Economy and Society*, 20 (2), pp. 138–72.

111 This is the "competition state" theory, as Luke Martell describes it. See: Martell, L. (2010). *The Sociology of Globalization*. Cambridge: Polity Press.

112 Gourevitch, P. (1986). *Politics in Hard Times: Comparative Responses to International Economic Crises*. Ithaca: Cornell University Press; Garrett, G., and Lange, P. (1991). 'Political responses to interdependence: what's "left" for the left'. *International Organization*, 45 (4), pp. 539–64.

113 Gourevitch (1986), p. 33.

114 Garrett and Lange (1991), p. 541.

115 Blair quoted in Callinicos (2001), p. 16.

116 Rosenau, J.N. (1990). *Turbulence in World Politics*. Brighton: Harvester Wheatsheaf.

117 For useful discussions see also: Camilleri, J. A. and Falk, J. (1992) *The End of Sovereignty? The Politics of a Fragmented and Shrinking World*, Aldershot: Edward Elgar; Dunn, J. (Ed.) (1995), *Contemporary Crisis of the Nation State?* Oxford: Blackwell.

118 Keohane, R. and Nye, J.S. (1987). 'Power and interdependence revisited'. *International Organization*, 41 (4), pp.725–53.

119 This undermines the notion associated especially with the transformationalists (or moderate globalists) that a solution to the "declinist" state is cosmopolitan democracy. See especially: Held, D. (1995). *Democracy and the Global Order: From the Modern State to Cosmopolitan Governance*. Cambridge: Polity Press; Held (1991a, 1991b); Beck, U. (2006). *Cosmopolitan Visions*. Cambridge: Polity Press; Beck, U. (2009). 'Critical Theory of World Risk Society: A Cosmopolitan Vision'. *Constellations*, 16 (1), pp. 3–21; Hayden, P. (2005). *Cosmopolitan Global Politics*. Aldershot: Ashgate Publishers.

120 Gilpin, R. (1981). *War and Change in World Politics*. Cambridge: Cambridge University Press

121 Harman, C. (1991). 'The state and capitalism today'. *International Socialism*, 2 (51), pp. 3–56; Stopford, J.M. and Strange, S. (1991). *Rival States, Rival Firms: Competition for World Market Shares*. Cambridge: Polity Press.

122 Bull, H. (1979).'The State's Positive Role in World Affairs'. K. Alderson and A. Hurrell (Eds.) *Hedley Bull on International Society*. London: Palgrave-Macmillan, pp. 139–56.

123 Harris (1987). *The End of the Third World: Newly Industrializing Countries and the Decline of an Ideology*. London: Penguin, p. 202. See especially: Harris, N. (1991). *National Liberation*. London: Bloomsbury.

124 Waltz (1979). *The Theory of International Politics*. New York: McGraw-Hill.

125   Waltz (1979), p. 185.
126   Harman (1996), p. 6.
127   Gordon, D. (1988). 'The global economy: new edifice or crumbling foundations'. *New Left Review*, 1 (168) (March/April), pp. 54–68. See p. 63.
128   Frontline (2014). *Timeline of the Panic*. PBS: Frontline (online).
129   Frontline (2014).
130   The final liability of the US government's rescue of its big banks in the aftermath of the 2007/09 financial crisis has retrospectively been estimated at between $498 billion and $4.6 trillion. See: Harbert, T. (2019). *Here's How Much the 2008 Bailouts Really Cost*. (21 February). MIT Management (online); Taibbi, M. (2019). 'Turns Out That Trillion-Dollar Bailout Was, in Fact, Real'. *Rolling Stone* (online). (18 March). The cost of the UK government's bailout of its own corporate-finance sector was estimated at £850 billion by the end of 2009, though part of this was repaid over the next few years. See: Grice, A. (2009). '850bn: official cost of the bank bailout'. *Independent*. (4 December).
131   The UK government, for example, launched the Covid Corporate Financing Facility (CCFF) in response to the pandemic. By April 2020, this had allocated £7.477 billion to the UK's largest companies. This was in sharp contrast to the much lesser monies distributed to businesses under the Coronavirus Business Interruption Loan Scheme (CBILS). The amount of funds provided to companies under CCFF was seven times greater than those provided under CBILS. The CBILS allocated government funds to the banks to loan to smaller businesses. But the banks then refused four-fifths of the applications and levied excessive interest rates as conditionalities on the successful ones. See: Barmes, D. (2020). 'Bank of England Provides £7.5 billion in Big Business Bailouts – Hidden from Public View'. PositiveMoney (online). (April). The US government, for example, committed $500 billion to corporate bailouts to be funded by taxpayers in response to the pandemic's first wave. See: Eisinger, J. (2020). 'How the Coronavirus Bailout Repeats 2008's Mistakes: Huge Corporate Payoffs With Little Accountability'. *ProPublica* (online). (7 April 2020). By October 2020, more than half of the US government's total pandemic relief budget of $4 trillion ($2.3 trillion) had been spent on subsidizing businesses, and only 16 percent of it had been devoted to coping with the health crisis and 25 percent to financially assisting workers and their families. This included "$651 billion in business tax breaks that often went to companies unaffected by the pandemic and others that laid off thousands of workers. Billions more went to the Federal Reserve to help stabilize markets, and those efforts enabled many companies – including Wells Fargo, AT&T and Carnival, the cruise company – to borrow at lower rates while also laying off thousands of workers". See: Whoriskey, P., MacMillan, D., and O'Connell, J. (2020). '"Doomed to fail": Why a $4 trillion bailout couldn't revive the American economy'. *Washington Post*. (5 October).
132   Callinicos (2001), p. 109.
133   Argentina defaulted in December 2001, in response to the Latin American slump that was triggered by the Southeast Asian financial crisis of 1997/98.
134   In Argentina, in response to the recession of 2000/01, FDI flatlined. But this was restored in 2002, despite the December 2001 default. This averaged 2.28 percent of GDP from 2002 to 2008, topping the average (of 1.96 percent) from 1991 to 1996. See: World Bank (2021). *Foreign direct investment, net inflows (% of GDP) – Argentina* (online).
135   In Argentina, from almost 30 percent in 2002 to 4.4 percent in 2004. See: Knoema (2020). *Argentina – average consumer prices inflation rate* (online).
136   GDP growth in Argentina was almost nine percent in 2002 and this level was maintained until the Great Financial Crisis of 2007/09. See: World Bank (2021). *GDP growth (annual %) – Argentina* (online).

137 Van Voris, B. and Porzecanski, K. (2016). 'Argentina Wins Court Ruling Letting Bond Sale Proceed'. Bloomberg (online). (13 April); DeFotis, D. (2016). 'Argentina Debt Outlook Improving, Moody's says'. Barron's (online). (16 March).

138 Ruigrock, W. and van Tulder, R. (1995). *The Logic of Economic Restructuring: The Management of Dependencies in Rival Industrial Complexes*. Cambridge: Cambridge University Press, p. 218.

139 Harman, C. (1995). *The Economics of the Madhouse: Capitalism and the Market Today*. London: Bookmarks, pp. 64, 65–66; Harman (2009), pp. 233–34.

140 Stopford and Strange (1991); Harman (1991), pp. 8, 12, 34–35.

141 Ruigrock and van Tulder (1995).

142 Harman (1991), pp. 33, 35.

143 Stopford and Strange (1991), p. 1.

144 Harman (1991), p. 13.

145 Harman (1991), pp. 12–13.

146 Ruigrock and van Tulder (1995), p. 164. My emphasis.

147 Harman (1996), pp. 14–15, 19; Harman (2009), pp. 258–59.

148 Globalism acquires a superficial plausibility especially by virtue of the massive expansion of FDI since the 1980s, this increasing from four percent of the value of world output in 1982 to 36 percent by 2007 (Harman, 2009, p. 255).

149 de Brunhoff, S. (1999). 'Which Europe Do We Need Now? Which Can We Get?' R. Bellofiore (Ed.) *Global Money, Capital Restructuring, and the Changing Patterns of Labour*. Cheltenham: Edward Elgar, p. 50.

150 Bryan, D. (2001). 'Global Accumulation and Accounting for National Economic Identity'. *Review of Radical Political Economy*, 33 (1), pp. 55–77.

151 Bryan (2001), p. 61.

152 Creaven (2024), Ch.1. (Forthcoming).

153 Creaven (2024), Ch.1.

154 See especially: Martell (2010).

155 Castells, M. (1996). *The Rise of the Network Society. The Information Age: Economy, Society, and Culture*. Oxford: Blackwell, p. 147.

156 Creaven, S. (2005). 'Recovering Marx for the Twenty-First Century'. *Journal of Critical Realism*, 4 (1), pp. 128–66. See p. 158. See also: Anderson, P. (2000). 'Renewals'. *New Left Review*, 2 (1), pp. 11–14; Callinicos (2001), p. 7; Castells (1996), pp. 135, 137, 140.

157 Birchall, I. (1985). *Bailing Out the System: Reformist Socialism in Western Europe 1944–1983*. London: Bookmarks.

158 Cliff, T. and Gluckstein, D. (1996). *The Labour Party: A Marxist History*. 2nd edition. London: Bookmarks; Miliband, R. (1961). *Parliamentary Socialism: A Study in the Politics of Labour*. London: Merlin Press.

159 Keohane, R. (1984). *After Hegemony: Cooperation and Discord in the World Political Economy*. Princeton: Princeton University Press, p. 32.

160 Mearsheimer, J. J. (2001). *The Tragedy of Great Power Politics*. New York: W.W. Norton.

161 Gilpin (1981), p. 29.

162 World Bank (2021). *GDP (current US $) – US, Japan* (online); World Bank (2021). *GDP (current US $) – European Union* (online).

163 Duffin, E. (2021). *U.S. military spending from 2000 to 2020*. Statista (online). (10 November); Spirlet, T. (2021). 'EU countries spend record €198B on defense in 2020 as joint spending slumps: report'. *Politico* (online). (6 July).

164 Kindleberger, C.P. (1973). *The World in Depression: 1929–1939*. Berkeley: University of California Press, p. 305.

165 Posen, B.R. (2003). 'Command of the Commons: The Military Foundation of U.S. Hegemony'. *International Security*, 28 (1), pp. 5–46.

166 Layne, C. (2006). *The Peace of Illusions: American Grand Strategy from 1940 to the Present*. Ithaca: Cornell University Press, p. 4.
167 Gilpin, R. (1987). *The Political Economy of International Relations*. Princeton: Princeton University Press, p. 87.
168 Keohane (1984), pp. 34–35.
169 Gilpin (1987), p. 72.
170 Keohane (1980), p. 132.
171 Gilpin (1981); Gilpin (1987); Gilpin, R. (2001). *Global and Political Economy: Understanding the International Economic Order.* Princeton: Princeton University Press; Kindleberger (1973); Kohout, F. (2003). 'Hegemonic Stability Theory'. *International Political Science Review*, 24 (1), pp. 55–56.
172 Gilpin (1987), p. 89.
173 Gilpin (2001), pp. 99–100.
174 Keohane (1984), pp. 39–41.
175 Gilpin (1987), p. 73.
176 Keohane (1984), p. 34.
177 Gilpin (1981).
178 Krasner, S. D. (1983). 'Structural Causes and Regime Consequences: Regimes as Intervening Variables'. S.D. Krasner (Ed.) *International Regimes*. Ithaca: Cornell University Press, p. 2.
179 Krasner (1983), p. 2.
180 Keohane (1984), p. 46.
181 Keohane (1984), p. 46.
182 The US's per capita income in 2020 was $63,413 compared to China's £10, 434. See: World Bank (2021). *GDP per capita (current $US) – United States, China* (online).
183 Kohout (2003, pp. 55–56) notes that consequences of a hegemon's decline may include the collapse of the international system into depression, war and banditry, or its replacement by a new hegemonic power.
184 In 2020, China spent $252.3 billion on arms. See: SIPRI (2021). *Military expenditure by country, in constant (2019) US$: 1988–2020*. Stockholm International Peace Research Institute (online).
185 The literature on US-enacted "regime change" *alone* (political destabilizations, covert operations, complicity in human rights abuses, military interventions) is vast, leaving aside literature addressing the other coercive aspects of US foreign policy, and indeed that on the equally significant phenomenon of "regime preservation". This includes support for drug oligarchs, neo-fascists, and terrorists in no fewer than 35 countries in the postwar period. Nicolas Davies helpfully chronicles these cases by way of indictment alphabetically. See: Davies, N.J.S. (2014). *35 countries where the U.S. has supported fascists, drug lords and terrorists*. Salon (online). (8 March). Indeed this aspect is so voluminous that a large encyclopaedia is dedicated to cataloguing it all.
   For a good sample of a range of excellent critical studies and reports on US imperialism in the period see: Ameringer, C.D. (1990). *US Foreign Intelligence: The Secret Side of American History*. 2nd edition. New York: Lexington; Bert, W. (2016). *American Military Intervention in Unconventional War: From the Philippines to Iraq*. Springer; Blakeley, R. (2009). *State Terrorism and Neoliberalism: The North in the South*. London: Routledge; Blum, W. (2014a). *Killing Hope: US Military and CIA Interventions Since World War II*, 3rd edition. London: Zed Books; Blum, W. (2014b). *Rogue State: A Guide to the World's Only Superpower*, 4th edition, London: Zed Books; Chomsky, N. (2006). *Imperial Ambitions*. Harmondsworth: Penguin; Chomsky, N. (2000). *Rogue States: The Rule of Force in World Affairs*. London: Pluto Press; Chomsky, N. (1999). *Profit Over People: Neoliberalism and the Global Order*. New York: Seven Stories Press; Chomsky, N. (1992). *Deterring Democracy*. London: Verso, esp. pp. 19–33, 139–77, 215–51; Chomsky, N. (2003). *Hegemony or Survival: America's Quest for Global Dominance*.

New York: Metropolitan Books; Curtis, M. (1998). *The Great Deception: Anglo-American Power and World Order*. London: Pluto Press; Esparza, M., Huttenbach, H.R., and Feierstein, D. (Eds.) *State Violence and Genocide in Latin America: The Cold War Years*; London: Routledge (esp. Chs 1–5); Fouskas, V. and Gökay, B. (2005). *The New American Imperialism: Bush's War on Terror and Blood for Oil*. Westport CO: Greenwood; German, L. and Marcetic, B. (2020). 'The CIA's Secret Global War Against the Left'. Jacobin (online). (30 November); McPherson, P. (2016). *A Short History of U.S. Interventions in Latin America and the Caribbean*. New York: John Wiley; Maurer, N. (2013). *The Empire Trap: The Rise and Fall of U.S. Intervention to Protect American Property Overseas, 1893–2013*. Princeton NJ: Princeton University Press; Musicant, I. (1990). *The Banana Wars: A History of United States Military Intervention in Latin America from the Spanish – American War to the Invasion of Panama*. New York: MacMillan; Schmitz, D.F. (1999). *Thank God They're on Our Side: The United States and Right-Wing Dictatorships, 1921–1965*. Chapel Hill NC: North Carolina Press; Sullivan, M. (2008). *American Adventurism Abroad: Invasions, Interventions, and Regime Changes since World War II*. 2nd edition. San Francisco CA: Wiley-Blackwell; Wilford, H. (2013). *America's Great Game: The CIA's Secret Arabists and the Shaping of the Modern Middle East*. New York: Basic Books; Woodward, R. (1987). *Veil: The Secret Wars of the CIA*. New York: Simon and Schuster.

186 Callinicos, A. (1994). 'Imperialism Today'. A. Callinicos, Rees, J., Harman, C., and Haynes, M. (Eds.) *Marxism and the New Imperialism*. London: Bookmarks, p. 27.

187 See esp. Chomsky (1992), pp. 19–33, 139–77, 215–51. See also Chomsky (2003).

188 The White House (1990). *National Security Strategy of the United States*. (1 March). National Security Strategy Archive: Washington DC, pp. 15, 26, 6.

189 See esp. Blakeley (2009) and Blum (2014a, 2014b). See also: Chomsky (2000).

190 Quoted in Chomsky (1992), p. 49.

191 Schoultz, L. (1981). *Human Rights and United States Policy toward Latin America*. Princeton: Princeton University Press, p. 7. Cited in Chomsky (1992), p. 51.

192 Callinicos (2009), p. 15.

193 Callinicos (2009), p. 17.

194 $19.39 trillion in 2017 compared to $17.28 trillion for the EU and $4.87 trillion for Japan. Worldometer (2020). *Population Comparison: China, EU, USA, and Japan* (online).

195 Callinicos, A. (2003). *The New Mandarins of American Power*. Cambridge: Polity Press, pp. 93–98; Klare, M. (2003). 'The Policies: Resources'. J. Feffer, (Ed.) *Power Trip: US Unilateralism and Global Strategy After September 11*. New York: Seven Stories Press, pp. 50–60.

196 Bromley, S. (2005). 'The United States and Control of World Oil'. *Government and Opposition*, 40, pp. 253–54.

197 Almost 70 percent of "defence" (that is, military) spending by NATO's 30 member states is by the US. The US makes by far the biggest contribution (22.4 percent) to NATO'S military and civilian budget compared to 14.7 percent by Germany and 10.5 percent each by France and the UK.

198 Harvey, D. (2005). *A Brief History of Neoliberalism*. Oxford: Oxford University Press, pp. 54–55; Callinicos (2009), pp. 169–70, 176; Wade, R.H. (2003). 'The Invisible Hand of the American Empire'. *Ethics and International Affairs*, 17 (2), pp. 77–88.

199 Callinicos (2009), p. 193.

200 Akrill, R. (2000). *The Common Agricultural Policy*. Sheffield: Sheffield Academic Press; Amadeo, K. and Boyle, M.J. (2021). 'Government Subsidies (Farm, Oil, Export, Etc. What are the Major Federal Government Subsidies?' *The Balance* (online). (30 April); Barakou, A. (2020). 'Dirty Subsidies: How Europe sabotages its climate goals'. *Investigate Europe* (online); Brown, D., Chow, H., Hanna, T.M., and McDonald, D. (2019). *Democratic public ownership in the UK pharmaceutical*

sector. Global Justice Now (online). (September); Chomsky (2000); Coats-Chaney, C.K. (2013). *State Aid to Car Companies: Were Government Responses to the Auto Industry Crisis Different in the United States and Europe?* Chapel Hill: University of North Carolina; Erskine, D. (2006). 'The United States – EC Dispute Over Customs Matters, and the Meaning of WTO Obligations', *Florida Journal of International Law*, 18, pp. 432–85; International Trade Administration (2020). *EU – Country Commercial Guide* (online). (24 August 2020); Lincicome, S. (2020). 'Examining America's Farm Subsidy Problem'. (18 December). Cato Institute (online); Meller A. and Ahmed, A. (2019). *How Big Pharma Reaps Profits While Hurting Everyday Americans*. Censer for American Progress (online). (30 August); Wallace, A. and Mason, G. (1995). *R & D Subsidies in the European Union: A Competitiveness Issue for US Firms?* Knowledge Media Institute (online).

201 Chomsky (1999), p. 21.

202 Chomsky (2000) reports that 80 percent of the total of UN sanctions imposed on countries in the period from the end of World War Two up to the start of the twenty-first century were tabled by the US government.

203 According to Chomsky (2012a), the US economy's share of global GDP fell by a quarter between 1945 and 1970. See: Chomsky (2012a). 'Losing the World: American Decline in Perspective'. (Part 1). *Guardian*. (14 February).

204 Todd (2004); Chomsky (2012a); Chomsky, N. (2012b). 'The Imperial Way: American Decline in Perspective'. (Part 2). *Guardian*. (15 February).

205 Mann, M. (1986). *The Sources of Social Power*, Vol. 1. Cambridge: Cambridge University Press.

206 Martell (2010), pp. 279–82.

207 Todd (2004, pp. 14, 15, 21–22) describes the US's recent "dramatized militarism" (wars or threats of war against minor adversaries dubbed as "rogue states" (Afghanistan, Iran, Iraq, North Korea, Cuba, etc.), as well as its declaration of eternal war against universal terrorism, as attempts to mask its growing economic and political weakness. These represent, he says, symbolic attempts to demonstrate before its allies and major adversaries that it retains superpower status, is indispensable to world security, and thus retains also the right to govern world affairs.

208 See especially: Callinicos (2003).

209 Cited in: Martell (2010), p. 81.

210 White House (1990), p. 26.

211 Martell (2010), p. 281.

212 Vine, D. (2015). *Base Nation: How U.S. Military Bases Abroad Harm America and the World*. New York: Metropolitan Books.

213 Rees, J. (1996). 'The New Imperialism'. Callinicos *et al*. (Eds.), p. 69.

214 Vine (2015).

215 Vine (2015). Harvey (2005), pp. 16–25; Klare, M. (2005). *Blood and Oil: The Dangers and Consequences of America's Growing Petroleum Dependency*. Harmondsworth: Penguin, pp. 40–41, 26–55, 74–112; Klare (2003), pp. 50–60; Harvey, R. (2003). *Global Disorder*. London: Robertson, pp. 117–21; Callinicos (2003), pp. 80–98.

216 Klare (2005), pp. 113–45.

217 Callinicos (2003), pp. 63–64; Callinicos (2009), pp. 191–93; Cohen, S. F. (2006). 'The New American Cold War'. *The Nation*. (10 July); Rees, J. (1999). 'NATO and the New Imperialism'. *Socialist Review* (June); Brzezinski, Z. (1998). *The Grand Chessboard: American Primacy and Its Geostrategic Imperatives*. New York: Basic Books, p. 74

218 Mearsheimer, J.J. (2015). *The causes and consequences of the Ukraine Crisis*. Uncommon Core Lecture: University of Chicago (online). (4–7 June).

219 Rohde, D. and Mohammed, A. (2014). 'How the U.S. made its Putin problem worse'. *Reuters* (online). (18 April).

220 Cornwell, S. (2008). 'U.S. to announce over $1 billion in aid for Georgia'. *Reuters* (online). (3 September); Henney, M. (2019). 'US aid to Ukraine: How it's changed under Trump, Obama and Bush'. *Fox Business* (online). (12 October).

221 Rohde and Mohammed (2014).

222 Mearsheimer (2015).

223 Mearsheimer, J.J. (2014). 'Why the Ukraine Crisis Is the West's Fault: The Liberal Delusions That Provoked Putin'. *Foreign Affairs* (online) (September/October).

224 The Monroe Doctrine was formulated as an article of US foreign policy in 1823. Its original intention was to deter specifically European colonial-motivated interferences in the Americas. Under this guise, the doctrine legitimized the annexation of Hawaii in 1842, the attempted annexation of the Dominican Republic in 1870, and the military occupation of Cuba following the American-Spanish war (1895–1902), which turned the country thereafter into a virtual US colony. Emboldened by the "Roosevelt corollary", which sanctioned the exercise of force also against "flagrantly" and "chronically" misbehaving Latin American nations, in order to protect US economic interests, the Monroe doctrine was extended far beyond its supposed original purpose – to defend the Americas from Old World colonialism. Instead, as the US began to consolidate itself as a great power, the doctrine was invoked and applied to assert the US's own regional hegemony and its own imperial projects. This was much in advance of the Cold War period. As US Secretary of State, Richard Olney, expressed the matter in 1895: "The United States is practically sovereign on this continent, and its fiat is law upon the subjects to which it confines its interposition" (Herring, 2011, p. 307). See Gilderhus, M.T. (2006) 'The Monroe Doctrine: meanings and implications'. *Presidential Studies Quarterly*, 36 (1), pp. 5–16; Herring, G.C. (2011). *From Colony to Superpower: US Foreign Relations Since 1776*. New York: Oxford University Press.

Subsequently, in the Cold War era, the Monroe Doctrine was asserted to justify a large number of military and other interventions in the Americas in the 1970s and 1980s to destabilize governments that were perceived as threats to free trade, capitalist enterprise, corporate ownership, or liberal democracy – those in Cuba, Chile, Nicaragua, and Panama being the main examples. Alternatively, it has been invoked to stabilize those US-compliant authoritarian right-wing regimes in the Americas (such as those in El Salvador, Guatemala, and Honduras) that were threatened by domestic opposition or popular insurgency under "communist influence". See especially: Chomsky (1992, 2003); Dominguez, J. (1999). 'US-Latin American Relations During the Cold War and Its Aftermath'. J. Dunkerley *et al.* (Eds.) *The United States and Latin America: The New Agenda*. David Rockefeller Center for Latin American Studies; Institute of Latin American Studies. Smith, G. (1995). *The Last Years of the Monroe Doctrine 1945–1993*. New York: Hill and Wang.

In the post-Cold War era, under the present Trump administration, the Monroe Doctrine has been invoked to justify possible military action against Venezuela's populist left-wing government and as necessary to deter Chinese "trade imperialism" (that is, China's efforts to cultivate Sino-Latin American commercial relations) in the Americas. See: Taylor, A. (2019) 'What is the Monroe Doctrine? John Bolton's justification for Trump's push against Maduro'. *Washington Post*. (4 March); Gramer, R. and Johnson, K. (2018). Tillerson Praises Monroe Doctrine, Warns Latin America of "Imperial" Chinese Ambitions'. *Foreign Policy*. (2 February).

225 Funajole, M.P. *et al.* (2021). *Unpacking the Russian Troop Buildup along Ukraine's Border*. CSIS: Center for Strategic and International Studies (online). (22 April); Siebold, S. and Emmott, R. (2021). 'NATO warns Russia over Ukraine military build-up'. *Reuters*. (15 November).

226 Rees, (1999), pp. 174–78; Klare (2005), pp. 150–61; Klare (2003), pp. 53, 57–58; Harvey (2003), pp. 118–21.

227 Callinicos (2009), pp. 215–16, 218.
228 Harvey (2003), pp. 145–55.
229 Callinicos (2009), p. 171.
230 History Editors (2010). *Europe's Common Market founded in major step toward economic unity*. History.com (online). (9 February).
231 Ross, E. (2019). *How the US influenced the creation of the EU*. The World (online). (28 January); Callinicos (2009), p. 172–73; *Al-Jazeera* (2017). *1950s: Birth of the European Project* (online); Milward, A. S. (2006). *The Reconstruction of Western Europe 1945–51*. Berkeley: University of California Press, p. 46.
232 Editorial of US *Marine Corps Gazette* (May 1990) cited in Chomsky (1992), p. 31.
233 As correctly diagnosed by the theorists of dependency and underdevelopment (Andre Gunder Frank, Samir Amin, Immanuel Wallerstein, etc.).
234 Giles, C. (2006). 'Warning over cost benefits of emerging economies'. *Financial Times*. (3 October); Harman (2009), pp. 213, 221–22, 242, 251–53; Harman (1999), p. 596. Even contemporary Japan shares certain of these features – with investments heavily concentrated in particular high-tech export-oriented industries at the relative neglect of investment in the rest of the economy and with average real wages that are only 60 percent of those in the US (Harman, 2009, p. 213).
235 Harman (2009), pp. 252, 337–41.
236 In China, only fractionally more workers are in the manufacturing sector (27 percent) than in the agricultural sector (25 percent), with the bulk of workers (47 percent) in "services" (where there is a heavy concentration in the casualized low-paid informal sector). The agriculture sector contributes seven percent to GDP. In India, 41 percent of workers are in agriculture compared to 26 percent in industry and 32 percent in services, with agriculture contributing 15 percent to GDP. In the EU, by contrast, only four percent of the workforce is in agriculture (contributing one percent to GDP), whereas in the US it is 11 percent (contributing 0.6 percent to GDP). See; Textor, T. (2020). *Distribution of the workforce across economic sectors in China 2019*. Statista (online). (29 July); Plecher, H. (2020). *India: Distribution of the workforce across economic sectors from 2010 to 2020*. Statista (online). (20 October); Eurostat (2018). *Farmers and the agricultural labour force – statistics*. Statista (online). (November); USDA (2020). *Agriculture and Food Sectors and the Economy* (online). (16 December).
237 Callinicos (2009), pp. 183–84; Harman (2009), pp. 218–19, 243–45; Harman (1984), pp. 94–97; Harris (1987), pp. 30–69.
238 According to OECD data, only one of the NICs (South Korea) was among the top 35 countries for hourly labour productivity (in 30th place), whereas all of the top 20 places (bar one – Japan, ranked 20th) were filled by the advanced countries of the Global North. See Johnson, D. (2017). 'These Are the Most Productive Countries in the World'. *Time Magazine* (online). (4 January).
239 Callinicos (2009), pp. 199–201.
240 China's GDP is $12.24 trillion compared to the US's $19.39 trillion and the EU's $17.28 trillion. These are statistics for 2017. See; Worldometer (2020). *Population Comparison: China, EU, USA, and Japan* (online).
241 Callinicos (2009), p. 219.
242 Aliyev, N. (2020). *Military Cooperation Between Russia and China: The Military Alliance Without an Agreement?* International Centre For Defence and Security (online). (1 July); Atalaya (2020). *The US considers China's enemies as allies in the region* (online). (27 October); Dwivedi, S.S. (2012). 'North Korea-China Relations: An Asymmetric Alliance'. *North Korean Review*, 8 (2), pp. 76–93; Simes, D. (2020). 'China-Russia alliance on horizon as nuclear arms treaties crumble'. *Nikkei Asia: Asia Insight* (online). (21 April); Enoa, A.J. (2019). 'China: Cuba's latest benefactor'. *Dialago Chino* (online). (5 November); Fassihi, F. and Myers, S.L. (2020). 'Defying U.S., China and Iran Near Trade and Military Partnership'. *New York Times*. (11 July);

Friedman, U. (2020). 'America Is Alone in Its Cold War With China'. *Atlantic*. (17 February); Smith, J. (2020). 'China's Xi says intends to deepen relations with North Korea: KCNA'. *Reuters* (online). (9 October); Standish, R. (2020). *China, Russia Deepen Their Ties Amid Pandemic, Conflicts With The West*. RadioFreeLiberty (online).

243 Chomsky (2000, 2003, 2006).

244 Gurr, R. (1994). 'Peoples Against States: Ethnopolitical Conflict and the Changing World System'. *International Studies Quarterly*, 38 (3), pp. 347–77. See p. 347.

245 Henderson, E.A. and Singer, J.D. (2000). 'Civil War in the Post-Colonial World, 1946–92'. *Journal of Peace Research*, 37 (3), pp. 275–99. The researchers found that "semi-democracy is associated with an increased likelihood of civil war, while greater economic development reduces the probability of civil war". They "also found that militarized post-colonial states are more likely to experience civil war" (p. 275). Both are unsurprising results. Economic weakness exacerbates conflicts over allocative resources, whereas economic growth may potentially diminish them. Militarization of the state may be an indicator of inner social division and discord in a society, hence of political instability (itself perhaps resulting from economic imbalances) and of reliance on coercion in order to manage the divisions and imbalances.

246 Allen, C. (1999). 'Warfare, Endemic Violence and State Collapse in Africa'. *Review of African Political Economy*, 26 (81), pp. 367–84; Emmanuel, N.G. (2012). 'Self-Help and Africa's Collapsed States'. *ASPJ Africa and Francophonie* (2nd Quarter) (online), pp. 76–96; Matthews, S. and Solomon, H. (2001). 'The Challenges of State Collapse in Africa: The case of the Democratic Republic of the Congo'. *Africa Insight*, 31 (3), pp. 24–31; Quaranto, P.J. (2008). *State Collapse and Security in Somalia*. Institute For Security Studies. (May).

247 Crawford, B. (1990). 'The Causes of Cultural Conflict: An Institutional Approach'. B. Crawford and D. Lipschutz (Eds.) *The Myth of 'Ethnic Conflict': Politics, Economics, and 'Cultural' Violence*. Berkeley: University of California, pp. 4–5.

248 For example, by Amy Chua (2003), who presents a comprehensive and acclaimed version of the theory.

249 Quaranto (2008).

250 Callinicos (2009), p. 185.

251 Bevins, V. (2017). 'What the United States Did in Indonesia'. *Atlantic*. (20 October); Budiardjo, C. and Liem, S.J. (1984). *The War against East Timor*. London: Zed Books; Defert, G. (1992). *East Timor: The Forgotten Genocide*. Paris: Editions de l'Harmattan; Kiernan, B. (2003). 'The Demography of Genocide in Southeast Asia: The Death Tolls in Cambodia, 1975–79, and East Timor, 1975–80'. *Critical Asian Studies*. 35 (4), pp. 585–97; O'Brien, A. (2005). *The US-Indonesian Military Relationship*. Council on Foreign Relations (online). (4 October); Pilger, J. (2003). *The New Rulers of the World*. London: Verso, pp. 17–47; Scott, P.D. (1985). 'The United States and the Overthrow of Sukarno 1965–1967'. *Pacific Affairs*, 58 (2), pp. 239–64; Simpson, B. (2018). *US Promoted Close Ties to Indonesian Military as Suharto's Rule Came to an End in Spring 1998*. National Security Archive (online). (24 July).

252 OECD (2019). *OPEC share of world crude oil reserves, 2018* (online).

253 Council on Foreign Relations (2021). *Oil Dependence and US Foreign Policy 1850–2017*. SFR: Timeline (online).

254 Callinicos (2003), p. 94.

255 Mills, R. (2019). 'The US isn't protecting oil supplies from the Middle East, it wants to control prices as foreign policy'. EURACTIV (online). (23 May); USEIA (2021). *Petroleum and Other Liquids*. (online).

256 NEP (2001) cited in Callinicos (2003), pp. 94–95.

257 Council on Foreign Relations (2021).

258 Yergin, D. (2013). 'Congratulations America, You're (Almost) Energy Independent'. *Politico* (online). (November); USEIA (2020). *Oil and petroleum products explained* (online). (27 April).
259 Council on Foreign Relations (2021).
260 Center on Global Energy Policy (2020). *The US isn't energy independent. Middle East oil still matters.* New York: Columbia University (online). (10 January).
261 Mills, R. (2019); Telhami, S. (2002). *The Persian Gulf: Understanding the American Oil Strategy.* Brookings Institute (online). (1 March).
262 Bromley, S. (1991). *American Hegemony and World Oil: The Industry, the State System, and the World Economy.* Cambridge: Polity Press, p. 86.
263 Sampson, A. (1976). *The Seven Sisters: The Great Oil Companies and the World They Made.* London: Coronet.
264 Callinicos (2003), p. 98.
265 Council on Foreign Relations (2021).
266 Rose, J. (2003). *Israel: The Hijack State*, 3rd edition. London: Larkham Publishing, pp. 44–45.
267 Rose (2003), p. 6.
268 Sharp, J.M. (2020). *US Foreign Aid to Israel.* Congressional Research Service. Report RL33222. (16 November).
269 Rose (2003, p. 6.
270 Sharp (2020), p. 8.
271 Chomsky, N. (1983). *The Fateful Triangle: The United States, Israel and the Palestinians.* London: Verso, p. 19; Chomsky, N. (1977). 'Oil Imperialism and the US-Israel Relationship'. *Leviathan*, 1 (3) (Spring), pp. 6–9.
272 Cited in Rose (2003), p. 21.
273 Hurst, D. (1977). *The Gun and the Olive Branch.* London, pp. 128–29, 138; Morris, B. (1986). 'The Causes and Character of the Arab Exodus from Palestine: The Israeli Defence Forces Intelligence Branch Analysis of June 1948'. *Middle Eastern Studies*, 21 (1), pp. 5–19; Bonds, J. *et al.* (1977). *Our Roots Are Still Alive: The Story of the Palestinian People.* San Francisco: People's Press, pp. 65, 74; Morris, B. (2001). 'Revisiting the Palestinian Exodus of 1948'. E.L. Rogan and A. Shlaim (Eds.) *The War for Palestine: Rewriting the History of 1948.* Cambridge: Cambridge University Press, pp. 37–59.
274 Bowen, J. (2003). *Six Days: How the 1967 War Shaped the Middle East.* New York: Simon and Schuster; Morris, B. (2001). *Righteous Victims: A History of the Zionist-Arab Conflict.* London: Vintage; Smith, S.C. (2016). *Reassessing Suez 1956: New Perspectives on the Crisis and Its Aftermath.* London: Routledge.
275 Ritter, S. and Pitt, R.W. (2003). *War On Iraq.* London: Allen and Unwin; Esposito, J. (1997). *Political Islam: Revolution, Radicalism, or Reform.* Boulder Co: Lynne Rienner, pp. 56–58; Cockburn, A. and Cohen, A. (1991). 'The Unnecessary War'. V. Brittain (Ed.) *The Gulf Between Us: The Gulf War and Beyond.* London: Virago Press, p. 5; Phythian, M. (1997). *Arming Iraq: How the U.S. and Britain Secretly Built Saddam's War Machine.* Boston: Northeastern University Press; Hiro, D. (1991). *The Longest War: The Iran-Iraq Military Conflict.* New York: Routledge. (See chapter on "Outside Powers").
276 Pilger (2003), pp. 62–63. An estimate of 500,000 is based on a study by UNICEF in cooperation with the Iraqi government. See United Nations International Children's Emergency Fund and Government of Iraq (1999). *Child and Maternal Mortality Survey 1999: Preliminary Report.* New York: UNICEF. See also: Global Policy Forum (2002). *Iraq Sanctions: Humanitarian Implications and Options for the Future* (online). (6 August). Zaida and Fawzi estimated child mortalities as high as 567,000. See Zaida, S. and Smith-Fawzi, M.C. (1995). 'Health of Baghdad's Children'. *Lancet*, 346 (8988). (2 December), p. 1485.

277 Garfield, R. (2000). 'The Public Health Impact of Sanctions'. *Middle East Report*, 215 (Summer), p. 17. Garfield subsequently re-calculated child-under-five deaths between 1991 and 1999 at 350,000, however. See: Richman, S. (2004). *Iraqi Sanctions – Were They Worth It?* Global Policy Forum (online). (January). See also: Garfield, R. (1999). *Morbidity and Mortality among Iraqi Children from 1990 through 1998: Assessing the Impact of the Gulf War and Economic Sanctions*. New York: Columbia University (online).

278 Garfield (1999).

279 Depleted uranium (DU) coated munitions were expended on a massive scale by US forces in the 1991 war. It has been estimated that between 315 and 350 tonnes of it were scattered across the Iraq warzones in microscopic particles. See: Energy Solutions (2015). *History Of Depleted Uranium and What It Is Used For*. Wayback Machine Internet Archive (online). (21 July).

280 Brittain, V. (1991). 'Introduction'. Brittain (Ed.), p. ix; Chomsky, N. (1996). *Power and Prospects: Reflections on Human Nature and Social Order*. Boston: South End Press, p. 35; Cockburn, A. and Cockburn, P. (1999). *Out of the Ashes: The Resurrection of Saddam Hussein*. New York: Harper-Collins; Frank, A.G. (1992). 'Third World War: A Political Economy of the Gulf War and the New World Order'. *Third World Quarterly*, 13 (2), pp. 267–82; Morrison, L. (1991). 'The NHS and Its Patients: Casualties of the Gulf War'. Brittain (Ed.), p. 117; Pilger (1999), pp. 48–52.

281 Brittain, V. (1991). 'Introduction'. Brittain (Ed.), p. ix; Morrison (1991), p. 117. US commander of the "Allied" war, General "Stormin'" Norman Schwarzkopf advised US congress that he thought that the war had killed at least 100,000 Iraqi combatants (Pilger, 1999, p. 51).

282 Ian Lee's study (cited in Pilger, 1999) estimated the number of civilian deaths resulting directly from the war as being as high as 250,000. See: Lee, I. (1991). *Continuing Health Cost of the Gulf War*. Medical Educational Trust: London. "This confirmed American and French estimates of 'in excess of 200,000 civilian deaths'" (Pilger, 1999, p. 53).

283 Foreign Affairs Select Committee (1991). *The Economic Impact of the Gulf Crisis on Third World Countries*. (March 1991). London: FASC; Lee, I. (1991). *Continuing Health Cost of the Gulf War*. Medical Educational Trust: London.

284 Bowcott, O. (2004). 'Was the war legal? Leading lawyers give their verdict'. *Guardian*. (2 March); Burkeman, O., and Borger, J. (2003).'War critics astonished as US hawk admits invasion was illegal'. *Guardian*. (20 November); Curtis, M. (2004). *Unpeople: Britain's Secret Human Rights Abuses*. London: Vintage, pp. 33–46; Falk, R. (2004). 'The Iraq War and the Future of International Law'. *Proceedings of the Annual Meeting (American Society of International Law)*, 98, pp. 263–66; Hirsch, A. (2010). 'Iraq invasion violated international law, Dutch inquiry finds'. *Guardian*. (12 January); Lobe, J. (2003). 'Law Groups Say US Invasion Illegal'. *One World News Centre* (online). (21 March); Kramer, R., Michalowski, R. and Rothe, D. (2005). '"The Supreme International Crime": How the U.S. War in Iraq Threatens the Rule of Law'. *Social Justice*, 32 (2), pp. 52–81; Norton-Taylor, R. (2003). 'Law unto themselves'. *Guardian*. (13 March); Lorenz, J. (2003). *The Coalition of the Willing*. Ethics of Development in a Global Environment. Stanford University (online). (5 June).

285 Iraq Body Count (2021). *Documented civilian deaths from violence* (online). Accessed: 28 March 2021; Iraq Body Count (2021). *Analysis: from the numbers* (online). Accessed: 28 March 2021.

286 Mills (2019).

287 Mills (2019).

288 Chulov, M. and Safi, M. (2020). '"We're poor people": Middle East's migrant workers look for way home amid pandemic'. *Guardian*. (9 June).

289 Baker Institute (2019). *The Politics of Rentier States in the Gulf.* Baker Institute: Project on Middle East Political Science. Washington DC; Beblawi, H. (1987). 'The Rentier State in the Arab World'. *Arab Studies Quarterly*, 9 (4), pp. 383–98; Crystal, J. (1990). *Oil and Politics in the Gulf: Rulers and Merchants in Kuwait and Qatar.* Cambridge: Cambridge University Press; Gause, F.G. (1994). *Oil Monarchies: New York: Domestic and Security Challenges in the Gulf States.* New York: Council on Foreign Relations Press; ILO (2020). *Arab States: Labour Migration* (online); Lewis, B. (2000). 'Monarchy in the Middle East'. J. Kostiner (Ed.) *Middle East Monarchies: The Challenge of Modernity.* Boulder CO: Lynne Rienner Publishers; Winckler, O. (2000). 'Gulf Monarchies as Rentier States: The Nationalization Policies of the Labor Force' in Kostiner (Ed.).

290 Achcar, G. (2018). 'The Saudi Predicament'. *New Socialist* (online). (20 April).

291 Chomsky (1977), pp. 6–9; Chomsky (1983), p. 463.

292 Gold, D. (2004). *Hatred's Kingdom: How Saudi Arabia Supports the New Global Terrorism.* Washington DC: Regnery Publishers; Pipes, S. (2015). 'The Scandal of US-Saudi Relations'. S. Pipes (Ed.) *Nothing Abides: Perspectives on the Middle East and Islam.* New York: Routledge; Posner, G. (2005). *Secrets of the Kingdom: The Inside Story of the Saudi-U.S. Connection.* New York: Random House; Stern, S. (Ed.) (2011). *Saudi Arabia and the Global Islamic Terrorist Network: America and the West's Fatal Embrace.* New York: Palgrave-Macmillan (esp. Chps. 2, 4, and 5).

293 Chomsky, N. (2002). 'Terror and Just Response' in M. Rai (Ed.) (2002). *War Plan Iraq.* London: Verso, pp. 34–35.

294 Creaven (2024), Ch. 1.

2 The pandemic in international relations

In the previous chapter, I analyzed the international state system. Key failings with regard to the politics of the pandemic (including with regard to public health management policy) cannot be grasped without comprehending the constitution and dynamics of this system. Nor can the peculiar and radical susceptibilities of contemporary modern civilizations to pandemic events (such as the present one) or their inability to cope with them economically (that is, prevent them from causing catastrophic harm everywhere to people's livelihoods) be grasped without relating these causally to the zombified corporate mode that is parasitic on the world economy. The task of this chapter is to situate the gross inadequacies (in terms of radical global asymmetries in the allocation of jabs) of the UN's vaccination "effort" in the framework of world politics as imperial and interstate rivalries in the service of mega-capitalism.

Capitalist world economy and international state system

I will start by summarizing the analysis contained in the previous chapter and linking this to Critical Realism's (CR) ontology of social systems – or critical-realist social theory (CRT) – and realist international relations theory (RIRT). The capitalist world economy and international state system are parallel but intersecting systems. These are also closely aligned systems of domination (in the political sphere) and of exploitation (in the economic sphere) owing to the structural interdependence of state and capital at the level of each country and worldwide. The interstate system is the bearer and defender of the world capitalist economy. This is by virtue of its command of powers of authorization (political, military, and juridical) by means of which law and order are more or less maintained worldwide. The world capitalist economy bankrolls the interstate system and the protections of capitalist property and commerce (normative and otherwise) that this provides.

This is hardly an integrated or harmonious systemic totality, however. This is exactly because both of its constituents are indeed systems of competition. Moreover, the logics of interest and competition in the two systems are not identical so tensions can arise between them. Capitals compete with other capitals for markets and profits in the economic sphere. This competition consolidates and often widens wealth and income differences by social class internationally and within national borders – as has been the pattern of recent decades. This is because

DOI: 10.4324/9781003437208-3

capitalist success depends on reducing labour costs, driving up labour productivity, and increasing the surplus value extracted from the workers in production. States compete with other states in the political sphere to further the interests of their own home-grown capitals against others in the world market and to attract the inward investments of foreign capitals. This dynamic is what establishes the structural interdependence of state and capital locally and internationally.[1] Capitals and states everywhere share common interests in the subordination and exploitation of labour at home and abroad. They are united on one side of the class divide.

Yet structural interdependence is not *functional* integration of state and capital because, despite the mutual dependence of state and capital, their interests are not identical. Nationalism requires state managers to prioritize the interests of their own home-based and home-grown capitals against those of rival states and to assist these in their competition with foreign capitals overseas. This is because states must rely on their own national economies to resource their own operations of governance. Every national state authority must draw on within-border economic resources (taxation of wealth and income of its own citizens and residents) to sustain its own offices and functions. A nation-state must defend as a matter of first resort a *national capitalism* – even though the national capitals in question may also be internationally facing and competing with others on the world stage. This ensures that any state must relate to other states as rivals. This is to ensure economic success at home and to deny business opportunities to other states that would disadvantage it economically. But this ensures as well that any state must also relate to the capitals that grew up in other states as rivals of its own capitals.[2] This is because the security and stability of any state depend on the competitive success of those capitalist enterprises from which it derives the bulk of its income.

The capitalist world economy and interstate system, like all social systems, is not composed simply of human agency embedded in social practices. This is, as critical-realist social theory (CRT) establishes, not merely an "interactional order" stretching out over space and time. Rather, the social practices that reproduce these systems day-to-day are embedded in the emergent structures generated by previously materialized social interaction.[3] These emergent structures are always the antecedent or anterior conditions of social practices that people find "ready-made" and which they are compelled to reckon with. These are basically "action-environments" in which people must act and relate to each other in response to the situational logics these confront them with. Structural emergence is what makes social life systemic. Social systems exist and are reproduced because they have structural properties. If this was not so, definite and particular regularities of social interaction over time, by consequence of which one can speak of its institutional or organizational forms or delineate specific types of society or social order, would not exist. Without structural properties, social life would be unsystemic, since social interaction would be endlessly, relentlessly, and randomly transformative so that societies were radically ephemeral, unstable, and shapeless.

Structural emergence renders social life systemic because structures not only contextualize social practices but also situate these practices within a framework of constraints and enablements that impart to the human agency that animates them directional guidance. This is what makes possible societal evolutionism rather than random chaotic historicity in the free play of events. However, the directional guidance that structures impart to social practices is not structural determinism. This is because constraints and enablements operate on the basis of the involuntary placement of people within social relations *vis-à-vis* resource distributions generated by structures and in accordance with the vested interests in specific kinds of social agency that are fixed by these involuntary placements. The structural conditioning of human agency within social practices is not such that people are programmed to respond to it in specific ways. Behavioural and attitudinal flexibility is allowed by structural emergence since this manifests as a framework of fetters and facilitators within which lives must be lived rather than as cultural hydraulics that permits only one response to these fetters and facilitators.[4]

Structural conditioning cannot be structural hydraulics as well because of the nature of the objects of conditioning – people. The situational logics of human agency and social interaction (of involuntary placement and attendant vested interests) that are given by structures may be disregarded or misdiagnosed or resisted or subverted by those under their sway. This is possible because people make and remake structures, whereas structures do not make or remake people. Rather, structures merely influence or condition the people who do the making and remaking of social systems. Structures are not agents, only people are. And people are agents of societal reproduction and/or transformation because they, unlike structures, have needs (biological and social) that animate the pursuit of interests, just as they have causal powers of intentionality and subjectivity by which they recognize these needs as their own and are incentivized to act on them socially.

This is the basic critical-realist ontological theory (CRT) of social systems, or critical-realist social theory. This, I contend, provides the most elementary abstract model of the constitution of the international state system and world capitalist economy. The world order that exists at any time reflects the distribution of powers in the two systems. The distribution of powers at every point in the history of the systems is the outcome of structural emergence arising from hitherto processes of social interaction in the two systems. These result from success or otherwise in the processes of competition between the actors (states and capitals) up to that point to consolidate and extend their powers of authorization and their control of marketable assets. This renders world order a hierarchically or asymmetrically structured one, because competition begets winners and losers, and success or failure in the competition of states and capitals is itself shaped (in the sense of constrained and enabled) by the structural emergence of previously materialized processes of competition.

Patterns of domination and subordination or of advantage and disadvantage are established by structural emergence. Hierarchized structural properties in the two systems sustain relations of asymmetrical interaction among the human agents that make or remake them, just as relations of asymmetrical interaction reproduce the hierarchized structural properties of the two systems. This developmental ratchet transports forward in time the structurally given patterns of domination/subordination and advantage/disadvantage from one phase of social interaction to the next.

Processes of asymmetrical competition between capitals and states in the systems of world capitalist economy and international relations have, in other words, the directional tendency to reproduce and reinforce the hierarchical structures. This is owing to the prior uneven distribution of resources of and capacities for authorization and allocation among the agents of competition.

Moreover, since capitalism is a system that through business competition piles up ever more colossal resources for reinvestment rather than consumption, there is also a general tendency for money-power to become ever more concentrated and centralized in the hands of those already advantaged by or from previous cycles of business competition. Centralization and concentration of capital (owing to the dynamics of accumulation and of merger and acquisition) consolidates and extends the powers of authorization of those states that administer and serve the interests of the most advanced and developed capitals (the MNCs) in their rivalries with other states. This is because these states can draw disproportionately on the prodigious surpluses that are generated by corporate-monopoly capitalism as a whole. The winners of structurally conditioned asymmetric inter-capitalist and interstate competition tend to accrue greater concentrations of authoritative and allocative resources. Structural emergence in the systems is thus a story of chronically reproduced inequality of outcomes. The most powerful capital-state actors that dominate are those that have inherited their structural advantages and are therefore best placed in competition to pass them on.

This "inheritance of inequality" as structural emergence is manifest in global political economy. For historical reasons, which are connected to uneven but combined development – colonial exploitation, postwar under-development, asymmetrical dependency, and unequal exchange – the dominant players in both systems (whether capitals or states) are almost completely those of the Global North.[5] At the centre of this nexus of capital-state power actors are the Western powers and Japan, under the political hegemony of the US. The US enjoys political leadership over the Western Alliance and Japan and political hegemony over the "free" world of liberal democracy and market economy more generally. This is because its state managers can draw on vastly superior economic (and hence military and ideological) capacities than can its coalition competitor-partners, or indeed those of any other state that presently may aspire to challenge its hegemony.

Now, the structural relations of economic and politico-military domination and subordination between the US-led state-capital actors of the Global North and those of the Global South are those that establish the world system as *imperial*. These relations of basically unequal exchange fix the three domains – the developed, developing (or semi-developed), and underdeveloped worlds – of global political economy. These domains of world order relate to but do not exactly coincide with the chief geo-spatial division of the system into rival regional blocs of state-capital combines. These are the North American, European, and Southeast Asian hubs, which are the economic power-centres of world capitalism. As I discussed in the previous chapter, these centres are where the bulk of the commodity trade, sales, and capital investments of the MNCs are concentrated. This amounts to a triadic centralization and concentration of money-power and means of production in specific places. By contrast, vast swathes of Africa, Central Asia, and the Americas remained locked in conditions of chronic economic under-development, since they are relatively cut-off from the circuits of trade and investment that circulate within and across the triad.[6]

The imperial system of states is multiple but subordinated to the primary imperialism of the US. This is owing to the special role that the US state has taken on since World War Two – and which in the postwar era only it has been capable of delivering. This role is, as writers of the Realist International Relations Theory (RIRT) school rightly argue, that of acting as a guarantor of worldwide order and security (especially of the order and security of a world market fully open for corporate exploitation by American MNCs). Dominance in the interstate system of the high-income countries under US hegemony is secured and legitimized by virtue of supranational and reputedly multilateral political institutions of worldwide governance in which the rules and values of liberal markets are inscribed. These organizations – the UN, G7, WTO, IMF, World Bank, NATO, and so on – mobilize resources of command (whether political, ideological, or military) to reproduce the hierarchical structural properties of interstate polity and world capitalist economy.[7] This, of course, is their primary function.

Empire versus realism

The analyses of realist political science (RIRT) and of the critical realist or "emergentist" CRT in social ontology may be contrasted with a quite different kind of analysis of contemporary world order that has been highly influential on the Left. This is Michael Hardt's and Antonio Negri's account of the world system as an imperial "network society" (*Empire*). This theory establishes Empire as a much flatter and much more fluid (that is, relatively or comparatively far less vertically hierarchical) system of nation-states and capitals than does the realist account summarized above and discussed at length in a previous chapter. In its essentials, Empire is conceived as a horizontal network of capitalist transnationality that has basically subordinated the interstate system to its own imperatives. Empire is essentially the sovereignty of global capital. Hardt and Negri's perspective will be elaborated below.[8]

Empire, Hardt and Negri argue, is a complex web of exchange relations spanning the globe. This has undermined the old, centralized hierarchies and concentrations of economic power that once divided up the world between first and other worlds (or between developed, semi-developed and underdeveloped zones) and which established the pre-eminence of the North and West over the rest in world systems. By doing so, Empire has replaced structures of domination and exploitation that reproduce relations of subordination and dependency between the developed countries and the less developed ones. Instead, Empire generates everywhere a decentred patchwork economy of pockets of wealth and poverty, of privilege and dis-privilege, and of domination and subordination.

This means that Empire is not owned or controlled or dominated by any particular state (or constellation of states). It articulates no specific national interests.

It has no central headquarters and nor is it animated by any political intentionality. As Hardt and Negri put it, "the United States does not, and indeed no nation state can today, form the centre of an imperialist project".[9] This is because, for them, the powers of the individual state actors are insignificant compared to those of the network as a whole. Individual states (no matter how powerful they are in economic or political terms) cannot act alone in trying to secure their interests in the network society because none can assert themselves unilaterally. Each and all act in concert with the other network-actors to secure their goals. Rather than serving the imperial designs of the US, the West, or the Global North, Empire serves the interests of pure global commerce, of transnational network capitalism. The role of governments (at the national and supranational levels) is not to embark on imperial politics but to facilitate Empire and release it from all fetters. Empire is the commodification and commercialization of all things in the service of the self-expansion of capital.

Hardt and Negri establish their case by drawing out the distinction as they see it between modern and postmodern capitalism and their associated imperialisms. Modern capitalism, they tell us, was characterized by a number of key structural features. These were (1) Marx's fundamental class cleavage between exploiting owners and non-owing producers; (2) the centrality of material work (industrial production of material commodities by manual workers); (3) the geo-spatial or territorial concentration and centralization of industrial power in the leading Western nation-states, together with nationally organized and integrated capitalism (the fusion of economic and political power at the level of the nation-state); and (4) imperialist rivalries between the opposing state-capitalist blocs for control of territory and other resources outside the capitalist orbit, alongside a basic division of the globe between capitalist "inside" (centre) and non-capitalist "outside" (periphery).

By contrast, postmodern capitalism and its associated imperial mode are characterized by a rather different set of economic and political relations. These are (1) the fragmentation of both capital and wage-labour (the former of which is globally dispersed and the latter of which splits off into an informational core, on the one hand, and a vast "multitude", on the other); (2) the centrality of immaterial or virtual labour (in manufacturing and the new service industries); (3) the deterritorialization of capital, which escapes the control of the nation-state system as it is extended across the world by footloose multinational companies, globally integrated markets, and new supranational organs of corporate governance; and (4) the replacement of classical imperialism with a new imperialism without colonies – an imperial regime without an imperial centre and lacking a guiding imperial strategy.

Empire is thus the political and economic rule of capital in the new global age. In this sense, it is simply capitalist globalization in its political and economic aspects. Empire is "the rupture or shift in contemporary capitalist production and global relations of power … [which] makes perfectly clear and possible today the capitalist project to bring together economic and political power, to realize … a properly capitalist order".[10] This Empire, Hardt and Negri instruct, is quite different to any previous form of imperial rule. Under Empire, power is not extended through territorial sovereignty (the colonial system), but through postcolonial supranational forms of sovereignty. As Jamie Morgan summarizes: "Where imperialism was an extension of certain nation states imposing their will on others, Empire is an internalised system to which all are subject, including the former imperial states".[11]

This is an order that no longer depends on the interstate system but is genuinely borderless and decentred since it is borne by transnational companies (TNCs), as Hardt and Negri see it, and globally integrated capital flows organized around their activities. Globalization, for Hardt and Negri, has "overcome all national borders" and "rendered the very notion of national corporations ... and a national economy and labour force meaningless".[12]

> The transnational corporations directly distribute labour power over various markets, functionally allocate resources, and organise hierarchically the various sectors of world production. The complete apparatus that selects investments and directs financial and monetary manoeuvres determines the new geography of the world market, or really the new biopolitical structuring of the world ... They [TNCs] tend to make nation-states merely instruments to record the flows of the commodities, money and populations they set in motion.[13]

According to Hardt and Negri, Empire is without geo-spatial limits. Rather, it comes from and extends everywhere and embraces everything. Whereas classical imperialism was parasitic on a non-capitalist "outside" to exploit (in order to ease tendencies towards under-consumption and over-production "inside" the system), "Empire is truly global without any spaces outside its domain".[14] By contrast with imperialism, for Hardt and Negri, "Empire establishes no territorial centre of power and does not rely on fixed boundaries or barriers".[15]

Yet, despite its multiform nature, and despite the fact that it has no "all-seeing plan",[16] Empire is nonetheless totalizing in its effects, since it functions to self-reproduce capitalist social relations, along with sharp polarizations between affluence and poverty everywhere, in ever-shifting configurations. According to Hardt and Negri, "transnational" capitalism has totally absorbed every corner of the globe, leaving nothing outside its domain, and generating uniform effects (the reproduction of its own network) everywhere. Under Empire, all nation-states (including the former imperial states) are absolutely "penetrated" by the imperatives of supranational capital.[17] Under Empire, imperialism based on colonies and imperial states disappears to be replaced by the seamless imperial sovereignty of the total network, at the centre of which are the so-called TNCs and new supranational organs of corporate-capitalist governance that represent them. Since, under Empire, the purpose of the nation-state in the interstate system is to uphold "bourgeois right" – the freedoms of capital and the market – this means that political authorization serves interests and goals that are indistinguishable from those of commerce. Political domination loses its distinctiveness from economic exploitation, just as the distinction between state and capital is undermined.[18]

In this network society, since individual nation-states are completely subordinated to the logic of globalized capitalism (as these are transformed into mere instruments of the TNCs and international finance capital), this explains why none can be at the centre of an imperial project or exercise dominance in the interstate system. The interstate system ceases to be a hierarchized system in which those of the West or Global North can preserve their special powers and advantages in relations of unequal exchange or unfair competition with those of the Global South. The domination and exploitation of the semi-developed and underdeveloped countries by the developed ones, along with clear-cut divisions between these different "worlds", is substantially undermined. Not even the US (the most powerful of the world's nation-states) can maintain unilaterally an imperial project on the world stage. And so

> conflict and competition among several imperial powers has in important respects been replaced by the idea of a single power that over-determines them all, structures them in a unitary way, and treats them under one common notion of right that is decidedly postcolonial and postimperialist.[19]

Thus: "Empire ... is sovereignty as a materially inscribed idea ... or global order, logic, and structure of rule that manages and produces the grounds on which all other activity occurs – the activity of nation states, business, cultural transactions ... everything".[20] For Hardt and Negri, as we have seen, Empire is organized around various supranational power-centres, which nonetheless function together automatically as a kind of machinery of uniformity (for the reproduction of capitalist sovereignty on a global scale):

> It ... progressively incorporates the entire global realm within its open, expanding powers. Empire manages hybrid identities, flexible hierarchies, and plural exchanges through modulating networks of command. The distinct national colours of the imperialist map of the world have merged and blended in the imperial global rainbow.[21]

At the summit of this pluriform transnational power network are "monarchical" institutions and organs of overall governance (the US state, the G7, NATO, the IMF, the World Bank, the WTO, and the EU). The US state is placed in this category because it is regarded as "holding hegemony over the global use of force – a superpower that can act alone but prefers to act in collaboration with others under the umbrella of the United Nations".[22] At the second level are clustered "aristocratic" institutions: "the networks of transnational capitalist corporations" which articulate "the single and univocal pinnacle of world command".[23] Here too are those nation-states that control collectively "global monetary instruments" and various other "associations". At the base level are various "democratic" and other lesser organs and bodies, such as the UN general assembly, NGOs, churches, and "subordinate and minor states".[24]

The network of Empire is over-determined by the unitary ideology of liberal-market democracy that keeps the chief states in line and legitimizes the multilateral deployment of force against the occasional "rogue" state that threatens to destabilize the system. This integrates the entire network by providing it with its legitimations. The sovereignty of Empire is based on norms and values (that is, those of cultural pluralism and liberal democracy) that are represented as universal because they supposedly articulate trans-cultural human rights and liberties. These ideological legitimations increasingly justify and allow the mobilization of supra-national military capacities – e.g. under the auspices of doctrines of "humanitarian intervention" – to neutralize the emergence of any challenges to the hegemony of Empire or to sweep away surviving leftovers from the modern age of rival impe-rialisms (such as UN-sanctioned military interventions against Iraq in 1990–1, against Yugoslavia in 1999, against Afghanistan in 2001, and against Iraq in 2003). "Empire is formed not on the basis of force itself but on the basis of the capacity to present force as peace".[25]

This is Hardt and Negri's account of the global political economy in the net-work age. This is commendable in that it places imperialism at the centre of the analysis. That is wholly justifiable, as I myself have shown: the neoliberal order of world capitalism supports and is supported by a neoimperial interstate system. But, despite the brilliance of specific insights, Empire is untenable overall, as my analy-sis of the capitalist world economy and of the international state system in the pre-vious chapter ought to demonstrate, since this has considerable empirical support.

The chief problem is that it is simply false to assert, as Hardt and Negri do, that network power is deterritorialized, operating uniformly everywhere, meaning that "there is no longer a first, second and third world of dependencies but an inter-mingling of cells of affluence and poverty".[26] World systems are, as I have shown, characterized by radically asymmetrical distributions of political and economic power and by highly uneven patterns of development within and between different geographical zones. Power and wealth are highly centralized and concentrated in particular hands and in specific places – and these hands and places include the same ones as in the age of classical imperialism. Structured inequalities between developed, developing, and developed regions remain absolutely pertinent, though their dimensions have altered over the past 50 years. There are, contrary to Hardt and Negri, very few TNCs, under any definition of the term. Rather, it is MNCs that are the dominant economic mode of corporate power. And most of the biggest MNCs hail from the Global North (with US corporations disproportionately repre-sented among them). The bulk of their commerce is situated in their home regions with virtually all of the remainder within the triad. The bulk of consumption of commodity goods and services takes place within developed countries.

There are, of course, enclaves of poverty in the most developed countries, just as there are (much smaller) enclaves of affluence in the least developed countries, as Hardt and Negri observe. But this does not invalidate or disprove the reality of the hierarchical core–periphery divisions of global political economy. There are still relatively few rich countries, which are largely situated in developed regions, just as there are still poor countries which are situated almost entirely in chroni-cally underdeveloped regions. Owing to that, the experience of poverty is quite different for the poor depending on where they are geographically situated. A land-less labourer in underdeveloped Honduras or a sweatshop worker in developing

Indonesia has significantly fewer life chances than an unemployed person or a gig worker in developed countries such as the UK or US, for example.

This shows that the notion of Empire as a multiform yet smooth web of domination – a form of power embracing everything in equal measure, homogeneous and uniform in its distribution, generating equal subordination everywhere – simply effaces the potentially malintegrative instabilities and conflicts of world economy and polity. Because all the powers of the various agents of the system are simply expressions of the normalizing disciplinary power of the total network, the system is evacuated of dialectical pathways towards an alternative system. This holistic super-functionalism is implausible. Those agents (whether workers or nation-states or local elites) experiencing these "imbalances" from different sides cannot possibly relate to the legitimations of Empire in the same way. The vast asymmetries of wealth and income along class or other lines, the split of the world into advantaged and disadvantaged regions, and the combined but uneven development of world capitalism overall mean that the effects of power can never be homogeneous or uniform. There will always be structural contradictions and attendant social malintegrations that work themselves out in different ways in different parts of the systems. These potentially could develop in such ways that the reproduction of Empire is threatened.

But at least Hardt and Negri are fully alive to the fact that network power is far from random in its effects. This renders their theory of network society rather less apologetic than, for example, Manuel Castells' version.[27] Yet the logic of any form of analysis of world systems couched in terms of network theory is an uncritical theory in fundamentals. This is shown to be the case where Hardt and Negri deny that inter-imperialist wars between "civilized states" are any longer a remote possibility under Empire, where notions of "bourgeois sovereignty" administered by supranational organs integrate the system ideologically.

Liberal democracy and liberal economics may be virtually hegemonic today in "official" politics, in bodies such as the UN the EU and the G7. And NATO (underwritten especially by the US state) may function to police the system on behalf of liberal-democratic capitalism (justifying "corrective" measures against "off-message" states under the rubric of "humanitarian intervention" or "global security"). But beneath the pristine liberal ideologies of corporate capitalism and its institutions of supranational governance, the complex realities of geopolitical rivalries between states are real and threaten to destabilize the economic and political systems. As Alex Callinicos rightly says:

> Not simply do the existing international institutions reflect the hierarchical nature of global power, in that they are dominated by the leading Western capitalist powers, but they are shaped by the conflicts that divide these powers, setting in particular the US against Japan and the EU (itself a far from homogeneous entity). Interlaced with these primarily economic and political forms of competition is the developing structure of geopolitical conflict that pits the US against both China and Russia … War is certainly highly improbable within the Western capitalist bloc … But the spy plane crisis that pitted

China against the US in the South China Sea in April 2001 is a symptom of a military build-up and developing geopolitical tensions ... Outside the advanced capitalist world, war shows no sign of disappearing – the war in the Democratic Republic of Congo alone has cost, on one estimate, 2.5 million lives since 1998.[28]

Contrary to network theory, as Jamie Morgan correctly notes, states "are not simply products of the system of Empire [but] ... are participants in the constitution of given characteristics of systems".[29] This is what makes instability and conflict possible in the international state system. There are numerous other indicators that such tensions are building in the post-Cold War political setup, which indicates that Empire is far from being a totalizing system of power.

For a start, the US state's doctrine of "pre-emptive self-defence", whichwas used as justification for the revenge-attack on Afghanistan's Taliban government in response to 9/11 (for allegedly harbouring and supporting Al-Qaeda) and the later US-led invasion of Iraq (to topple Saddam Hussein's Ba'ath state), is longstanding. This is irrespective of the fact that it is rarely deployed.[30] This is in the sense that the US has acted unilaterally to assert its own imperial interests throughout the postwar period, especially though not exclusively in its "backyard" of Latin America, under the rationale of defending national security interests. The US's military assault on Iraq in 2003 was not backed by the UN or by international law, even though approval was sought for it. The US did not even see fit to obtain international backing at all for its attack on Afghanistan in 2001. Rather, the US government simply notified the UN of its intentions.[31]

The Iraq war revealed the willingness of the US government under certain circumstances to remove by military force unfriendly governments without (if necessary) multilateral backing and outside the framework of international law. Indeed, to do so in the face of opposition from most member states of the UN. Not only that, the doctrine of pre-emptive self-defence that has supported these kinds of ventures itself is of dubious validity under international law.[32] The US state under the Bush Junior and Trump presidencies has also demonstrated a willingness to flout multilateral agreements on environmental protection for the benefit of specific American corporate interests.[33]

Of course, the US typically prefers to secure UN backing for its various imperial moves, because this secures the illusion of international consensus and of might as based on normative right. And the dominant players of the UN (and most of the lesser ones) are for the most part prepared to acquiesce. This is because, as we have seen, the developed countries shelter under the umbrella of US power that preserves the capitalist world economy from which they obtain the benefits of unequal exchange, whereas the subordinate ones can be browbeaten (e.g. through aid or trade sanctions) or bribed (e.g. through aid or trade incentives) into compliance. Without the active agency of US diplomacy in trying to win multilateral support for its various imperial interventions of the postwar period, these would not have had even the semblance of being consensual or justifiable under international law.

This establishes that Empire is no mere effect of capitalist "transnationalism", but is very much a project designed by the US state that serves the interests primarily of its own corporate elite and MNCs. (As I have said, there are, contrary to Hardt and Negri, very few TNCs in world economy). Only secondarily does the system serve the interests of US allies or "partners" in the rest of the developed world. This (US unilateralism and US-dominated multilateralism) is plainly inconsistent with Hardt and Negri's Empire. For it is clear that the world's sole superpower is quite capable of placing itself at the centre of an imperial project and pursuing this quite independently of the "powers of the network". The second war on Iraq, for example, was intended to enhance the US state's strategic geopolitical control over the entire oil-rich Middle East region, as well as to privatize Iraqi oil for the benefit of especially US corporations.[34] This imperial capability is derived from the fact that the US is, as Susan Strange rightly says, dominant still internationally in the four fundamental structures of power – security, production, finance, and knowledge.[35]

As Callinicos observes: "Not to recognise the depth of ... antagonisms between rival centres of capitalist power is badly to misunderstand the nature of the contemporary world".[36] The PIR Realists are undoubtedly correct to assert against the utopian globalists that the formation of supranational organizations of political governance demonstrates not the obsolescence of the nation-state but of how nation-states are cooperating strategically to better empower their own vested interests faced with the internationalization of markets.[37] But there are limits to interstate cooperation – which are sometimes underplayed by certain IRR analysts, though not by others. These stem from the fact that consensus-building is motivated by national self-interest and benefits the stronger states and their capitals much more than the others. Such renders interstate cooperation a force that is inextricably tied to interstate competition and perpetually vulnerable to destabilization by it.

These interstate rivalries arguably are encouraging an arms build-up among states that are insecure, vulnerable, "off-message", or politically marginalized in the US-dominated interstate system. As I have pointed out, states such as China, Russia, Iran, and North Korea are incentivized to acquire weapons of mass destruction (WMD) and to forge new alliances in order to discourage the kinds of US-orchestrated military intervention that has been seen in recent times in former Yugoslavia, Afghanistan, and Iraq. There is also the ebb and flow of tensions elsewhere – for example, between India and Pakistan over sovereignty over Cashmere (both of these states possessing nuclear weapons).[38] Meanwhile, in the Middle East, the potential for war between Israel (armed to the teeth with nuclear weapons) and certain of its Arab neighbours (especially Iran which undoubtedly wishes to acquire its own nuclear arsenal) remains very real.[39] Indeed, US diplomats reportedly had to restrain the Israeli state from getting involved in the US-led "coalition's" war against Iraq in 1991 and its unilateral follow-up in 2003, with potentially disastrous regional consequences.[40]

But the logic of Hardt and Negri's Empire also leads them into a kind of economic hyper-globalization whereby the complete deterritorialization of capital is seen as an accomplished fact, and nation-states are portrayed as helpless registers of the imperatives of highly mobile "global" corporations (TNCs, as they see them) and international finance institutions:

The informatization of production and the increasing importance of immaterial production have tended to free capital from the constraints of territory, and capital can withdraw from negotiations with a given local population by moving its site to another point in the global network … Entire labouring populations, which have enjoyed a certain stability and contractual power, have thus found themselves in increasingly precarious employment situations.[41]

Hardt and Negri are, of course, right to note the growing internationalization of capitalism over the past 40 years. Nonetheless, it is necessary to reject their notion (shared with innumerable other theorists of a postmodern or hyper-modern orientation) that so-called globalization has decisively undermined the economic power of the nation-state and especially of the capacity of the elected legislature of the advanced states to intervene against capitalism in support of domestic policy goals.

The reasons for rejecting this proposition are set out in detail earlier in this chapter. Here it is enough to reiterate my argument that globalization myths of the powerless state function to mask the strategic alliance of neoliberal governments and capitalist elites for mutual advantage that was forged in the 1980s and 1990s. First, as I have elaborated, "globalization" is largely mythical. And it is the myths of globalization that distort a real understanding of the relationship between the world capitalist economy and the interstate system as one in which the latter is simply subordinate to the former. Second, as Manuel Castells has shown, the conversion of most nation-states to neoliberalism since the 1980s was not forced on them by the inexorable pressure of global markets that insisted on surrender and would suffer no refusal. Rather, this was conceded because it was positively endorsed by political powerholders in some of the neoliberal "pioneer" states of the Global North (notably, the US, UK, and Australia). State power from this point onwards, far from passively falling into line with capitalist economic power, has aggressively acted to cultivate and extend it, by means of policies of deregulation, trade liberalization and privatization.[42]

The conversion of the US into a neoliberal state was crucial to the worldwide success of the enterprise, owing to its hegemonic imperial status in world systems. Without the agency of the US state, the neoliberal revolution would have foundered. Thus, neoliberalism did, contrary to Hardt and Negri, have a headquarters, and this was in Washington DC. In any case, to grasp neoliberal ascendancy in the language of "concession" renders it passive and reactive rather than, as it was, positive and initiative-taking. As I have said, neoliberalism was and is class warfare from above waged by state power in the service of monopoly capital. This was class warfare from above, which in response to a period of worldwide recession in the 1970s, fought to roll-back a social-democratic settlement that was considered incompatible with profit-fuelled economic competitiveness upon which state power ultimately rested.[43]

This means that the "simple identity" of the interests of state and capital posited by the authors of Empire is simply implausible. The interests of state and capital are certainly strategically and instrumentally aligned, but nonetheless, these are not simply synonymous. States have capacities for acting in ways that place limits on corporate enterprise (indeed capacities for causing harm to their own economic bases in capitalist production) and they may sometimes have impelling reasons for exercising those capacities. Such is theoretically licensed by the concept of structural *interdependence* of state and capital. For this is the interdependence (and hence relative autonomy) of two distinct modes of social power – of authorization and allocation. Especially when a state is formally committed to parliamentary democracy, this must place certain checks on its capacity to accommodate corporate demands or expectations under circumstances where doing so would risk damaging its legitimacy. No liberal-democratic state, no matter how absorbed by economic liberalism (neoliberalism), can afford to disregard the polls and the risks of electoral harms, because those harms are not simply to the electoral viability of the ruling party but to the legitimacy of the liberal state form itself.

Moreover, as I have shown, "globalization" is in any case an unfortunate term, since this supports the neoliberal fantasy that capital is genuinely borderless. In fact, most of it is, as we have seen, regionalized within the most industrially developed zones of the world economy – the biggest share of it in the Global North and virtually all of it in the triad. A greater part of the investment and trade flows of the MNCs also circulate even more narrowly within their home nations. As Chris Harman notes, although money-capital may be relatively mobile in the informational age of high-speed communications, productive capital is far less so.[44] And capitalism cannot live on finance alone but has to translate this to and from value-adding productive investment in means of production and labour power if it is to reproduce itself.

The interstate system, nationalism, and the pandemic

The political events of the pandemic, I contend, validate the concept of structural interdependence of state and capital, and hence of the lack of strict or simple identity between the interests of economic and political powerholders, in favour of a strategic alignment of interests between them. This means that there is space for dissonance between state power and capitalist power. Capital nowhere welcomed the lockdowns, for obvious reasons.[45] Yet virtually everywhere, states brought in lockdowns (sometimes repeatedly) and in many cases wound these down rather less quickly and recklessly than in the UK. Employers tended to agitate for the government to ease work-at-home and physical distancing restrictions quickly as the first and second waves abated so that they could get employees back on site for at least part of the week in what was dubbed by some as "hybrid models" of homeworking and site-working. This was even though many were able to adapt in whole or in large part to homeworking.[46]

The CEO of Goldman Sachs, David Solomon, doubtless voiced the views of many business leaders when he described virtual working as an "aberration" that was to be ditched at the earliest opportunity. This was on the grounds that remote working lost the benefits of mentoring and controlling employees.[47] In the UK, in the summer of 2020, the Confederation of British Industry (CBI) warned the government of dying high streets and of "ghost towns", if they did not more pro-actively encourage office returns than it was in fact doing. This was even though 61 percent of employers had by then brought workers back on-site at least in part, with this hardly being discouraged by the government. Yet, notably, the then UK Health Secretary Matt Hancock (and the wider Westminster government) was at the time prepared to resist those calls for a stronger "return to work" steer.[48]

Various manifestations of pandemic-management policies of governments vir-tually everywhere are, I will argue, striking confirmation of the primacy of interstate competition over interstate cooperation and bilateral consensus-building in world politics. As such, this is also a vindication of the key arguments of Marxist politi-cal economists, as well as those of certain leading scholars of the realist school of PIR. This is also consistent with my own reading of critical-realist systems theory (CRT). Before discussing the international politics of pandemic control, however, I will summarize the key theoretical positions derived from the above (which have been discussed at length elsewhere) that will substantiate them.

Firstly, the nation-state retains in the present age its old classical-modern status as the primary power container of political and judicial authority, despite "globali-zation". The bulk of political authority and legitimacy resides still at the national rather than supranational level, despite the bilateral political organizations that sup-posedly establish the "united nations" as the basis of the world political order. Secondly, nationalism remains a tenaciously fertile source of local social and cul-tural affiliations. Predictions of the decline of nationalism and of national identi-ties are not new. Wolfram Hanrieder responded to such claims back in the 1970s, before globalization became fashionable: "Nationalism ... is alive and well", he opined. "Far from being secondary or obsolete, the nation-state, nationalism, and the ideas of the national interest are central elements in contemporary world poli-tics".[49] And so this has continued. Can this be convincingly disputed today in a world of resurgent right-wing populist nationalisms (such as Trump's "America First" and Johnson's "Brexit Britain")?

The latter reflects two opposing dynamics. On the one hand, this reflects the fact that the nation-state still is (and for the foreseeable future) the primacy political unit of the modern world and retains a considerable degree of relative autonomy of decision-making on internal matters, despite "globalization". This is certainly the case for those nation-states of the developed world. For those of the poor countries, this autonomy is considerably reduced, however. But in the former case at least, national affiliations or identities have a rational basis. On the other hand, this also expresses the fact that the nation-state is nonetheless placed under greater pressure than ever before by the internationalization of capital and the ramping-up of world-wide market competition. This is pressure placed on governments to preserve the economic security of their own nation-states by aligning these more closely to the needs of capital and neoliberalism.

These needs are opposed to those of most people for a politics of interventionism that would build a fairer society. "Globalization" has therefore legitimized world-wide convergence of state policy on matters of economic management and social welfare. This has generated an international consensus, as Peter Gourevitch puts it, "to curtail state spending and interventions" as far as possible.[50] In the developed countries, policies of full employment were done away with in the 1980s, along with public ownership and expansive welfare states. This was as governments interpreted these as undermining the international competitiveness of their own capitals. Nationalist affiliations reflect in part people's discontent over the negative impacts of international forces (sometimes interpreted as the cultural imperialism of cosmopolitans) that have, in their interpretation, dishonoured their own country or nation, and that threaten its autonomy. As Kobena Mercer points out: "Identity ... becomes an issue when it is in crisis, when something assumed to be fixed, coherent and stable is displaced by the experience of doubt and uncertainty".[51]

Now, pandemic politics worldwide manifestly contradict globalization theory's most cherished claims, for reasons I will elaborate. These are that the various processes connected to or identified with "globalization" (including and especially the economic) are undermining both nationalist identifications and nationalist expectations. As the narrative goes: nationalist identifications are eroded especially by the impacts of global economic integration. But other corrosive forces include international travel and tourism, the worldwide diffusion of lifestyle consumerism and cosmopolitan one-world values through the internet and global media and communications, and so on. Nationalist expectations are radically challenged because, in the famous words of Daniel Bell, the "nation-state is too small for the big problems of life, and too big for the small problems of life".[52] This reflects, for globalists, the basic crises of *autonomy*, *competence*, and hence of *legitimacy*, which are faced by nation-states.

Back in the real world, however, whatever the limitations of state responses to the pandemic, what cannot be in doubt is that, with rare exceptions, it was nation-states that erected the COVID-barricades (of lockdowns and other NPIs) and that supported these with furloughs that kept people in home-isolation. These measures, notwithstanding their greater or lesser commitment or efficiency, did suppress the virus, and by doing so did save a million plus lives across the world in the pre-vaccine context – and will perhaps continue to save millions more until vaccination is globalized. So too did nation-states coordinate the vast nationwide vaccination rollouts that within two months (in the case of the UK) had offered protection to all of the vulnerable and elderly cohorts, and which by the end of the first year had extended that coverage to include even young adults, with boosters for over 50-year olds. Or, rather, it was the nation-states at the core of the world system that did that, followed by those in the more or less developed countries of the triad, drawing upon comparatively well-resourced and well-organized public healthcare systems to deliver assembly-line inoculations.

The administrative "competence" of the vaccine operations can hardly be questioned – and this was a competence that the public simply took for granted. Nor can the "autonomy" of those who ran them be questioned. This was no international aid operation coordinated by the World Health Organization (WHO) or UN. Humanitarian aid organized at the supranational level is reserved for those countries that are regarded under the Western gaze as lacking in autonomy and competence. These are those who are too poor to sustain stable nation-states and functional healthcare systems.

Moreover, taken together, the experience of lockdowns and mass vaccinations demonstrated that nation-states commanded enough "legitimacy" in the public mind for a majority of people to acquiesce to them. Citizenries more or less and for the most part accepted that their national governments and underlying supporting machineries of state administration were, however reluctantly, committed to saving lives, defending healthcare services, and providing reliable public health guidance, and were competent in delivering these goals. This was in spite of these in some places (such as the UK and US) falling far short of the highest standards and delivering suboptimal outcomes.

The politics of vaccine nationalism especially evidences the realist case (in politics and international relations theory) for upholding the primacy of interstate competition over interstate cooperation and bilateral consensus-building in world politics. There are two main elements to vaccine nationalism. Firstly, there has been interstate rivalries among the developed countries to procure vaccine supplies for their own residents and citizens, which has translated into asymmetrical allocations. This led in certain cases to threats of "vaccine wars" (e.g. in the dispute between the UK and some of the leading EU states). This also demonstrated the national advantages of adopting a competitive lone-state procurement strategy (as the UK did) rather than a cooperative multi-state one (as did the EU). Secondly, there has been interstate competition for access to vaccines between the developed nations and those of the semi-developed and especially underdeveloped worlds. This has generated exactly the radical inequalities of worldwide coverage to the detriment of the latter that one might suspect. Indeed, competition among the developed nation-states for vaccine supplies has further contributed to the chronic shortages elsewhere, since this has led them to accumulate surpluses much in excess of local demand. I will now explore these developments further.

Vaccine nationalism and the UK–EU dispute

The UK government claimed national success in its "vaccine wars" with the EU as a Brexit bonus. The context of this was the UK's much faster and smoother rollout of the vaccines (starting from December 2020) compared to the EU's. Towards the end of January 2021, only two vaccine doses per 100 people had been delivered across the EU compared to ten per 100 in the UK (and seven per 100 in the US).[53] At the start of March, the situation had improved, but not by much. By then the UK had delivered 32.3 jabs per 1,000 of the population compared to the EU's 8.1 per 1,000. The US was also still streets ahead of the EU having by then delivered 24.3 jabs per 1,000 of the population.[54]

By the spring of 2021, the EU had recovered from its slow start to begin matching the UK's rates of vaccination and surpassing those in the US. Even so, at that point, the union's overall rate of vaccination was still languishing. By 20 May, 33 percent of the EU's adult population were vaccinated compared to 54 percent of the UK's and 48 percent of the US's.[55] Such provided an opportunity in the UK for much jingoistic triumphalism courtesy of Tory Brexiters.[56] This attributed UK vaccine success to early contract signings with the pharmaceutical companies to procure vaccines in comparison with the EU's slower signings and its faster-tracked regulatory clearance for the vaccine rollout compared to everywhere else.

According to Brexiters, the early vaccine procurements and quick regulatory clearance for mass distributions resulted from the dynamism of a neoliberal business state that was set free from excess normative controls to pursue its own best national interests. These benefits were, as the story goes, to be contrasted with the stultifying bureaucratic rules of the European "superstate", which precluded speedy decision-making on all things concerning vaccines.[57] As Mark Francois, of the Conservative party's almost comically misnamed European Research Group, put it, "one of the side effects [of the pandemic] has been it has brutally exposed the weakness in the EU project, from protectionism to excessive bureaucracy".[58] Or, as Matt Hancock would have it, although the UK carried out "the same [vaccine] safety checks and the same processes ... we have been able to speed up how they're done because of Brexit". The same view was expressed more succinctly by Jacob Rees-Mogg, Leader of the House of Commons: "We could only approve this vaccine so quickly because we have left the EU".[59] This euphoric English vaccine nationalism even found its way into journalistic commentaries in the quality press lamenting the descent of the world into this self-same vaccine nationalism.[60]

But, contrary to this view, fast-tracking of vaccine regulatory clearance was permissible under EU law. So, red tape was not the explanation for the EU's supposed tardiness in giving vaccines the green light. Rather, at the time, the EU states were by-and-large making a better fist than the UK of suppressing the pandemic by means of NPIs and test-and-trace systems. This provided the EU's leaders with incentives to exercise caution over clearing the vaccines for use until more data was in with regard to possible side-effects. Johnson's government, by contrast, beleaguered by its terrible COVID-19 record up until that point, had impelling motives to cast caution to the winds.

The EU's European Medical Agency (EMA) rebuked the UK government for its fast-tracked approvals on the grounds that insufficient data-checking had been conducted by the UK's regulator, the Medicines and Healthcare Products Regulatory Agency (MHRA). Professor Anthony Fauci, of the US's National Institute of Allergies and Infectious Diseases, repeated this claim. He stated that the US regulator, the Food and Drug Administration (FDA) was proceeding "correctly", whereas the UK regulator "did not ... as carefully".[61] Fauci later retracted his claim. This may have been because he became convinced it was wrong. Or he may have decided to retract his claim because, though true, he considered it as potentially harming the UK rollout.

However, more haste certainly risked less careful scrutiny. The UK government (along with those of the US and Canada) gave permission for the vaccines to be deployed as basically an unlicensed product under emergency measures. By contrast, in the EU, under the auspices of the EMA's approval process, the vaccines needed to earn licensing approval, renewable after a year, which commits provider companies to submit more trial data on an ongoing basis.[62] Vaccine approval under the EMA, arguably, draws on a wider body of evidence than the fast-tracked emergency approvals of the UK.

The approval process may have been slower in the EU as well because the 27 member countries all had to give their approval to the European Commission (EC) before the vaccines were licensed.[63] Nonetheless, under EU law, "individual countries can use an emergency procedure that allows them to distribute a vaccine for temporary use in their domestic market".[64] At the time, the UK was still bound by the EU rules as part of the post-Brexit transition process. The fact that none of the EU's 27 member states activated emergency use powers for local vaccination approvals may be read reasonably as evidence that they considered the pandemic sufficiently under control from the NPIs and test-and-trace programmes to err on the side of a safety-first approach to the vaccines.

Nor were the restrictions on member states under the EC's centralized vaccine procurements system (which the UK declined to join) responsible for the initial slowness of the rollout or the supply shortages that soon manifested which delayed further its progress. This was because even though the terms of the EU scheme were that member states must "agree not to launch their own procedures for advance purchase of [any] vaccine with the same manufacturers"[65] that were already contractual providers under the scheme, this clause certainly did not prevent participant states from disregarding it and signing their own deals with the pharmaceutical companies independently. Germany, for example, signed its own agreement with Pfizer for 30 million doses other than those already committed through the EU's central procurements system in September 2020.[66]

Yet the UK did secure vaccine-procurement contracts from the pharmaceutical companies faster than was achieved by the EC on behalf of the EU. In doing so, the UK outcompeted a powerful confederation of states so that it had first call on supplies that were not yet plentiful because of productive under-capacity. This, again, demonstrated the very real autonomy of action of the individual nation-state in the "global" world – so long as the state in question was one of the dominant ones. But, again, this also evidenced the primacy of national competition over cooperation in the complex dialectic of the two in the interstate system, in the sense that this was consistent with the response of most states to vaccine procurements, and in most cases by necessity. For most other countries (unlike the UK), there were simply no cooperative supranational alternatives to reliance on narrow vaccine nationalisms. I will discuss this issue later.

But this primacy of interstate competition over cooperation in world systems was also revealed by the fact that Brussel's collective procurements strategy was itself necessitated by the need to prevent interstate rivalries for vaccine supplies within the bloc fracturing the union. This strategy was adopted to pre-empt the EU's leading states queue-jumping in negotiating contracts that prioritized their own national self-interest over that of the other member states.[67]

This was further motivated to undermine "Russian and Chinese vaccine diplomacy in Europe".[68] That is, it was intended to ensure that the vaccine marketplace in the EU was dominated by its own pharmaceutical industries and, to a lesser degree, those of the US (rather than those of China and Russia – the US's and EU's biggest potential geopolitical rivals), and to prevent vaccination offers being used by Russia and China to build political and economic influence in

Europe.[69] Pandemic nationalism had already threatened EU unity at the start of the crisis. This was because France and Germany undermined the single market by barring exports of Personal Protective Equipment (PPE) to other member countries. This trade ban was lifted only after the EC capitulated to Germany's demand to restrict exports of PPE outside the bloc.[70] The crisis exposed fissures between the free trade politics of the EC's neoliberal utopians and the politics of national self-protection favoured by governments of the most powerful member states. The nationalists won this particular tussle.

The centralized vaccine-procurement strategy was proposed not by the weaker EU states but by the stronger ones, at the centre of which were France and Germany. Initially, France and Germany assembled the so-called "Inclusive Vaccination Alliance". This was a select group of core EU states (Germany, France, Italy and the Netherlands) to organize their own vaccine procurements. But they were later persuaded by the EC to hand these over to the new EU-wide procurements system and cease seeking out new contracts on their own behalf. The EC's procurements system thereby superseded the Alliance, and in doing so inherited a deal struck by the Alliance with AstraZeneca for 400 million doses of the "Oxford" vaccine.

Berlin's and Paris's conversion to the EU policy was primarily motivated by their national self-interest since this was best served within the framework of the EU, which would be placed under stress by the pursuit of competitor vaccine nationalism within the bloc. They were sufficiently convinced by EC's president Ursula von der Leyen's argument that centralized procurements on behalf of all of the member states would allow a magical convergence of narrow national self-interest and general altruism.[71] Von der Leyen lauded the EU scheme as transcending the vaccine nationalism of other states, such as the US and UK, and hence as showing world leadership on how a collective cooperative supranational response to the pandemic could be mobilized. This was to be quickly exposed as fantasy by subsequent events.

The tardiness of the EU's procurements process was likely a function of the greater complexity of negotiations when these were on behalf of 27 nation-states rather than one. These negotiations would be fraught precisely because the EU's partner-states are simultaneously *competitor*-states bound together only by collective self-interest against those states and confederations of states ranged against them outside Fortress Europe. As the EU's vaccine rollouts ran into trouble right from the start,[72] the interstate rivalries within the union were radicalized. So much so that these widened into vaccine antagonisms between members that threatened to further diminish the effectiveness of the programme. Mistrust was sowed among the weaker states by the fact that the leading states with their own pharmaceutical industries responded to the problems by continuing to make their own independent procurements. The problem was then exacerbated by the fact that the initial delivery of vaccines among the member states was asymmetric. Some did better than others.[73] This gave a boost to Chinese and Russian vaccine diplomacy that the collective approach was intended to undermine, especially among the more fringe EU states of southern and eastern Europe, some of which struck their own deals for vaccines produced by the Chinese and Russian manufacturers.[74]

Competition of a different kind also obstructed the speed of the EU's vaccination effort. This was price-competition as the EC sought to wield the vast collective political and economic power of the bloc to negotiate with the pharmaceutical companies "competitive" financial terms for delivery of the vaccines. Negotiations were animated by a fundamentally business-led or commercially driven concern to ensure that the "price was right".[75] This was presumably in the sense that certainly no more and ideally much less would be paid out for the vaccines than by international competitors. This was obviously a peculiarly neoliberal concern – to treat vaccine contracts as an opportunity for commercial bidding rather than as simply the means to secure the quickest resolution of a public health emergency. Yet it was also motivated by a sense of protecting the public interest in that a motive was to divest the drug companies of the opportunity to drive up prices by negotiating terms with each member state individually, with these terms unknown to the others owing to confidentiality clauses. The evidence indicates that the EU did squeeze from the drug corporations much lower prices than the go-it-alone states (US and UK) which fast-tracked safety clearance and contract signings.[76] But the process that delivered this result was protracted.

But, in fairness to Brussels, this tardiness in signing contracts may not have been decisive in causing slowness in the actual vaccine rollout across the member states. This was because the contracts signed by the EU committed providers to deliver supplies to the member states on the same timescales as for honouring their UK deliveries. The fact that the UK government signed its own contracts much earlier (by up to three months on some accounts) arguably did not provide it with contractual privilege over the EU in terms of delivery dates. This was despite the fact that apparently UK negotiators, in a classic play of vaccine nationalism, got written into their contracts that the drug companies must deliver in full on their UK commitments before honouring others. In the case of the UK's deal with AstraZeneca, this not only committed the company to turning over all vaccine production in the UK to serving exclusively UK needs but also to diverting output from its European factories for UK use in the event of shortages.[77]

AstraZeneca CEO Pascal Soriot's defence of the company's "UK first" policy was thus probably bogus. As he put it: "The contract with the UK was signed first and the UK, of course, said 'you supply us first', and this is fair enough".[78] Yet this was not fair enough. The company's prioritization of UK deliveries was unlikely to have been settled simply by the logic of first come-first served. Rather, the decisions of the vaccines companies generally to honour commitments to the UK prior to honouring the equivalent commitments to the EU were quite possibly taken owing to the fact that there were penalties for lateness written into the UK contracts but not into the EU ones.[79] The absence of penalty clauses in the latter reflected differences in contractual custom between the UK and the EU. Whereas the latter regarded contracts as mechanisms for building trust between business partners, the former reflected a view of the contract negotiators as potentially untrustworthy because they were business antagonists. This again evidences the complex dynamics of competition-cooperation rivalries within the interstate system that ended up distributing the benefits of vaccination unevenly.

The consequences of this were clear enough in the EU's dispute with AstraZeneca over the company's failure to deliver the promised volumes on the contracted time-scales. Gareth Davies noted at the time that the UK contracts required the suppliers to deliver "preferentially if necessary" (and with strict sanctions in the event of not meeting deadlines). "By contrast, the EU contract is said to be somewhat less detailed and more conciliatory, providing for informal discussions in the event of disagreement, and no penalties beyond withholding of payment". And so, as Davies says, "having promised to supply the UK preferentially, and the EU fairly, AstraZeneca simply cannot do both, and so has made a commercial decision to breach the contract that will cost it less". So, this was likely a pragmatic voluntary decision of corporate self-interest, not one that AstraZeneca was coerced into by the primacy of the UK's exclusivity clause. For an "exclusivity clause in one contract does not justify a failure to supply in another one – to achieve that AstraZeneca should have put in a 'UK priority' clause in the EU contract too".[80]

By the end of March 2021, the UK had administered 30 million doses of the various vaccines. This meant that 40 percent of Britons had received a first dose at that point. Yet locally produced vaccines were by then sufficient to offer a jab to only 20 percent of the UK population. Now, on the same timescale, as little as one-third and certainly less than half of the UK's vaccine supply was produced by local plants, with most of the rest imported from the EU. This was the case for all of the UK's 13 million doses of the Pfizer jab,[81] as well as undisclosed volumes (likely several million) of the AstraZeneca jab – that is, from the Halix plant in the Netherlands,[82] and of a further five million doses of AstraZeneca from the Serum Institute in India.[83] By contrast, European plants had by then produced around 110 million doses of the various vaccines, which was sufficient to offer a first jab to a little more than 20 percent of the EU's population. As for the EU's vaccine-producing countries, these

> have made enough to vaccinate about half their population with a first jab (the 100 million jabs were made in EU states with a combined population of about 200 million – Germany, Belgium, the Netherlands, Spain and Italy). If they had kept this for themselves, they would be far ahead of the UK – which would have had to make do with its own more limited production – and at around the same stage as the US.[84]

Yet, by the end of March, only 12–14 percent of the EU population had received a first dose.

There is therefore good evidence that the fundamental reason for the slowness of the EU's vaccine rollout, especially compared with those of the UK and US, had little to do with delayed procurements or drawn-out regulatory clearance – not in any direct sense. Rather, the cause was simply that those select European countries in which the drug companies had (heavily EU-subsidized) vaccine-manufacturing facilities were exporting much of their output to various destinations overseas as well as across the bloc. The European producers had by then exported a third of doses to the other EU member states, whereas a further 35 percent of their output was exported beyond the EU, with some of that international trade going to the US, but with by far the biggest chunk of it going to the UK.[85] As was reported by the EC on 11 March 2021:

> The main export destinations include the United Kingdom (with approximately 9.1 million doses), Canada (3.9 million), Mexico (3.1 million), Japan (2.7 million), Saudi Arabia (1.4 million), Hong Kong (1.3 million), Singapore (1 million), United States (1 million), Chile (0.9 million) and Malaysia (0.8 million).[86]

Thus, as Davies rightly concludes, rollout problems did not explain the big discrepancies in vaccination rates in the UK compared to the EU.

> Rather, that difference is to do with supply: the UK is getting more … The overwhelming reason why the UK is so far ahead with its vaccination programme is that it has received so many vaccines from the EU.[87]

The drug companies, of course, would claim that the reason that the UK (rather than the EU) had reaped the benefit of European vaccine production supplies in the first few months of 2021 was simply that its contracts were signed sooner so that supply-chain or production-capacity issues could be sorted out in advance. As we have seen, this was AstraZeneca's explicit self-defence. But the fact is that the companies themselves did not foresee such problems arising to blow off-course the EU contracts, despite their earlier contract signings with the UK. If they had they would not have signed off on the delivery timeframes that they did.[88]

Moreover, as we have seen, if there were privilege or priority clauses in the UK contracts, which appears likely, these provided no obligation for AstraZeneca to act on them since doing so would break the EU contracts. Nor did these clauses provide legal justification for the company to evade its equivalent contractual obligations to the EU. AstraZeneca, for example, was not contractually debarred from responding to its manufacturing under-capacity issue by adopting a more even-handed approach to supplying the EU and the UK. An even-handed approach would mean both clients taking some of the hit, rather than the EU taking all of it. This would not be an attractive prospect for AstraZeneca, however, because it would spell double the liability, as two contracts rather than one would be broken.

This was almost certainly the genuinely held interpretation of the crisis in Brussels and among the EU's leading statespersons. This was also, in my judgement, the correct one. The sense of consternation, bewilderment, and moral outrage among EU leaders over the conduct of AstraZeneca in particular appears undeniable. These sentiments – as well as the magnitude of the dangers posed to public health and economic renewal by the problems of the vaccine programme – provoked a robust response to the company from Commission officials and from leading EU governments. This response demanded that AstraZeneca meet its obligations to the EU and warned of legal proceedings against the company if it did not.[89] Legal proceedings indeed followed.[90] This was in all likelihood no mere smokescreen to deflect attention from the EC's supposed vaccine-procurement failings (as British media commentators claimed),[91] although an element of blame-shifting before the court of public opinion could not be ruled out.[92]

As the Commission's boss Ursula von der Leyen responded: "These are binding orders and the contract is crystal clear". AstraZeneca's defence of its own conduct – that is, that the contracted delivery times to the EU was a commitment to only "best effort" – was vehemently denounced by von der Leyen and other EU diplomats, and rightly so, since "best effort" was also written into the UK contracts. This could not be otherwise because when the contracts were signed the product was theoretical rather than real. As von der Leyen also pointed out:

> "Best effort" was valid while it was still unclear whether they [AstraZeneca] could develop a vaccine. That time is behind us. The vaccine is there.[93]

But the most eloquent expression of the force of the EU's feelings was delivered courtesy of EC health commissioner, Stella Kyriakides, who led the EU's centralized vaccination-procurements. This was a remarkably powerful rebuke that is worth quoting at length:

> We are in a pandemic. We lose people every day. These are not numbers, they're not statistics. These are persons with families with friends and colleagues that are all affected as well ... We signed an advanced purchase agreement for a product which at the time did not exist and which still today is not yet authorised and we signed it precisely to ensure that the company builds a manufacturing capacity to produce the vaccine early so that they can deliver a certain volume of doses the day that it is authorised ... Pharmaceutical companies, vaccine developers have moral, societal and contractual responsibilities, which they need to uphold. The view that the company is not obliged to deliver because we signed a best effort agreement is neither correct, nor is it acceptable ... We reject the logic of first come, first served ... That may work in a butcher's shop but not in contracts and not in our advanced purchase agreements.[94]

The primary focus of the EU's ire was, of course, AstraZeneca – which, as Kyriakides pointed out, accepted €336 million from the EC in order to build up in advance of regulatory clearance the necessary production capacity to deliver on its EU contract, only to then fail to do so.[95] The company was accused of entering into agreements to sell vaccines at higher prices to other countries only to discover that it had over-committed as its commercial ambition outstripped its productive capacity.[96] But the EU's ire was perhaps not only for AstraZeneca's shortcomings but also for the lesser though real failures of the other drug companies to deliver the promised quantities on time.

There was also undoubtedly accompanying moral revulsion at the role of the UK government in the sordid affair. This was for insisting on inserting into its own vaccine contracts those special clauses that were certainly intended to commit the drug companies to delivering on every nook and cranny of the UK's orders before they could meet obligations to other clients. EU anger was particularly centred on the UK's contractual claim over AstraZeneca's UK production facilities for priority UK use and first-call privileges on the company's production facilities in Europe until its own contractual needs were met. This basically legitimized AstraZeneca's policy of turning over vaccine production in both European and UK plants to the task of completing the UK orders to strict deadline, to the detriment of hundreds of millions of Europeans, who were made to wait on their deliveries until the UK orders were delivered in full.

As von der Leyen opined, the company's factories in the UK as well as in the EU were legally obliged to deliver on the EU's contract. Exactly the same factories in the UK and on the continent were contracted to deliver on the UK and EU orders. Yet AstraZeneca's EU plants were exporting to the UK, just as its UK plants were *not* exporting to the EU. This was the opposite of interstate cooperation between trading "partners". In von der Leyen's words. "we haven't received anything from the Brits, although we are delivering to them".[97]

For the EC and the leading EU states, therefore, the vaccine dispute with AstraZeneca and the UK government was motivated primarily by a real sense of injustice faced with a basic disregard for parity in the delivery of contractual obligations rather than disingenuous buck-passing. Germany's demand of AstraZeneca for "fairness" of delivery was echoed repeatedly by the EC over the course of the dispute. As von der Leyen explained – as she threatened to trigger Article 122 of the EU treaty in mid-March 2021 (which would permit the Commission to seize control of vaccine production and distribution in the bloc) – parity was a question of

> reciprocity and proportionality in exports … making sure that Europe gets its fair share … It is hard to explain to our citizens why vaccines produced in the EU are going to other countries that are also producing vaccines, but hardly anything is coming back.[98]

The EC's principal demand of AstraZeneca was that the company divert some output from the UK-based plants to cater for European needs in accordance with the EU contract. As a senior EU official put it:

> Given that, according to several reports, Britain was supplied with AstraZeneca vaccines produced in the EU when its British factories faced production shortfalls a few weeks ago, it would only be logical now to deliver vaccines from Britain to the EU.[99]

However, that would require British PM Boris Johnson's go-ahead, given the penalties written into the UK's contract with AstraZeneca. And neither logic nor basic fair-dealing was likely to trump the UK government's own vaccine nationalism. This was not least because the UK's vaccine rollout was its government's only pandemic success story. The political capital of this self-declared "Brexit bonus" for Johnson's crew was not to be dimmed in the slightest by easing up on the vac-cination accelerator, especially since the competitor-advantage of an earlier return to capitalist normality in the UK than then seemed likely on the continent was beckoning. Thus, to say that Westminster's response to the European vaccine crisis was hardly an act of solidarity would be an understatement.

Six weeks after the EC's plea for "reciprocity" of vaccine deliveries, AstraZeneca's UK-based plants were still not exporting doses to the continent, even though Pfizer vaccine exports to the UK from the EU were continuing. (During that period ten million doses of European-manufactured Pfizer were imported into the UK). Instead, the response of Johnson and his ministers was to warn the EU states and the EC of the hazards of a protectionism motivated by self-defeating jingo-ism – and seemingly to do so without a hint of embarrassment at the hypocrisy of it all.[100]

In response to the Commission's threat to invoke Article 122, in order to pres-sure the UK government into giving permission for AstraZeneca to export doses from its English-based factories to the EU, foreign minister Dominic Rabb offered not the hint of a concession. Instead, he expressed his shock at the "brinkmanship" of the EC's move. This was the kind of thing to be expected of countries with "less democratic regimes", he said, not of civilized countries.[101] Such British intransi-gence in placing national self-interest as a matter of first and last resort, while lec-turing the EU on its duty to respect its close "friend" and "ally" (as Johnson did),[102] was sufficient to motivate accusations in Brussels that Westminster was even set on provoking a vaccine war with the bloc.[103]

The UK government's warning to Brussels was issued in the event that the EU would introduce export controls, in response to its vaccine shortages, which would threaten the UK's access to its European suppliers – including 40 million Pfizer doses from the company's Belgian plant. At the same time, Johnson's crew, bran-dishing its contract privileges, noisily self-congratulated on declining to join the EU's centralized vaccine-procurement scheme (since doing that would have been a "great pity", as Johnson said) and on being the European vaccination leader "by some way" (as Johnson also put it).[104] Ministers also announced that they would insist that AstraZeneca refrain from diverting any of its UK output towards meet-ing its contractual obligations with the EU – not until the UK order was completed. Only after the company's English plants had delivered their quota of 100 million doses for UK distribution would they be permitted to export vaccines to the EU.[105] There would be "no interruption" to UK supply so that the "schedule that has been agreed and on which our vaccine has been based goes ahead" – as cabinet office minister Michael Gove put it.[106]

This was just as the EC was incentivized to introduce its "vaccine transparency" policy to breathe life into its stalled vaccine rollout. According to this policy, all drug manufacturers in the union (which included Pfizer) must declare their vaccine exports before the EC for approval. This was in effect an export control policy, or rather it was turned into one, thanks to pressure from string-pulling member states such as Germany.[107] This granted the EC powers to restrict or block vaccine exports so as to overcome European shortfalls. These powers, however, though sometimes used, were rarely. As it transpired, they were not used to curtail exports to the UK, even though tensions with Westminster ensured that this was seriously entertained for more than a month.[108] But ominous talk of trade wars by senior Eurocrats receded as under-capacity issues in Europe were ironed out by the drug manufacturers by the start of the summer of 2021 and as the EU rollout began to outpace those in the UK and US.[109] Even so, since the new regulations demanded drug company accountability for and transparency over their vaccine exports, these inevitably were not well received. Pfizer complained that EU red tape was slowing down the (largely non-existent outside the developed world) vaccine rollout, for example.[110]

Before the EU's vaccine crisis began to recede, however, there was to be one big flashpoint of the EU–UK dispute. This was sparked by the EC's declaration of intent to head off the potential for unsanctioned vaccine exports passing from Europe to the UK by means of introducing emergency controls at the border between the Irish Republic and Northern Ireland.[111] This move would have been part of a strategy to prevent the UK from drawing on European vaccine-manufacturing capacity at the expense of the member states in response to if not in retaliation for Westminster's refusal to permit the diversion of UK-produced vaccine output to cater for European needs.

But such a policy would have "suspended" the terms of the Brexit deal and endangered the Good Friday agreement that ended "the troubles" in Ulster. For these reasons, and also faced with dissent from member states, the EC quickly U-turned.[112] By that decision, a major escalation of the crisis was averted, since if the EC had stuck to its guns, Johnson's government (animated as it was by populist Brexit nationalism and licensed as it would have been by an implacably anti-EU tabloid press)[113] was perfectly capable of retaliating.[114] Such retaliation would quite feasibly have consisted of blocking vaccine exports across the channel indefinitely, provoking a fully fledged trade war that would endanger the lives of hundreds of thousands.

But, even if tardy contracts in a first come-first serve world were the cause of the EU's vaccine woes (which as we have seen is disputable), there would be some mitigation for it. This is inasmuch as the reason for it was not simply commercial haggling. From the start of the process, the EC was committed to securing contracts that would also offer protection to consumers by making the drug-makers carry legal liability in the event of their vaccines causing health ill-effects in users. This was not an unreasonable demand, even under emergency conditions. Since all adults were to be inoculated, there could potentially be as many if not more people suffering adverse side-effects from the vaccines than were rendered ill by the virus. This was also a sensible precaution since vaccine scepticism was much higher in the EU than in the UK or US so legal de-responsibilization clauses could only strengthen vaccine resistance in the public.[115]

For the drug-makers, however, this was of course a major sticking point. They wanted immunity from prosecution in the event of unforeseen hazards affecting users. Responsibility and liability clauses were likely evaded in their fast-tracked deals with the US and UK governments, which would further incentivize resistance to EU demands. As a Commission negotiator put it: "They've [UK and US] clearly had to create the worst terms and conditions ... God knows what they've agreed to on liability and indemnification".[116] In the end, the EU had its own way. This was after the vaccine manufacturers' lobbying efforts to insert non-liability clauses had been media-exposed and thereby undermined. But this delayed the signing of contracts. Not only that, the EC's hard bargaining may have alienated the pharma capitalists, providing them with added motives for prioritizing deliveries to friend-lier clients, under circumstances where production shortfalls meant that supplies were insufficient to meet overall obligations.

As Deutsch and Wheaton rightly surmise: "At the very least, Europe's hard bargaining hasn't sufficiently motivated pharma to boost production". This was according to Guntram Wolff, director of the Bruegel Brussels thinktank.[117] Nor would the EC's insistence on placing liability clauses in their vaccine contracts have done anything to deter AstraZeneca's or Moderna's or Pfizer's prioritization of UK and US deliveries over EU ones. There was certainly foot-dragging and other "soft" resistances by the drug companies with regard to discharging their equivalent contractual obligations to the EU compared to others. Thus:

> Moderna's vaccine was approved by the EU on January 6 – ahead of the U.K., Commission officials like to point out privately. But while that offers another source of inoculations, the company will have a limited supply in the EU throughout the year, promising 10 million doses in the first quarter of 2021.

Moreover, although Pfizer and BioNTech "submitted their application for an emer-gency use authorization in the US ... on November 20" (2020), it took them almost another two weeks "to complete their submission with the European Medicines Agency". Despite the size of the EU's order for the Pfizer vaccine being twice as big as the US's, "Pfizer committed to delivering 200 million doses for Americans – produced on US soil – by the end of July [2021] ... while the EU ... [wasn't] ... assured that sum until September" [of that year].

As Deutsch and Wheaton continue:

> Pfizer hadn't taken money from Trump's Operation Warp Speed, but its part-ner, BioNTech, had received the EIB loan and cash from the German govern-ment. And yet Pfizer, headquartered in New York City, opted to coordinate closely with the FDA – rather than the EMA – as well as Germany's vaccines regulator, the Paul Ehrlich Institute, to design their clinical trials. Pfizer and BioNTech declined to explain why they prioritized the U.S. application.[118]

Of course, the priorities of Pfizer and Moderna can also be explained, pure and simple, by vaccine nationalism. These, as American corporations, may have sim-ply regarded American lives as more important than European lives. More plausi-bly, perhaps, such decisions may be explained simply by capitalistic self-interest. American pharma companies had been scaling down investments in production capacity in the EU owing to greater vaccine resistance among the Europeans compared to Americans. The US drug marketplace is not only vast but less regulated (and hence more profitable) than the EU's. Realizing those higher profits would also normally be easier and quicker than in the EU, owing to the greater complexity and volume of separate negotiations with the member states that are involved in entering these European markets compared to exploiting the US one.[119] Even though these typical advantages did not really apply to the COVID-19 vaccines (given that the EU had assumed central control of the procurement process), for Pfizer and Moderna, nonetheless, the usual ways of doing things may have simply been repeated by way of habit or custom.

Most plausibly, however, Pfizer's and Moderna's prioritization of the US market (though not the UK's) was probably simply the consequence of their close strategic-instrumental alignment with the US state. This would be simply the working out of a particular case of the structural interdependence of capital and state. This interpretation would be supported by the EU's biggest complaint against the drug companies; namely, that they were exporting large volumes of vaccines produced by European factories outside the bloc (hence generating shortages in Europe), in order to prioritize other unspecified needs. As we have seen, the charge was levelled explicitly at AstraZeneca (a British-dominated firm) in the context of the company's stated commitment to guarantee UK deliveries at the expense of the EU's, but was motivated by more general discontent.[120] But the Commission's introduction of new "transparency" regulations in response to the vaccine shortages, which compelled the drug companies to disclose in advance their export destinations for EU approval, showed that the complaint was not specific to AstraZeneca.[121]

Pfizer and Moderna, like all other MNCs, shelter under the patronage of their "own" state. For this reason, they owe their loyalty to that state in particular. The executives of these companies would have good reason to believe that an even-handed policy of vaccine distributions (that is, simultaneously to the US and EU) would not endanger their political alignment with the "parent" state. After all, states are incentivized to protect the commercial interests of their biggest corporations in their competition with those of other countries. This is because the success of any national economy upon which a corresponding state power is based depends on the competitiveness of its "own" enterprises. Yet structural interdependence is a two-way street so that states and capitals are bound by ties of loyalty as well as by those of mutual self-interest. In all likelihood, Pfizer and Moderna prioritized American lives over European lives because, hardly surprisingly, that is exactly what the US state demanded and expected of them, whereas they would have no pressing commercial interests in setting aside these ties of loyalty.

As we have seen, the EU entertained the idea of escalating its vaccine dispute with the UK government into a fully fledged trade war. This was by creating a "hard" border between the Irish Republic and Northern Ireland so as to block European-produced vaccines from crossing into the UK. Thankfully, there was no appetite for the move across the bloc, since this was likely to spell losses for everyone rather than clear-cut winners and losers. This would also have driven a horse and carriage through the EU's largely mythical self-representation as a force for international cooperation and as a redoubt against vaccine nationalism, and this would have incurred major reputational damage for the union. In any case, even though the EC and the leading EU states were certainly prepared to countenance invoking Article 122 of the EU treaty – in order to raise the possibility in Johnson's mind that this would lead to the diversion of doses bound for the UK to the EU and thereby encourage him to offer compromises – the rationality of raising the stakes in that way receded in the spring of 2021. This was as the production issues on the continent were ironed out and as supplies were sucked into the bloc from elsewhere.

If the EC had escalated the conflict with the UK, however, this would have undoubtedly been motivated by a keen sense of injustice among Eurocrats over the vaccine parity issue. From this perspective, or according to this narrative, even though the EU was exporting millions of vaccinations to the UK and across the world (hence acting as a beacon of global solidarity), it was receiving from the UK nothing in return. This was just as the UK (and the US) were hoarding their own enormous vaccine stashes for exclusively local use.

****

But it is now time to critically interrogate the EC's concept of vaccine "fairness" in the context of global political economy. Even though the EC noisily self-congratulated on its role in supporting the international vaccine effort, this effort was in fact far from impressive. By 13 July 2021, the EU had exported less than three percent of the doses that were promised to the poorer countries (four million out of 160 million).[122] Those donations that had been made were a classic case of "aid as imperialism", in that the bulk of the recipient countries were those with established links to the donors (often former colonies or protectorates) so that vaccine diplomacy was a mechanism for strengthening those ties and dependencies.[123] As for the EU's dispute with the UK, in the end, the Commission had insufficient cause to wage risky (because potentially counterproductive) vaccine wars with Johnson's government because, like the US and other developed countries of the Global North, the bloc occupied a highly advantaged position in the global vaccine marketplace *vis-à-vis* the overwhelming majority of countries of the Global South.

In this context, given the fact that the EU's vaccine troubles were not of procurement, but of delays in receiving supplies that would easily cater for its collective needs, radical self-protection measures were not spurred by a politics of desperation. These were seen as teething troubles and they were expected to be resolved in a few months. Without emergency incentives, embracing a form of protectionism that would have been at the expense of the UK was not worth the risk. This, after all, would work only if it succeeded in forcing concessions rather than retaliations from the UK government. And concessions did not seem likely owing to the peculiarity of the UK government's belligerent populist Brexit nationalism and the probable willingness of Johnson's crew to gamble on the EU being the first to blink in any standoff.

Vaccine imperialism and the international state system

Turning now to the international picture with regard to the rollout of the vaccines. The way this has unfolded from its start on the cusp of 2021 up until the present day (April 2023) perfectly reflects the asymmetries of authoritative and allocative resources generally across the interstate system and world capitalist economy. As Ryan and Nanda observe: "While the vaccine rollout has been impressive, it has also been unequal", with this "embedded in the global aspects of COVID-19 ... global power relations, trade wars, economic interactions".[124]

This also exposes the moral hypocrisy of European talk of "unfairness" under the impress of the EU–UK vaccine wars. For, even though vaccine nationalism in a world organized politically as competitor nation-states would typically be the rational course of action for an individual state (and for most the only one), this must also lead to suboptimal results internationally, due to the asymmetrical distribution of powers of authorization in the interstate system.[125] As Pilkington *et al.* rightly say:[126] "A nationalistic approach is not effective during a global pandemic. International cooperation is essential to achieve global goals against COVID-19".[127] Indeed. However, this flies in the face of *structural* reality: a global system of interstate and inter-capitalist competition between players with radically different powers of command over authoritative and allocative resources.

The biggest problem posed by vaccine nationalism for the poorer countries is that it has licensed the vaccine imperialism of the richer ones, under the spur of emergency politics. The UK's (and US's) go-it-alone pursuit of national self-interest, for example, could certainly be interpreted as much more egoistic, selfish, or just plain greedy than it needed to be.[128] This basically committed them to buying-up vast stockpiles of vaccines far beyond the wildest projections of national demand, even factoring in booster jabs and the inoculation of children, hence contributing to the radical supply shortages that were experienced elsewhere.[129]

For the governments of the developed countries, such as those of the US and UK, greater command of authoritative resources, underpinned by monopolization of allocative resources, enabled them to jump to the front of the queue in negotiating contracts with the aspirant vaccine manufacturers. These governments could much better shoulder the financial risk of having to write-off substantial sums from backing the wrong vaccine horses than the others could. They could also afford to back many different vaccine horses. By contrast, many governments of low-income countries were simply too poor to rustle up the finances to gamble on the results of the various vaccination trials through advance purchasing deals, whereas those of middle-income countries would have strained their exchequers unduly by attempting to outcompete those of their higher-income rivals for first call on the vaccines if or when they came on tap.

For middle-income countries, the attraction of playing a game of wait-and-see on the results of the various vaccine trials by the rival pharmaceutical companies would be much stronger than spinning the roulette wheel of vaccine speculation. Middle-income countries could not, after all, afford to back as many vaccine horses as the higher-income countries, so this, for them, would be a riskier game. In any case, since the vaccine producers were companies of the Global North, under the patronage of their home-base nation-states, these would always prioritize drugs-dealing with the patron governments rather than with those of developing countries. For the vaccine capitalists as well, selling to governments of the rich countries was always going to be more commercially appealing than trading with those of the poorer ones. The rich countries have been a cash cow that would pay out multiple times. And these multiple pay outs would each time yield bigger profits for pharma capitalism than could be made by catering for the primary needs of people in poor countries whose governments could not afford the same bulk-buys for saving lives as were tolerated by governments in the rich countries.

Pharma capitalism and vaccine nationalism

Although the US and UK were stand-out offenders and beneficiaries of vaccine nationalism (as was Canada),[130] they were not alone. The EC on behalf of the EU member states also placed its bets on many vaccine horses and for volumes of some of the more promising much in excess of reasonable demand.[131] By November 2020's end, AstraZeneca, Pfizer, and Moderna (those companies where trials were most advanced and seemingly offering the brightest prospects for vaccine success) were estimating "a total production capacity of 5.3 billion doses for 2021, which could cover between 2.6 billion and 3.1 billion people". Moreover, "a vaccine created at the Gamaleya National Center of Epidemiology and Microbiology in Moscow could cover another 500 million people per year outside Russia from 2021". However, the EC on behalf of the 27 EU member states plus the five next richest countries (including the US and UK), with just 13 percent of the world's population, had by then advance-purchased 50 percent of this estimated output. Even factoring in the next half dozen of the leading drugs manufacturers whose vaccines were less developed than those of the three frontrunners, these richest countries were at that point set to monopolize half of the expected supply owing to their advance purchase agreements.[132]

Other researchers confirmed these estimates. According to the Johns Hopkins Bloomberg School of Public Health in the US, 51 percent of doses set for production in 2021 were procured under advance purchase deals by governments administering territories in which less than one-sixth of the world's population lived.[133] Indeed, according to the People's Vaccine Alliance (an advocacy group made up of a number of international aid organizations), the imbalance in worldwide vaccine allocation generated by unequal international competition over the next 12 months was set to be even more precipitous. This was because, based on their estimates, 53 percent of the doses of the eight most promising candidates for a viable vaccine (including all of Moderna's and all but four percent of Pfizer-BioNTech's) were advance-purchased for 2021 by governments of the developed countries housing just 14 percent of people in the world.[134]

But the potential was for this imbalance to grow since this was written into the contracts that the governments of these countries had drawn-up with the drug companies, as far as this allowed for orders to be endlessly repeated and upscaled.[135]

Unequal exchange is, as we have seen, self-reproducing. And so it transpired. By mid-April 2021, high-income countries had increased their share of the world's vaccine supply to 87 percent of the total. This was a total of 4.6 billion doses. This left middle-income and low-income countries housing 85 percent of the world's population with just 670 million doses between them.[136]

By mid-July 2021, according to statistics gathered by *Our World in Data*, people in wealthy and "upper-middle-income" countries had received more than 80 percent of the total doses administered worldwide at that point,[137] whereas 75 percent of these were received by people in just ten countries. The WHO estimated that by then the ratio of jabs in rich countries compared to poor countries stood at 62:1.[138] Similarly, the organization "reported that, by November 2021, more than 80% of the world's vaccines had gone to G20 countries, whereas LICs had received just 0.6% of all vaccines".[139] This was despite the fact that developing countries were responsible for around two-thirds of global vaccine-manufacturing output, albeit outsourced by the US and European pharma corporations.[140]

Not only were the middle-income and low-income countries pushed aside by the rich ones in the scramble to acquire vaccines even before they were ready to be produced. They were also pushed aside at every stage after the vaccines came on tap. At a Group of Seven (G7) leaders' summit on 19 February 2021, vague commitments to tackle vaccine disparities worldwide were presented before the world's media. However, the vast bulk of the population of the Global South remained without vaccine protection thereafter, even as governments in the Global North began to vaccinate children and roll out booster jabs from the autumn of that year.[141] Oxfam released a press statement, based on data provided by the People's Vaccine Alliance, which reported that, by the spring of 2021, at rates of vaccination that were then current, it would take 57 years for the low-income countries to inoculate their populations.

> New calculations from the Alliance, which includes Health Justice Initiative, Oxfam, and UNAIDS, found that last month people living in G7 countries were 77 times more likely to be offered a vaccine than those living in the world's poorest countries. Between them, G7 nations were vaccinating at a rate of 4.6 million people a day in May, meaning, if this rate continues, everyone living in G7 nations should be fully vaccinated by 8 January 2022 … Of the 1.77 billion doses of COVID vaccines given globally, 28 per cent have been in G7 countries. In contrast just 0.3 per cent of COVID jabs have been given in low-income countries, despite the fact G7 and low-income countries have a fairly similar population size.[142]

Vaccine imperialism carried by unequal interstate competition was thereby responsible for a global state of vaccine apartheid. Sometimes this interfaced with local-level vaccine apartheid. This was, for example, the case for the Palestinians, who were at the wrong end of it. Israel's vaccine rollout may be considered the absolute world leader – until one considers that this was to the exclusion of the Palestinians in the occupied territories, in contravention of international human rights law and the terms of the Fourth Geneva Convention.

As was reported by the UN in January 2021: "Israel has not ensured that Palestinians under occupation in the West Bank and Gaza will have any near-future access to the available vaccines".[143] This was as Israel began vaccinating its own citizens in these territories, with 20 percent inoculated by the start of March.[144] The Palestinian authorities (PAs) would thereafter have to rely mostly on donations from the COVID-19 Vaccines Global Access programme (COVAX), with additionals from China and the UAE, having received up until February 2021 a few thousand doses of Sputnik courtesy of Russia. Eventually, in June, having vaccinated 85 percent of its own population, the Israeli government offered the PAs 1.4 million surplus doses of Pfizer. This was in exchange for receiving the same number of doses back from the PAs when they received supplies from COVAX. Such was simply Israeli opportunism, however, since the vaccination of Palestinians was still languishing at around 30 percent so the PAs were placed under pressure to accept a "new for old" deal. This collapsed because the Israeli government's Pfizer vaccines were so old they were on the cusp of their expiry date.[145]

Global vaccine apartheid was also aided and abetted by the commercial greed of the pharma capitalists.

> Instead of working together to support common sense proposals to vaccinate the world as quickly as possible, the G7, the EU and the pharmaceutical corporations have signed a "devil's pact" – wealthy countries hoard doses and break promises, while pharmaceutical corporations exploit their monopolies to earn record profits.[146]

The vaccine capitalists were, as we have seen, only too happy to service – in the first and last and every instance – the wants of those richer national clients who would generate for them the more lucrative contracts, pushing the poorer countries to the back of the line, placing hundreds of thousands if not millions of lives at risk outside the fortresses of the developed world.

But to describe this state of affairs as risking a human calamity would be radically under-selling it, since the calamity was an actual one. As was reported by Oxfam, more than a million people died from COVID-19 worldwide in the four months between the G7 leaders' February and June summits in 2021.[147] This was as, according to the People's Vaccine Alliance (in their report of 21 October 2021), almost

> half (49 percent) of the vaccines sold by AstraZeneca, Pfizer/BioNTech, Moderna, and Johnson and Johnson have been delivered to high-income countries, even though such countries only comprise 16 percent of the world's population ... None of the four companies or partnerships (AstraZeneca, Pfizer/BioNTech, Moderna, and Johnson and Johnson) have sold more than 25 percent of their vaccine supply (agreed through contracts) this year to COVAX. Pfizer/BioNTech sold only one percent of its contracted supply to the initiative, Moderna only 3 percent; and Johnson and Johnson and

AstraZeneca have sold 25 and 19 percent of their supply to COVAX respectively ... Moderna has delivered an estimated 84 percent of its supply to high-income countries while the company ignores low-income countries. To date, AstraZeneca, Pfizer/BioNTech, Moderna, and J&J have collectively delivered 47 times as many doses to high-income countries compared to doses delivered to low-income countries.[148]

By the end of May 2021, only 28 million Africans had been vaccinated – less than two percent of Africa's population. (Africa was almost entirely dependent on the WHO's and UN's COVAX programme. This was just one percent of the one billion vaccine doses administered worldwide at that point. Moreover,

> between February and May, African countries received only 18.2 million of the 66 million doses they had expected through COVAX ... And a little over 1% – a million people – are fully vaccinated, according to the WHO's Africa office.[149]

As for the international picture, on 10 April 2021, WHO Director-General Tedros Adhanom Ghebreyesus, reported in a press conference: "On average in high-income countries, almost one in four people have received a Covid-19 vaccine. In low-income countries, it's one in more than 500".[150] A month later, Ghebreyesus briefed the media that there was no sign of improvement in the international situation. By then, just 0.3 percent of the world's vaccine supply, he said, was going to low-income countries.[151] Of these, "the Democratic Republic of Congo (0.005%), Haiti (0.003%), Burkina Faso (0.01%), Vanuatu (0.03%), South Sudan (0.04%), Yemen (0.04%), Chad (0.04%), Syria (0.05%), Guinea Bissau (0.06%) and Benin (0.1%)", were, as the *Guardian* reported, the most neglected.[152] At the time of writing the first edit of this chapter (October 2021), the basic structure of global vaccine injustice remained as firmly entrenched as from when the vaccines became available since by then, 98 percent of adults in low-income countries were still unvaccinated.[153]

****

But what of trends or trajectories in global vaccination since October 2021? Unsurprisingly, for reasons discussed above (primarily unequal interstate competition on the basis of national self-interest and differential financial capacities to buy-up stockpiles of drugs, but also commercial self-interest by the pharmaceutical companies as this has been supported by their "home" states and governments in the West), there has been little change in the basic pattern of inequality. But there has been slow, fitful, uneven progress in the number of people who have been at least once-vaccinated in low-income countries. This pattern may even persist for several years, prolonging the life and danger of the pandemic, as governments of the high-income countries hoover up vaccine supplies to support ongoing booster programmes.[154] "Pressure on global supplies will continue as booster dose programs are rolled out, further diverting much needed doses from those countries struggling to complete even initial vaccine courses".[155]

By 2021's end, by which time the vaccines had been available for public roll-out for more than a year, 75–80 percent of people in high-income countries had received at least one jab, whereas only ten percent of people in low-income countries had done so.[156] By the spring of 2022, only 58 percent of the world's eligible population had received a first vaccination, whereas the number of once-vaccinated people in low-income countries had grown by a solitary percentage point since December 2021 (up to 11 percent).[157] By then, the WHO's target or rather exhortation of the previous year (later pushed back to mid-year 2022) of achieving 70 percent vaccination in every country had been "met by only 52 countries", while the "interim milestone of 40% coverage" was "yet to be achieved by 69 countries", 21 of them having "not yet achieved even 10% coverage".[158]

More recently, by mid-summer 2022, global vaccine inequities had been eased, albeit only marginally, with 15.8 percent of people once-jabbed in the low-income countries compared to 55 percent in the lower middle-income countries and 78.7 percent in the higher middle-income countries. At that point, just one in seven people had been immunized in the poorest countries.[159] By mid-March 2022, in comparison, 79 percent of the population of the high-income countries had received at least their first jab.[160] Progress since then towards the WHO's international target has continued to be painfully slow so that, based on current rates, this would take several years to accomplish, assuming that progress is maintained at all, which cannot be assumed given the instability and fragility of the world economy. Towards November 2022's end, a further four-and-a-half months further along the road, more than three-quarters of people in low-income countries remained without any vaccine protection.[161] Presently, at the time of updating this chapter (April 2023), 67.4 percent of people in the poorer countries are still unvaccinated, approximately 2.3 billion people worldwide.[162]

Africa retains the lowest rates of vaccination globally, despite substantial recent improvements. At the start of 2022, only five percent of Africans had received their first dose. This was in those of the continent's poorest countries that were providing data on vaccination rates. However, due to a two-year €16 million project funded by the EU, dramatic progress has since been made. This project involved WHO-mentored indigenous health workers providing jabs in settings outside vaccination centres (in towns, villages, outdoor markets, workplaces, refugee camps, displacement settlements, etc.) so that people who could ill-afford to travel, or who were prohibited from travelling, could receive the vaccine in their locales. Consequently, the rate of vaccination was elevated to close to 30 percent by the spring of 2023, in the 16 participating countries, which was almost on par with the average for the continent as a whole.[163] This was still at the tail end of vaccination rates globally, even for low-income countries. Nonetheless, the scheme showed what could be achieved, and with relatively modest resources, even if in so doing this threw into sharper relief the spectacular general failures resulting from the imperatives of the hydra of vaccine imperialism and pharma commerce.

Over-procurement in high-income countries generating supply-side problems elsewhere and driving up prices beyond the affordability of the poorer countries has remained a substantial part of the vaccine inequity problem throughout 2022 and beyond. Countries such as Canada, Australia, and the UK were, up to mid-year 2022, continuing to accumulate "enough ... doses to vaccinate their populations several times over: 11.1, 9.9 and 7.6 doses per person, respectively". By contrast, the African Union's (AU's) "purchase of 330m doses of Moderna and Janssen vaccines equated to just 0.2 doses a person across the bloc".[164] The problem of insufficiency of supply and inequality of allocation also continues to be exacerbated by the prohibitions placed on producing the vaccines freely across the world, owing to the pharma companies' continued exercise of their corporate property rights and the unwillingness of neoliberal governments (especially of countries to which these corporate interests belong) to waive or restrict those rights in the interests of global public health.

> Intellectual property (IP) rights allow the pharmaceutical companies involved in developing these vaccines to control the manufacture of vaccine supplies and therefore control pricing ... This means that vaccine supplies can only be manufactured when licensed and with the technology transfer overseen by these companies. This, in turn, results in prices set based on monopolistic access to a market, leading to prices that are well over the estimated costs of production.[165]

It has been estimated that the production costs of the vaccines vary from $1–3 per dose. However, the prices that are charged for them are typically several times higher. "For example, the UK is estimated to have overpaid $1.8 billion over the cost of production for the Pfizer and Moderna vaccines, the United States by $17.4 billion, and the EU by €31 billion".[166] The high-income countries can cope with the financial costs of this corporate price-fixing in rigged markets, whereas the low-income countries cannot. Indeed, for the latter, the problem is radicalized by the fact that they are charged higher prices for the vaccines than the former. For example: "In 2021, when the European Union was paying $3.50 (£2.70; €3.20) per dose of the Oxford-AstraZeneca vaccine, South Africa was being charged $5.25 and Uganda was being charged $7".[167]

Even if there was a level playing field globally in terms of the prices of the vaccines, and even if the prices of the vaccines reflected their manufacturing costs, the economic burden on the lesser and least developed countries of funding mass inoculation programmes would be punitive, if not prohibitive. These demands would be economically burdensome not only absolutely, but also relatively, in comparison with those financial demands placed on the public purse in the high-income countries.

> Data from the MI4A COVID-19 Vaccine Purchase Dataset shows that the average cost per COVID-19 vaccine dose ranges between US$ 2 – $ 40. The estimated delivery cost is US$ 3.70 per person vaccinated with two doses,

after accounting for vaccine wastage. This represents a significant financial burden for low-income countries, where the average annual per capita health expenditure amounts to US$ 41 ... While vaccination programmes will increase healthcare costs across all countries, it is especially the case in low-income countries as they would need to increase their health expenditure by a staggering 30–60 percent to reach 70 percent of their population under the current pricing and over a period of one year. High-income countries are expected to increase theirs by only 0.8 percent to achieve the same vaccination rate in one year.[168]

The point is especially pertinent when one considers that the COVAX scheme to vaccinate the world's poorest 92 countries – those which would struggle to self-vaccinate – made provisions only to inoculate 20 percent of their populations.

Little surprise, then, that governments of lower-income and some middle-income countries have been forced to take out major loans at high rates of interest to support their vaccine procurements, in the context of escalating monopolistic prices. Such price-exploitation of clients by the pharma capitalists also continues to be facilitated by the confidentiality clauses that they insist are built into the contracts offered to buyers, which are especially to the detriment of the poorer countries.[169] Confidentiality means a lack of transparency so that governments with weak bargaining power cannot negotiate terms based on an understanding of the "going rate" or "fair rate". Price inflation also has been ramped up by the decision of AstraZeneca (in November 2021) to abandon its pledge to provide doses "at cost" under emergency conditions in the service of global health. This was justified, perversely, on the grounds that the pandemic was over.[170]

Vaccine imperialism and the world economy

Vaccine inequity is likely to be hugely detrimental to a world economy that has been in the doldrums since long before the pandemic. In the shorter term at least, the failure to inoculate populations outside the developed countries will significantly contribute to the longstanding zombification of international capitalism I have discussed elsewhere.[171] The pandemic and lockdowns had already chalked off $16 trillion from the value of global output before 2020's end.[172] These caused world GDP to fall by "3.2 percent in 2020, by six percent in the EU, by 4.4 percent on average in the high-income countries, and by 3.4 percent in the US".

Nor have the predicted "robust bounce-backs" in economic performance after the lockdowns were lifted and the NPIs were scaled down since materialized. Aggregate output for the high-income economies was forecasted in 2021 to recover its pre-pandemic trajectory only by the end of 2022 and to exceed this only by 0.9 percent in 2024 ... Global GDP was just 3.5 percent higher by the end of 2021 than it was in 2019. The US's GDP was just 2.3 percent larger on that same timescale. The EU's GDP was 0.2 percent smaller by the close of 2021 than it was in 2019, whereas the GDP of the high-income countries taken as an aggregate was just 0.6 percent higher. As for the UK, recovery has been even slower. Here GDP was still 2.3 percent smaller by the close of 2021 than it was in 2019. Even prior to the Russia–Ukraine war, world GDP growth was predicted to slow down in 2022 (to 4.9 percent), languishing below the 2021 level (of 5.9 percent), and was predicted to slow further in 2023 and 2024 (to around 3.3 percent).[173]

Vaccine inequities are contributing to these economic doldrums. The Eurasia Group has estimated, that if vaccine equity worldwide is achieved, the high-income countries could obtain an economic boost by up to $466 billion by 2025.[174] Similarly, according to Çakmakli *et al.*, even though the lion's share of global financial losses from worldwide vaccine inequity will be incurred by middle-income and lower-income countries, these will not suffer alone. Rather, the high-income countries are projected to incur losses in sales revenues of anywhere between 13 and 50 percent unless vaccine inequity is overcome, depending on different scenarios, owing to reduced international trade and disruption of supply chains.[175]

However, the biggest losers from vaccine inequity economically are those countries that can lesser or least afford it. A report of mid-July 2021 by the WHO, Oxford University and the United Nations Development Programme (UNDP) estimated "that if lower-income countries had been able to vaccinate as quickly as high income countries, it could have added $38bn to their GDP forecasts" for 2021 and 2022.[176] According to the Economist Intelligence Unit, the "glacial" progress of the international vaccination rollout would chalk-off $2.3 trillion dollars from the value of global output between 2022 and 2025, with up to $1.7 billion of this being lost to the more dynamic "emerging" Asian economies. Such a scenario was probable unless 60 percent of the populations of the middle-income and low-income countries were inoculated by mid-2022, which at vaccination rates at the time had no prospect of being accomplished.[177] This indeed was not accomplished.

The WHO's pandemic and vaccine imperialism

These politics of vaccine nationalism and imperialism confirmed the irrelevance if not impotence of organizations or agencies of international political governance in the fight against the pandemic. This is clear enough from the WHO's role in the crisis – which was evident before the interstate vaccine rivalries got started. The WHO's formal mandate, according to its website, is to "direct international health within the United Nations and to lead global partners"[178] on public health emergencies. "We direct and coordinate the world's response to health emergencies". As the organization's formal constitution puts it, the WHO's role is to "act as the directing and coordinating authority on international health work".[179]

But, from the start of the pandemic, the WHO was restricted to an advisory role, just as few national governments actually adopted in full the organization's public health "directives".[180] This reflected an apparent paradox: the declining political influence and capacities for action of a supposedly international public health organization in the supposedly "global" age. Part of the problem is that the WHO is simply lacking in resources to support practical ongoing international interventions (including basic pandemic surveillance work).[181]

A further obstacle is that its world leadership role in public health has been challenged by the emergence of other private (or private-public) corporate health bodies. These include the US President's Emergency Plan for AIDS Relief (PEPFAR); the Bill And Melinda Gates Foundation; the World Bank; the Gavi Alliance; and non-governmental organizations (NGOs) such as Médecins Sans Frontières. This has also been compromised by the organization's penetration by commercial interests (including those of the pharmaceutical companies) and by its reliance on patronage by the leading states and corporate sponsorship. This means that the WHO is caught in the middle of interstate rivalries and tensions (most recently that of the US and China) and is under pressure to perform a delicate balancing act in accommodating them. Before then, the leading state actors had demonstrated that they would disregard or bypass the WHO's public health proposals if these were considered incompatible with the commercial interests of their own drug companies or those of other national industries.[182]

Owing to these factors, the WHO was reduced to a frustrated bystander as the pandemic's first wave spread across the world, and it was powerless to intervene to prevent subsequent waves. During the pandemic, the WHO's authority would be further undermined by hostility from the US government. In a blatant move of pandemic nationalism, faced with a COVID-19 crisis for which his government was ill-prepared, Trump accused the organization of being incompetent and anti-American (that is, beholden to China). The WHO, he claimed, had "covered up" the spread of the disease, owing to its dysfunctional bureaucratic inertia and close ties to China.[183] He announced the US's withdrawal from WHO membership and de-funding of the organization.[184] This was later retracted by Joseph Biden's successor Democrat administration in one of the opening shots of the new presidency.

The WHO, despite its apparent enthusiasm for China's lockdowns, spoke the language of globalization throughout the pandemic – that is, of the need for a coordinated international response to deal with the crisis. This was where all countries accepted the WHO's leadership in managing the pandemic. The pandemic policies that the organization recommended to the world were the full rafter of NPIs (physical distancing, self-quarantining, testing and contact-tracing) along with free movement of PPE for the supposed benefit of poorer as well as richer countries. By contrast, the WHO was set against border closures, international travel bans and trade restrictions on the movement of PPE across national turnstiles, precisely because it was penetrated by corporate interests and beholden to neoliberal governments.[185] Yet the major players of the international state system (the US, the UK, and the EU's leading states) often either paid little attention to much of the WHO's guidance or, where they accommodated aspects of it, did so partially, incrementally, and tardily, in accordance with local judgements of risk.

The more common response to the pandemic within the interstate system was various forms and degrees of local protectionism. Germany and France blocked exports of PPE at the start of the European crisis, for example.[186] The US, EU, and indeed virtually all other countries sealed their borders as the pandemic approached their shores, either proactively (as for example New Zealand did) or reactively (as for example the US and the EU countries did). The UK, of course, set as it was on British exceptionalism, resisted border closures for a long while, just as it disregarded almost every one of the WHO's recommended NPIs.[187]

Later on, the WHO would be reduced to futile handwringing in response to the various manifestations of vaccine nationalism. This was the organization's response to the EU's export controls on vaccines that was motivated by the UK government's vaccine nationalism, for example.[188] This was just as the success of the UK's vaccine nationalism compared to the EU's "vaccine socialism" appeared to demonstrate that this was a more viable strategy for developed countries which were well placed to outcompete the lesser developed ones for access to vaccines, especially under circumstances where demand massively exceeded supply.

COVID-19 Vaccines Global Access programme (COVAX)

The WHO's and UN's solution to protecting middle-income and low-income countries from losing out on interstate vaccine rivalries was by offering their support to COVAX. COVAX was patronized by the WHO and by UNICEF and led by the Gavi Alliance and by the Coalition for Epidemic Preparedness Innovations (CEPI). The scheme aimed to "facilitate global COVID-19 vaccine distribution" by operating "as a centralized vaccine buyer's club, either purchasing vaccines directly from pharmaceutical manufacturers or receiving donations" from high-income countries. "Sixty seven low-income countries (LICs) rely on COVAX for their COVID-19 vaccine supplies".[189] The scheme was primarily intended to procure vaccine supplies for use by governments of the world's least wealthy 92 countries, which would struggle to finance their own vaccine supplies. The relatively unambitious goal of COVAX was to provide sufficient vaccines to inoculate 20 percent of the population of these countries – these being key workers and those most vulnerable to being harmed by COVID-19.

How would COVAX actually work? The idea was that governments of the wealthier countries would finance the programme by virtue of being permitted to purchase vaccine supplies through it at reasonable prices (secured by the scheme's collective bargaining power) for their own use. These governments were permitted to buy enough doses to inoculate 20 percent of their own populations, in accordance with the scheme's goals and parameters, though this was quickly raised to 50 percent in order to motivate their involvement. As Yamey *et al.* describe:

> The incentive for these nations to buy doses from Covax, rather than only through bilateral deals with vaccine manufacturers, was as an insurance mechanism. If a high income country's bilateral deals were unsuccessful (that is, the candidates failed in trials), the country would still have access to vaccine doses from the wide portfolio of around a dozen Covax candidates.

As for the 92 lower-income countries that COVAX intended to support, vaccines would be provided for them by means of donation funding (if not actual donations) by the higher-income countries, in part exchange for the benefits they derived from the scheme. The architects of the scheme expected that

> a huge number of high and lower middle income countries would buy doses through the facility, which would have given Covax massive buying power to invest in research and development, fund manufacturing at risk, drive prices down through pooled purchases, and ensure that some of the supply would go to low income and lower middle income countries.[190]

However, COVAX's primary purpose – to pool vaccine procurement on behalf of the poorer countries so as to control costs and distribute equitably – quickly ran into the buffers of national self-interest. Very few governments of the high-income governments supported the scheme, instead acting unilaterally on their self-interest, by pursuing bilateral deals with multiple pharma companies for several vaccines. They also failed to honour their commitments to provide COVAX with donations or donor funding, as I will discuss later. Consequently,

> COVAX repeatedly failed to hit key targets. Projections were scaled back and … [there was] … a 25% reduction in anticipated volumes of vaccine available compared to initial forecasts in early 2021. African countries received only 18.2 million of the 66 million doses they had expected through COVAX in the first half of 2021, and most did not reach even 10% vaccination by the end of 2021.[191]

Futile handwringing was also the WHO's response to these issues, as COVAX was undone by a range of calamitous problems that were largely made by Western governments. In summary: (1) the buying-up and hoarding (as we have seen) of the vast bulk of vaccine supplies by the rich countries, which emptied the programme of doses available from the market; (2) the failure of the drug companies to deliver on their commitments to the scheme (in favour of servicing the needs of the wealthier countries); (3) the policy-decisions of most governments of the high-income countries to vaccinate children and young adults and roll out boosters rather than donate to countries where vulnerable and older populations were unprotected; (4) their delayed signing-ups to subsidize the programme in the first place (e.g. the EU and US procrastinated); (5) their failure to commit sufficient funds to get the scheme up and running; and (6) their failure to donate enough of their surplus or leftover doses to the programme, or even to deliver on these inadequate undertakings to donate surplus or leftover jabs on time.[192]

Yet COVAX was undermined not simply by lack of buy-in from and disregarded promises of those governments it relied on, but also by the agents of pharma commerce. Thus, it was confronted by the barriers of intellectual property rights (IPRs) imposed by the pharmaceutical companies and defended by their respective national governments that prevented local vaccine production, of confidential clauses in contracts (which allowed the drug companies to drive up prices by setting poor countries in competition with each other), and so on.[193] Of the major vaccine providers, only AstraZeneca pledged itself to providing doses to COVAX at prices which would be pegged at production costs rather than at those which would allow profits to be generated.[194] But it is doubtful that AstraZeneca ever did deliver on this commitment that was later formally abandoned.

COVAX intended to devote resources from buy-in by the high-income countries to the scheme to finance independent vaccine production facilities and technologies in lesser developed countries. But this too foundered on the reluctance of the pharma capitalists and their sponsor governments in the West to abandon their exclusive rights to the vaccine patents and technologies. As Pilkington *et al.* observe: "Whilst globally there is majority support for waivers of IP ... key opponents blocking this move include the UK and other European countries which host large domestic pharmaceutical industries".[195] President Joseph Biden's US government eventually sought to demonstrate its global leadership on the issue by declaring its willingness to waive the IPRs of its own vaccine-producing companies, so long as others agreed to do the same.[196] But this was likely done in the knowledge that the others would not agree to do the same.

COVAX had also barely got started when a particular manifestation of vaccine nationalism – that of India's ruling party – intervened to blow it off course. COVAX's main supplier of vaccines was India's Serum Institute. But a huge COVID-19 upsurge in the country in the spring of 2021 that was driving up hospitalizations and deaths incentivized the Indian government to block vaccine exports and devote the Institute's output to catering for exclusively local need. Set alongside these issues, the well-documented logistical problems encountered in delivering COVAX to poor countries without supportive infrastructure and weak public health systems,[197] and the difficulty of planning distribution owing to "ad hoc" deliveries (due to lack of supplies), though real, were secondary.[198] The logistical constraints, for example, could have been considerably ameliorated with additional aid alongside COVAX vaccine deliveries from the G7 and EU to ramp-up local delivery systems.

Vaccine hesitancy in certain communities of low-income countries has also undoubtedly played a role in obstructing COVAX's cause, as it has obstructed take-up elsewhere, though again this is only as a bit-player. I explore this matter in Chapter 4. But for now, it should be noted that this hesitancy is a rather different kettle of fish to the versions found among the citizenries of the Global North since here it is often strongly incentivized by the imperative to avoid economic penalties that would be *fundamentally* injurious to basic subsistence livelihoods. Taking up vaccines in the poorest countries often involves long and arduous travel to vaccination centres (often to find the supplies have not arrived or have run out), during which time income from employment (often based on cash-in-hand payments in the vast informal sector) simply ceases. Thus, the unreliability, unpredictability, and scarcity of vaccine deliveries here is an added incentive for people to avoid incurring these severe penalties.[199] As Maaza Seyoum, Global South convenor of the People's Vaccine Alliance, expresses it:

> The pandemic, and the economic issues that have come with it – some of the data we've seen shows that 100 million more people have been pushed into

poverty by this pandemic – make it difficult when you're asking people in that environment to take out a huge amount of time from their money making to stand in line for a vaccine. We have to imagine what we would feel like if we were trying to access a service that we were told was delayed over and over.[200]

Nonetheless, the sheer scale of the vaccine inequities between the high-income and upper-middle-income countries, on the one hand, and the rest of the world, on the other hand, are such that the overwhelming bulk of it cannot possibly be explained by hesitancy – however, impelled by adverse economic circumstances this may be for many. The key obstacle to vaccinating people in the "developing world" (especially the poor of the poor countries) is at the supply-side of things (lack of access to doses), not at the demand-side of things (people's reluctance to get jabbed). This is even though Africans, in particular, would have good reason to be suspicious of the machinations of White Western "vaccine paternalism", and indeed of the science behind it, owing to the colonial record and its legacy, and to the present-day rapacious profiteering of the corporate owners of the science. It has been mooted that "a history of colonial medical and vaccine research abuse in Africa diminishes trust in current vaccines".[201] Even so, this cannot account for why three-quarters of Africans are unvaccinated, or why rates of vaccination in the AU are especially low in the poorest countries and in the poorest communities.

Other critiques of COVAX accused it of Western-centric high-handedness, of not consulting with or involving experts or government officials from low-income countries, of poor planning, and of lack of knowledge or understanding of conditions on the ground in recipient countries that would obstruct vaccine distribution. These may also be considered germane in accounting for its problems.[202] But, again, these were not the primary cause of COVAX's failure, and these were not insuperable barriers to the scheme's success. Moreover, some of these problems were exacerbated by the pressures placed on the scheme from without. Thus, it was simply *not* the case, as was alleged by Fifa Rahman, a WHO representative, that COVAX's vaccination deliveries were "almost negligently late, because you've got a bunch of New Yorkers in a room making decisions about Africa".[203] New Yorkers may indeed have been making these decisions, but even if they were not, whoever was making them would still have to reckon with the radically adverse impacts on supplies generated by the vaccine imperialism of the leading state power actors and the commercial self-interest of Western pharma capitalism.

By the start of October 2021, only five percent of the world's vaccine supply was provided by COVAX, and the programme had delivered only 300 million doses to developing and underdeveloped countries. Thus, at the time of completing the first draft of this chapter (October 2021), COVAX's unambitious target of delivering two billion vaccines by the end of 2021 (inoculating 20 percent of the population of low-income countries) was set to be missed by a distance. Finding alternative suppliers to the Serum Institute also drove up prices from between 50–100 percent, further stressing the coffers of middle-income and low-income countries, as the vaccine capitalists exploited the opportunity of fierce competition among desperate governments for plunder.

Many governments of these countries, faced with non-delivery of promised supplies or clear information on when these would arrive, were forced to resort to making their own contractual arrangements with the drug companies. By doing so, they were in effect paying twice for the same vaccines, at higher prices, and from the back of the queue. Some governments of wealthy countries even siphoned off for local use large volumes of vaccines allocated under COVAX.[204] For example: "Despite extreme vaccine shortages in developing countries", the UK and Canada "took an estimated 1.5 million doses from COVAX this [2021] year".[205] This was, of course, permitted under the scheme. But, even so, this was, under the circumstances, ethically wrong.

These practices were greeted by moral exhortations and appeals by the WHO and by global justice groups to do better for the poor countries, but to no avail. Frustrated by the failure of COVAX to deliver on its contractual obligations, and of the G7 to honour its pledges of delivering surplus doses to the programme, the countries of the AU established their own collective procurements agency (the African Union Vaccine Acquisition Trust) in order to bulk-purchase vaccines directly from the pharmaceutical companies. However, the AUVAT's "vaccine socialism" has been much less successful than the EU's. By mid-October 2021, this had "been able to purchase 100 million doses from Pfizer-BioNTech and Johnson and Johnson", on behalf of more than 1.2 billion Africans, This was as, on the same timescale, the EC, on behalf of 447 million Europeans (including 355 million or so adults), had purchased "nearly 1.5 billion doses from AstraZeneca, Pfizer-BioNTech, Moderna, and Johnson and Johnson, or approximately 15 times the number of doses compared to the AU".[206]

Governments of the high-income countries pledged at the G7 summit in June 2021 to donate 785 million doses to COVAX.

> The centrepiece was a promise from US President Joe Biden to donate 500 million doses of the vaccine made by pharmaceutical company Pfizer of New York City and biotechnology company BioNTech in Mainz, Germany. This is in addition to 87.5 million previously pledged. The United Kingdom pledged 100 million, and France, Germany and Japan ... pledged around 30 million each.[207]

But, on the cusp of October 2021, only 18 percent of the promised vaccine aid had been delivered. The June summit was lobbied by an impressive array of former presidents and prime ministers who were demanding that the G7 leaders agree to a vaccine assistance package of $44 billion for the poor countries. This sum would have made up almost two-thirds of the $66 billion cost of vaccinating their populations. However, the G7 agreed to stump up only $7 billion.[208] Almost as if to add insult to injury, British PM Boris Johnson, who was hosting the summit in Devon (England), used the occasion to announce that his government would cut £5 billion from the UK's £15 billion overseas aid budget.[209]

Later, on 21 October 2021, the People's Vaccine Alliance report showed that of the 1.8 billion doses pledged to COVAX by the G7 and Team Europe (the EU plus Norway and Iceland), only 261 million had been delivered – or just 14 percent of the total. Japan had delivered on 31 percent of the assistance it had promised at the July summit; the US had delivered on 16 percent of its commitments; and the UK and Europe had delivered on just 10 percent. Moreover, the pharma corporations had delivered on just 12 percent of the doses they had agreed to offer to COVAX – or 120 million out of 994. Moderna and Johnson and Johnson had delivered on none of their pledges. AstraZeneca had delivered on 14 percent of theirs. Pfizer-BioNTech, on the same timescale, had done best. By late October, they had delivered on 39 percent of their pledges.[210]

This was despite a massive upscaling and diversification of manufacturing vaccine capacity by the drug companies that had basically done away with the supply shortages that had dogged the early rollouts. By September 2021, 1.5 billion doses were being produced each month, with this projected to surpass two billion per month by the year's end.[211] Yet grotesque vaccine apartheid persisted and showed no sign of easing even though, according to a report by the research group Airfinity, there would be sufficient manufacturing output to vaccinate 70 percent of the population of all middle-income and low-income countries by the spring of 2022.[212] Indeed, by June 2022, as was predicted by Airfinity, "the number of doses will reach 27 billion, enough to fully immunise the world's population twice over".[213]

Not only that, the stockpiling of vaccines in the developed countries (which simply could not be used because these were superfluous to national needs) raised the scandal of imminent wastage of doses on a gargantuan scale.[214] Airfinity calculated that there were 500 million surplus doses hoarded by the G7 by September 2021's end, with this number projected to exceed 1.2 billion by the end of the year.[215] As former UK Prime Minister Gordon Brown put it:

> Until recently, western leaders could defend holding supplies in reserve because they feared interruptions to the manufacturing supply chain. Now there is sufficient capacity to guarantee a rising flow of vaccines for the months ahead. So many doses are being produced that the bigger risk is now that millions may go to waste.[216]

In fact, the risk was an imminent and actual reality. In the US alone, 15 million doses had already passed their expiry date and been binned between March and September 2021.[217] The People's Vaccine Alliance estimated that over a billion doses would go unused in the G7 by the end of the year. Of these:

> At least 100 million vaccine doses could … expire in G7 countries in 2021, and the number of wasted doses could reach up to 241 million. Furthermore, based on their current donation pledges, the number of wasted doses could rise to 800 million by mid-2022 due to expiration.[218]

This, for Airfinity, raised the spectre of between 1 and 2.8 million lives worldwide being lost to the pandemic in 2022 unless the rich hoarder-nations broke open their vaccine treasure chests and began redistributing in earnest.[219]

But, as we have seen, the global disparities in vaccine supplies and procurements to the advantage of the Global North and to the detriment of the poorer countries of the South have persisted throughout 2022 and up until the present. So too has the problem of hoarding or stockpiling of the drugs in these countries beyond the wildest projections of national need so that astronomical waste is inevitable as other peoples in other places are denied. In the US, for example, it has been estimated that around 82 million doses of the vaccines had to be discarded because they had passed their use-by date in the period from December 2020 through to May 2022.[220] The US, of course, is not a sole offender. "The COVID GAP project estimated in November 2021 that, by the end of 2021, the Group of 7 (G7) and EU countries had 834 million excess doses, even after accounting for boosters, child vaccinations, and contingencies".[221] These surplus doses did not get reallocated to countries or populations in need. Moreover, hundreds of millions of other doses that did end up getting donated towards the end of the year were unusable because these were on the cusp of their expiry dates.[222]

The consequences of this in terms of lost or damaged lives are clear enough. The WHO has calculated that up to 70 percent of the world's population has to be vaccinated if the protections from COVID-19 afforded by herd immunity are to be globalized. That is, if "global immunity" from the virus is to be accomplished.[223] Presently, this is a pipedream. Yet this is actually necessary to end the pandemic, which is otherwise perpetuated, perhaps for years. As Kavengo Matundu, of the Global Call to Action Against Poverty (GCAP) advocacy group, rightly says: "Unless we achieve equitable action in addressing this pandemic, it will always remain with us in the world".[224] As for the foreseeable future,

> mathematical modeling suggests that when HICs [high-income countries] preferentially obtain the majority of the available vaccine doses at the expense of lower income countries (LICs), this could result in 900 additional deaths per million of the world population, equating to millions of excess deaths globally. Médecins Sans Frontiers (MSF) have estimated that, if available vaccine doses were steadily redistributed, nearly one million deaths would be averted by mid-2022 compared to the current scenarios.[225]

This is why, coinciding with the global inequities of vaccine coverage, the number of people killed worldwide by the pandemic remains at high scales, albeit this is occurring at a lesser rate than during the first two years of the crisis. According to the Worldometer dashboard, almost 1.3 million lives were lost to the virus in 2022, during a time in which, according to politicians in the West, the pandemic was defeated by the vaccines. In 2021, the number of people killed by the pandemic worldwide numbered more than 3.5 million, up from almost 2 million in 2020.[226]

This was during a period when the high-income countries were steadily building their vaccine walls and mortalities and hospitalizations were tumbling there in response. Pandemic years two and three thus constitute a different stage in the evolution of the crisis, inasmuch as since then the burden of COVID-19 mortalities has increasingly shifted away from the high-income countries and onto the lower-income countries whose populations are at best only partially vaccine-protected. These public health harms endured mostly by the non-Western Other have been accompanied by escalating losses from vaccine wastage especially in the over-procuring countries.

Yet these pandemic harms may return to plague the high-income countries as well. As Seyoum rightly points out:

> Rich countries keep thinking that if they just protect themselves, they're going to get out of the pandemic, but that is, on a public health front, completely ridiculous. It sounds trite, but as the head of WHO said last year: none of us is safe until we're all safe.[227]

Despite the fact that governments of the West and of the North have been declaring the pandemic as over for them, owing to the vaccine walls they have built around their own populations, these are fragile and uncertain gains. This is because these are in danger of being undermined by the lack of "global immunity", which is due to the vaccine inequities worldwide and the dismantling of all other public health controls (that is, NPIs) by these governments other than the drugs fix.

> Inequities in COVID-19 vaccine access do not just impact those who are unable to get immunized, they affect all of us. Millions of new cases are reported every day worldwide, bringing with them the possible emergence of more infectious variants, as seen with Omicron.[228]

COVID-19 has shown itself to be highly flexible and adaptable. The point is that this property of the virus is radicalized or accelerated under conditions in which NPIs that would contain transmission are set aside and where unvaccinated populations can act as incubators of new strains that will better evade vaccines and which may have greater virulence.

COVID-19 Technology Access Pool (C-TAP)

Aside from its support for COVAX, the WHO's big idea for getting the world vaccinated was the COVID-19 Technology Access Pool (C-TAP) initiative. This was its proposal of "a patent pool offering patient-free licences of anti-COVID drugs to whoever wants to manufacture them". But this initiative was supported by only 40 UN member states and hardly any of the bigger players. This too was basically undermined by an alliance of vaccine nationalism and zombie commerce. "Most high-income states prefer to have their own national strategies and bet on specific substances through advance purchase agreements". International cooperation among the leading state actors on the distribution of vaccines (through the COVAX scheme) was for them only a "supplementary" matter.[229] The WHO and advocacy groups agitated for the temporary waiving of IPRs over the manufacture of the vaccines and for technology transfers so that these could be produced independently in middle-income and low-income countries to address local needs. But this move was rejected by the four biggest drug companies (AstraZeneca, Pfizer-BioNTech, Moderna, and Johnson and Johnson):

> All four corporations have refused to share their know-how and intellectual property with the WHO's COVID-19 Technology Access Pool (C-TAP), set up expressly for increasing access to vaccines and other lifesaving tools. Furthermore, bilateral partnerships, especially those signed by Johnson and Johnson and AstraZeneca, have been accompanied by restrictions and obligations that limit the total number of suppliers and dictate where each manufacturer can sell its product.[230]

The vaccine capitalists claimed that waiving IPRs and the abandonment of their monopolies on manufacturing technologies and restrictions on where the vaccines would be produced or distributed and by whom were matters of commercial necessity rather than of choice to optimize profits. This was especially the case when it came to resisting knowledge transfer and preserving ownership rights. Jealously guarded monopolies here were supposedly integral to the commercial "risk-taking" and industry-specific investment of resources needed to develop the vaccines. Without these privileges of private ownership and capitalistic self-interest, it was argued, there would be no COVID-19 vaccines, and there would be little incentive to produce others in the future.

Yet the private property in question (the vaccine commodity) and the "risky" commercial enterprise that generated it were supported by massive public subsidies courtesy of governments of the developed countries, access to a range of other public resources and facilities, and advance goods procurements by those same governments that guaranteed sales even if the product was useless.[231] Where, then, was the risk? Where, for that matter, was the unilateral role of private enterprise and of the corporate-capitalist mode in generating the vaccines that would even justify their appropriation as wholly private property? As Pilkington *et al.* make clear, there was none:

> In the United States alone, the Biomedical Advanced Research and Development Authority (BARDA) has awarded more than $10 billion of public funds to the development of COVID-19 vaccines … In the UK, public and charitable funders accelerated the development of the AstraZeneca vaccine and the European Union has spent an estimated €93 billion on public sector investment in COVID-19 vaccines and therapeutics R&D. Public investment was instrumental in accelerating COVID-19 vaccine discovery, with technologies often being based on decades of academic research. Public investment also supported vaccine development through clinical development stages, with the use of government facilities, research grants, and by accelerating regulatory approval. Public investment was then used to underwrite the risk of production costs, with advance purchase schemes.[232]

This alignment for mutual advantage of neoliberal-supported zombie capitalism and vaccine imperialism was confirmed as governments of the leading nation-states – including Trump's in the US and Johnson's in the UK – blocked proposals that would compel the drug companies to suspend their vaccine IPRs.[233] If the IPRs had been temporarily waived, the door would have been opened for large volumes of vaccines to be produced locally in the poorer countries, at lower costs, and for local use where the need was greatest.

Hardt and Negri revisited

The politics of pandemic nationalism and vaccine imperialism – and the manner of their interface with the economics of corporate "zombie" capitalism – simply do not square with Hardt and Negri's theory of Empire. Empire affirms the decentring of interstate rivalries under the uniform rule of "bourgeois right". Since this is so, Empire ought to predict a systemic or "network" political response to the pandemic under the auspices of the "monarchical" supranational authorities of global capital. This response certainly has not been evident in the response of national governments to the pandemic. There was no uniform strategy or policy. Some governments (such as those of the UK, the US, Brazil, and Sweden) were, for example, much less proactive in the cause of public health protection than others (such as New Zealand's and many of those of the Southeast Asian countries).

As for the international vaccine rollout, there was no supranational body (certainly not the WHO, nor the UN or OECD) which assumed or rather was handed the authority and funds to deliver the necessary results. With the main exception of the EU's collective vaccine-procurement programme, representatives of nation-states made their own negotiations and signed their own deals with the pharmaceutical companies. Hardt and Negri affirm that Empire is the decentred imperial design of postmodern network capitalism. But what kind of global imperial system totally absorbed or "penetrated" by commerce would tolerate the chronic disruption and curtailment of markets worldwide by vaccine-unprotected majorities in a vast swathe of countries beyond its developed centre? For that matter, what Empire of capital would ever have overseen the politics of lockdown in virtually every country in response to the pandemic? The relative autonomy of the imperial interstate system from the capitalist world economy (as well as the structural interdependence of the two) is upheld.

The relative efficacy and competence of the leading nation-state actors in administering NPIs and mass vaccination rollouts within borders contrasts sharply with the radical inefficacy of their collaborative bilateral proposals for bringing under control the present pandemic and safeguarding against future pandemics. Again, the gap between national-level and supranational-level policy action could hardly be more pronounced. Yet only the latter stands any chance of averting future global pandemics or foreclosing on the current one in the foreseeable future. This is clear enough as we consider the response of the G7 to the pandemic. The outcome of the G7 summit in Carbis (Cornwall, England, UK), in June of 2021, was the unveiling of the "historic" (as it was hailed) Carbis Bay Declaration.[234] This was an abbreviated health-policy-focused distillation of the larger and rangier Carbis

Communique.[235] This was, as I have noted already, presented as the G7's global anti-pandemic strategy.

The future of pandemic management – the Carbis Declaration

The Communique, according to the Confederation of British Industry (CBI), "reignited a belief that the international community can come together in a spirit of collaboration to tackle the big issues of our age".[236] If so, this belief was unfounded. Although the Communique expended plenty of rhetoric, much of this was tangential to the pandemic. This included the undertaking to promote "freer, fairer trade" (as if the two were identical),[237] a "more resilient global economy, and a fairer global tax system".[238] This also included a promise to harness the "power of democracy" and the "rule of law", to "strengthen partnerships" (including with Africa), and to support the "green revolution".[239] Naturally, the G7 were all for abolishing the scourge of injustice and inequality everywhere, "so that no place or person, irrespective of age, ethnicity or gender is left behind". Acting on such lofty aspirations, as the Communique candidly noted, "has not been the case with past global crises", but this time people should be reassured that it would be different.[240]

All of this reads as a neoliberal wish list rather than a statement of real goals to be delivered by actual plans. How exactly these spectacular results would be accomplished was not explained – unless one was supposed to assume that these would grow spontaneously from the worldwide promulgation of liberal values and open markets (which mysteriously have not yet delivered on them after several decades of "globalization"). The possibility of more economic assistance for Africa was mooted by means of the IMF, which would mean presumably more loans tied to Structural Adjustment Programmes (SAPs) for already debt-ridden countries. The pledge to "green" the world economy was simply a reiteration of longstanding, unambitious, and insufficient sustainability targets that were unlikely to be delivered. "We commit to net zero no later than 2050, halving our collective emissions over the two decades to 2030, increasing and improving climate finance to 2025; and to conserve or protect at least 30 percent of our land and oceans by 2030".[241]

As for the pandemic: "Our immediate focus", the Communique stated, "is beating COVID-19 and we set a collective goal of ending the pandemic in 2022".

> The COVID-19 pandemic is not under control anywhere until it is under control everywhere. In an interconnected world global health and health security threats respect no borders. We therefore commit both to strengthen global action now to fight COVID-19, and to take further tangible steps to improve our collective defences against future threats and to bolster global health and health security.[242]

Needless to say, the pandemic did not end in 2022 (which saw 1.3 million COVID deaths worldwide), nor yet in 2023 (which in its first four months has seen 143,132 people killed by it).[243] However, this has not deterred governments of the North from decreeing it as such. Indeed, the UK government was the world leader in declaring the pandemic over, on exactly 19 July 2021.[244] Since that date, on the official undercount (data derived from death certification paints a far worse picture), 66,644 Britons have been killed by the virus, up to and inclusive of 23 April 2023.[245]

But how would these commitments to defeat the pandemic be delivered? The "global action to fight COVID-19" would, the Communique affirmed, be "an intensified international effort, starting immediately, to vaccinate the world by getting as many safe vaccines to as many people as possible as fast as possible". Including the February G7 summit commitments, "a total of over two billion vaccine doses" were pledged, including "one billion over the next year" (that is, for 2022).[246] Alas, beyond the dazzle of political rhetoric, the February commitments had not yet been operationalized by the time the June summit came along, and those added by the Carbis Communique (and Declaration), as I have noted before, showed no sign of being honoured deep into the autumn of 2021. Action by the "international community" was verbal rather than actual. And so it has remained ever since.

As for future international pandemic defence strategy, this rested on pledges that were few and for the most part empty of specificity or detail. This was merely the language of goals and aspirations without underlying policies to support them:

> This includes strengthening the World Health Organization (WHO) and supporting it in its leading and coordinating role in the global health system ...
> At the same time we will create the appropriate frameworks to strengthen our collective defences against threats to global health by: increasing and coordinating on global manufacturing capacity on all continents; improving early warning systems; and support science in a mission to shorten the cycle for the development of safe and effective vaccines, treatments and tests from 300 to 100 days.[247]

This was all rather vague inasmuch as it was disconnected from the articulation of plans that would show how these outcomes would be delivered and on which timescales. How would the WHO be strengthened, for example?

Aspects of the Communique also smacked of a naïve idealism that the politicians who penned it could scarcely have believed in. This was a legitimatory ideology of a "globalization" that did not exist, represented as "policy" before an uncritical media. Increasing and coordinating global manufacturing capacity on all continents? How could this be done without challenging the pharma capitalists' monopoly on advanced technologies and IPRs or their control over who produces vaccines and where? The summit that produced the Carbis Communique (and Declaration) failed to overturn these obstacles. As Patrick Watt, director of public affairs and campaigns at Christian Aid, rightly observed, the summit also failed to overturn other obstacles: debt relief for the poor countries; substantial financial aid to support vaccination; and so on.[248] As we have seen, the pledges of the G7 leaders to donate surplus jabs to COVAX would also be largely unmet. Again, the rhetoric of internationalism was at odds with the practices of national and corporate-capitalist self-interest.

As I have noted elsewhere, the solutions mooted for future pandemics were reductionist and technocentric rather than social and cultural, confined as they were within the narrowly pragmatist and instrumental frameworks allowed by power-holders.[249] This was also the opportunity for nationalist posturing. Thus, the UK government's declaration of intent at the summit to place itself at the centre of the bioscientific and technological system of pandemic surveillance management and disease control by establishing the Animal Vaccine Manufacturing and Innovation Centre at the Pirbright Institute in Surrey certainly fits that mould. This would operate supposedly on behalf of the world to find cures for zoonotic diseases (that is, those which could cross species barriers to infect humans), fast-tracking vaccines for newly-emerging viruses – and all of that on a start-up budget of just £24 million (with £10 million of that pledged by the UK government).[250]

26 October 2021 (updated March 2022 and April 2023)

Notes

1 See especially: Harman, C. (1991). 'The state and capitalism today'. *International Socialism*, 2 (51), pp. 3–54.
2 See especially: Stopford, J. and Strang, S. (1995). *Rival States, Rival Firms: Competition for World Market Shares*. Cambridge: Cambridge University Press.
3 Archer, M. (1995). *Realist Social Theory: The Morphogenetic Approach*. Cambridge: Cambridge University Press; Bhaskar, R. (1998). *The Possibility of Naturalism: A Philosophical Critique of the Contemporary Human Sciences*. [1979]. 3rd edition. London: Routledge; Creaven, S. (2000). *Marxism and Realism: A Materialistic Application of Realism in the Social Sciences*. London and New York: Routledge.
4 Archer (1995); Creaven (2000); Creaven, S. (2007). *Emergentist Marxism: Dialectical Philosophy and Social Theory*. London and New York: Routledge.
5 For reasons elaborated in my *Contagion Capitalism* (Routledge, forthcoming)
6 Callinicos, A. (2009). *Imperialism and Global Political Economy*. Cambridge: Polity Press.
7 Callinicos (2009).
8 Hardt, M. and Negri, A. (2000). *Empire*. Cambridge MA: Harvard University Press.
9 Hardt and Negri (2001), p. xiv. (Emphasis removed).
10 Hardt and Negri (2000), pp. 8–9.
11 Morgan, J. '*Empire* inhuman? The social ontology of global theory'. *Journal of Critical Realism*, 2 (1), pp. 95–127. See p. 100.
12 Hardt and Negri (2000), p. 51.
13 Hardt and Negri (2000), pp. 139–40.
14 As August Nimtz puts it. See Nimtz, A. (2002). 'Class struggle under *Empire*: In defence of Marx and Engels'. *International Socialism* (online), 2 (96) (Autumn).
15 Nimtz (2002).
16 Hardt and Negri (2000), p. 3.
17 Hardt and Negri (2000), p. 9.
18 Hardt and Negri (2000), pp. 5–9, 65–68.
19 Hardt and Negri (2000), pp. 9–10.
20 Morgan (2003), p. 99.
21 Hardt and Negri (2000), pp. xii–xiii.
22 Hardt and Negri (2000), p. 5.
23 Hardt and Negri (2000), p. 310.

24 Hardt and Negri (2000), pp. 310, 347.
25 Hardt and Negri (2000), p. 15.
26 Morgan (2003), p. 104. See Hardt and Negri (2000), pp. xiii, 295.
27 Castells, M. (1996). *The Rise of the Network Society: The Information Age – Economy, Society and Culture* (Volume 1). Oxford: Blackwell-Wiley.
28 Callinicos (2001). *Against the Third Way*. Cambridge: Polity Press, p. 53
29 Morgan (2003), p. 125.
30 See O'Connell, M. (2002). *The Myth of Preemptive Self-Defense*. The American Society of International Law Task Force on Terrorism (online). (August).
31 O'Connell (2002).
32 Callinicos, A. (2002). 'The grand strategy of the American empire'. *International Socialism* (online), 2 (97). (Winter); Callinicos, A. (2003). *The New Mandarins of American Power*. Cambridge: Polity Press.
33 McGrath, M. (2020). 'Climate change: US formally withdraws from Paris agreement. *BBC News* (online). (4 November); Borger, J. (2001). 'Bush kills global warming treaty'. *Guardian*. (29 March).
34 Bromley, S. (1991). *American Hegemony and World Oil: The Industry, the State System, and the World Economy*. Cambridge: Polity Press; Callinicos (2003), Chs 3, 4, and 5; Feffer, J, (Ed.) *Power Trip: US Unilateralism and Global Strategy After September 11*. London: Seven Stories Press, pp. 117–72; Chomsky, N. (2006). *Imperial Ambitions*. Harmondsworth: Penguin; Klein, N. (2005). 'Baghdad Year Zero'. N. Klein, Mealer, B.; Watkins, S. and W. Laquer (Eds.) *No War: America's Real Business in Iraq*. London: Gilbert Square Books; Telhami, S. (2002). *The Persian Gulf: Understanding the American Oil Strategy*. Brookings Institute (online). (1 March).
35 Strange, S. (2009). 'The persistent myth of lost hegemony'. *International Organization*, 41 (4), pp. 551–74.
36 Callinicos (2001), p. 52.
37 See for example: Keohane, R. (1984). *After Hegemony: Cooperation and Discord in World Political Economy*. Princeton: Princeton University Press.
38 *BBC News* (2019). 'Kashmir: Why India and Pakistan fight over it'. (8 August).
39 Avis, D. (2021). 'Understanding the Shadow War Between Israel and Iran'. *Bloomberg* (online). (4 August).
40 Dowd, M. (1991). 'War in the Gulf: The President; Bush Urges Israeli Restraint In Phone Appeals to Shamir'. *New York Times*. (1 February); Friedman, T.L. (1991). 'War in the Gulf: Washington; U.S. Says Israel Is Signaling A Limit to Restraint on Iraq'. *New York Times*. (1 February); Robbins, C.A. and Leggett, K. (2003). 'How the U.S. Plans to Keep Israel on Iraq War Sidelines'. *Wall Street Journal*. (23 March).
41 Hardt and Negri (2001), p. 286.
42 Castells, M. (1996). *The Rise of the Network Society*. Oxford: Blackwell, pp. 135, 137, 140.
43 Anderson, P. (2000). 'Renewals'. *New Left Review*, II (1), pp. 11–14; Callinicos (2001, p. 7; Castells (1996), pp. 135, 137, 140; Harvey, D. (2005). *A Brief History of Neoliberalism*. Oxford: Oxford University Press.
44 Haman (1991, 1996).
45 This was especially for those in the leisure, retail, travel, and hospitality sectors, of course, who could not survive lockdowns without government aid. But this was also true of the employers of office workers. From the perspective of most capitalist employers, on-site working would be preferable to homeworking, because this would allow tighter surveillance-monitoring and technological control of the labour process to build productivity gains. This would especially be the case for the employers of lower-grade routine manual service-sector workers since these workers are less psychologically invested in their work roles than those who command higher status and monetary rewards from their labours.

46 See for example: Iyengar, R. (2021). 'Uber expects employees to spend at least three days a week at the office'. *CNN Business* (online). (14 April).

47 McKeever, V. (2020). 'Goldman Sachs CEO Solomon calls working from home an "aberration"'. *CNBC News* (online). (25 February).

48 *BBC News* (2020). 'Coronavirus: Campaign to encourage workers back to offices'. (28 August).

49 Hanrieder, W.F. (1978). 'Dissolving International Politics: Reflections on the Nation State'. *American Political Science Review*, 72 (4), pp. 1276–87.

50 Gourevitch, P. (1986). *Politics in Hard Times: Comparative Responses to International Economic Crisis*. Ithaca and London: Cornell University Press, p. 88.

51 Mercer, K. (1990). 'Welcome to the Jungle: Identity and Diversity in Post-Modern Politics'. J. Rutherford (Ed.) *Identity: Community, Culture, Difference*. London: Lawrence and Wishart, p. 90.

52 Bell, D. (1987). 'The World and the United States in 2013'. *Daedlus*, 116 (3), pp. 1–32. See p. 14.

53 Editorial Board (2021) 'Vaccine protectionism by the EU will backfire'. *Financial Times*. (26 January).

54 *BBC News* (2021). 'Covid: What's the problem with the EU vaccine rollout?' *BBC News*. (4 March).

55 De Maio, G. (2021). *EU learns from mistakes on vaccines*. Brookings Institute (online). (20 May).

56 As the UK's ruling Conservative Party boasted on its Twitter account on 28 January: "We are No.1 in Europe and third in the world for vaccination doses … We've administered more vaccine doses than Italy, France, Germany and Spain COMBINED!" See Colson, T. (2021). 'Ugly vaccine fights are emerging as rich countries battle for doses while poorer countries miss out completely'. *Business Insider* (online). (28 January).

57 *BBC News* (4 March, 2021).

58 *BBC News* (2021). 'EU demands UK Covid vaccines from AstraZeneca to make up shortfall'. (27 January).

59 Morris, C. (2021). 'UK vaccine approval: Did Brexit speed up the process?'. *BBC News*. (2 December).

60 For a classic example of this see Lynn, M. (2021). 'Vaccine wars: the global battle for a precious resource'. *Spectator*. (30 January). Having correctly noted "how quickly our globalised world collapses when push comes to shove", as "the major powers of the world are … descending into a fierce, increasingly nationalistic competition", the real object of Lynn's polemic quickly became apparent – the EU as a "failed state". Thus, whereas "Britain … wrote into its contract with Oxford-AstraZeneca a stipulation that vaccines made in Britain would be offered to Britain first", and signed-up this contract in May, the "EU dithered for an extra three months and didn't agree terms until the end of August. It failed to extract similar promises on delivery. It will now wish that it had". As Lynn's heroically selective interpretation of vaccine conflict continues:

> The EU hijacked the vaccination programme, wildly overpromised and then failed to deliver. It ordered too few vaccines, made some bets that went wrong (including the failed Sanofi vaccine) and didn't put down enough money upfront to allow companies to prepare for mass production. Like any cornered bureaucracy, and in a manner eerily reminiscent of a failed state, Brussels has lashed out, blaming everyone else. At the start of the week, the Italian Prime Minister, Giuseppe Conte, and the EU Council President, Charles Michel, threatened the drugs companies with legal action to ensure supplies. The saga took a darker twist when, on Tuesday, the EU said it would need to be notified before the export of any vaccines from the EU. Its commitment to internationalism seemed to have gone completely out of the window. There appears to be an underlying belief that somehow the perfidious Brits were siphoning off Pfizer and Oxford supplies that instead should have been reserved for Europe.

61 Boseley, S. (2020). 'How vaccine approval compares between the UK, Europe and the US'. *Guardian*. (4 December).

62 McCaffrey, D. (2021). 'Why does the EU take longer than the UK to approve a COVID-19 vaccine?' *Euronews* (online). (27 December).

63 Morris (2021).

64 Morris (2021).

65 European Commission (2020). *Annex to the Commission Decision on approving the agreement with Member States on procuring Covid-19 vaccines on behalf of the Member States and related procedures* (online), p. 2.

66 Newkey-Burden, C. (2021). 'Germany "violates" EU joint vaccine scheme by buying 30 million extra doses. *Week*. (11 January).

67 Deutsch, J. and Wheaton, S. (2021). 'How Europe fell behind on vaccines'. *Politico* (online). (27 January).

68 De Maio (2021).

69 Deutsch and Wheaton (2021). The strategy was not entirely successful. See Gosling, T. (2021). 'Russia and China Are Exploiting Europe's Vaccine Shortfalls'. *Foreign Policy* (online). (31 March).

70 Vela, J.H. (2021). 'Europe faces identity crisis over vaccine trade war'. *Politico* (online). (26 January).

71 Deutsch and Wheaton (2021).

72 AstraZeneca announced that they would be able to deliver only 40 percent of the vaccines that they were contracted to deliver to the EU in the first quarter of 2021 owing to "supply chain difficulties". This was 60 million jabs fewer than was promised. But, on some estimates, only 25 percent of the EU's order would be delivered in the first quarter of 2021. This was just as the company guaranteed its UK deliveries in full and on time. Almost simultaneously, Pfizer-BioNTech announced that they would suspend deliveries to the EU for several weeks to allow work to take place on re-calibrating a Belgian production plant. Some EU countries (e.g. Germany, France, Italy, and Spain) also reported that Moderna had not delivered on the expected volumes of vaccine doses at the start of the rollout. See *BBC News* (2021). 'Coronavirus vaccine delays halt Pfizer jabs in parts of Europe'. (22 January); *BBC News* (2021). 'Covid: What's the problem with the EU vaccine roll-out?' (4 March).

73 Deutsch and Wheaton (2021).

74 Leigh, M. (2021). 'Vaccine diplomacy: soft power lessons from China and Russia?' *Bruegel* (online). (27 April); Economist Intelligence Unit (2021). 'Vaccine diplomacy boosts Russia's and China's global standing'. *Economist*. (22 April); Juncos, A.E. (2021). *Vaccine Geopolitics and the EU's Ailing Credibility in the Western Balkans*. Carnegie Europe (online). (8 July).

75 Apuzzo, M., Gebrekidan, S., and Pronczuk, M. (2021). 'Where Europe Went Wrong in Its Vaccine Rollout, and Why'. *New York Times*. (5 May).

76 As Deutsch and Wheaton (2021) point out:

Israel, the world leader in vaccinations, has made no secret of the fact that its whatever-it-takes approach to vaccine procurement involved shelling out more. Likewise, the U.K. almost certainly had to pay more per dose than the EU. Published figures suggest that the EU is paying less than $2 for a Oxford/Astrazeneca vaccine, while the U.S. is paying around $4. The U.S. negotiated a $20 price tag with Pfizer. The EU's price is less than $15.

77 Choonora, J. (2021). 'Pandemic politics: year two'. *International Socialism* (online), 170 (Spring).

78 Peel, M., Fleming, S., Mancini, D.P., and Parker, G. (2021). 'EU demands UK Covid vaccines from AstraZeneca to make up shortfall'. *Financial Times*. (27 January).

79 Davies, G. (2021). *Has the UK really outperformed the EU on Covid-19 vaccinations?* London School of Economics (online). (25 March).

80 Davies (2021).

81 Davies (2021).

82 Deutsch, J. (2021). 'Breton: No AstraZeneca jabs exported from the Netherlands after EU export controls'. *Politico* (online). (3 March).

83 *BBC News* (2021). 'Covid vaccine: UK supply hit by India delivery delay'. (18 March).

84 Davies (2021).

85 Davies (2021).

86 European Commission (2021). *Commission extends transparency and authorisation mechanism for exports of COVID-19 vaccines*. Press release. (11 March). European Commission (online).

87 Davies (2021).

88 AstraZeneca, in announcing the EU delays, stated that it was running "two months behind" on its production schedule. See *BBC News* (2021). 'Coronavirus: EU and AstraZeneca seek to resolve vaccine supply crisis'. (28 January).

89 *BBC News* (2021). 'Coronavirus: EU and AstraZeneca seek to resolve vaccine supply crisis'. (28 January); Casert, F. (2021). 'EU pressures AstraZeneca to deliver vaccines as promised'. *AP News* (online). (25 January); Cunningham, E. and Morris, L. (2021). 'EU threatens drug companies with legal action if it doesn't get its vaccines'. *Washington Post*. (26 January); Gye, H. (2021). 'AstraZeneca vaccine: France and Germany threaten to sue if firm doesn't boost number of jabs for EU'. *I-News* (online). (31 January).

90 Amaro, S. (2021). 'EU prepares legal action against AstraZeneca over vaccine delivery shortages'. *CNBC News* (online). (2 April); Deutsch, J. and Barrigazi, J. (2021). 'EU preparing legal case against AstraZeneca over vaccine shortfalls'. *Politico* (online). (21 April); Guarascio, F. and Vagnoni, G. (2021). 'EU sues AstraZeneca over breach of COVID-19 vaccine supply contract'. *Reuters* (online). (26 April); *ITV News* (2021). 'Covid: EU sues AstraZeneca in Brussels court for millions over "promised" vaccine deliveries'. (26 May); *Sky News* (2021). 'COVID-19: Ireland joins possible legal action against AstraZeneca over vaccine supplies'. (22 April).

91 As we have seen, Lynn (2021) eloquently affirms this one-sided view.

92 Ursula Von der Leyen, the EC's president, later conceded a measure of EU responsibility for the slowness of the vaccine rollout: "We were late to authorise. We were too optimistic when it came to massive production and perhaps too confident that what we ordered would actually be delivered on time". See *BBC News* (2021). 'Covid: What's the problem with the EU vaccine rollout?' (4 March).

93 *BBC News* (2021). 'Covid: EU-AstraZeneca disputed vaccine contract made public'. (29 January).

94 Boffey, D. and Sabbagh, D. (2021). 'Britain and EU clash over claims to UK-produced Covid vaccine'. *Guardian*. (27 January).

95 Deutsch, J. and Herszenhorn, D.M. (2021). 'EU commissioner: AstraZeneca logic might work at the butcher's, but not in vaccine contracts'. *Politico* (online). (27 January).

96 Deutsch and Wheaton (2021).

97 *Al-Jazeera* (2021). 'EU threatens to ban AstraZeneca exports if vaccines not delivered'. *Al-Jazeera* (online). (20 March).

98 Henley, J. and Sabbagh, D. (2021). 'EU threatens to halt Covid vaccine exports to UK unless it gets "fair share"'. *Guardian*. (17 March).

99 Peel *et al.* (2021).

100 *BBC News* (28 January); Colson (2021).

101 Henley and Sabbagh (2021).

102 As he put it: "The UK has legally-binding agreements with vaccine suppliers and it would not expect the EU, as a friend and ally, to do anything to disrupt the fulfilment of these contracts". See *BBC News* (2021). 'EU vaccine export row: Bloc backtracks on controls for NI'. (30 January).

103 Woodcock, A. (2021). '"Maybe the UK wants to start a vaccine war". EU official stokes up row over jabs'. *Independent*. (29 January).

104 *BBC News* (2021). 'Coronavirus: EU demands UK-made AstraZeneca vaccine doses'. (27 January); Boffey and Sabbagh (2021).

105 Boffey and Sabbagh (2021).

106 *BBC News* (28 January, 2021).

107 *BBC News* (2021). 'Coronavirus: WHO criticises EU over vaccine export controls'. (30 January); Boffey, D. (2021). 'EU threatens to block Covid vaccine exports amid AstraZeneca shortfall'. *Guardian*. (25 January).

108 Colson (2021); Deutsch and Wheaton (2021). The Commission again threatened to block vaccine exports to the UK on behalf of the EU in mid-March having initially proposed to do so towards January's end. See Henley and Sabbagh (2021); Fortuna, G. (2021). 'EU leaders cautiously back vaccine export controls; claim to be world's main exporter. (26 March). *EURACTIV* (online).

109 Calcea, N. (2021). 'How the EU has overtaken the US on Covid-19 vaccines'. *New Statesman*. (26 July); De Maio, G. (2021). *Order from Chaos: EU Learns from Mistakes on Vaccines*. Brookings Institute (online). (20 May); *BBC News* (21 June 2021); Henley, J. (2021). 'Six EU states overtake UK Covid vaccination rates as Britain's rollout slows'. *Guardian*. (6 August); Mount, I., Walt, V., Meyer, D. and Werner, G. (2021). 'Operation Overtake: How Europe surpassed the U.S. in its COVID vaccination push'. *Fortune*. (1 July); Oltermann, P., Giuffrida, F. and Wilsher, K. (2021). '"It's such a relief": how Europe's Covid vaccine rollout is catching up with UK'. *Guardian*. (19 June).

110 Skopeliti, C. (2021). 'EU rules holding back Covid vaccine production, Pfizer says'. *Independent*. (1 April).

111 Campbell, J. (2021). 'Brexit: EU introduces controls on vaccines to NI'. *BBC News*. (20 January).

112 *BBC News* (30 January, 2021).

113 Colson (2021). The prospect of the EU blocking European vaccine exports to the UK was met with tabloid fury. In response, the *Daily Mail's* banner front-page headline ran: "NO, EU CAN'T HAVE OUR JABS!" Or, as the *Daily Express* headline of the same day put it: WAIT YOUR TURN! SELFISH EU WANTS OUR JABS".

114 Retaliation was certainly hinted at. This was accompanied by incendiary language – such as Northern Ireland first minister's Arlene Foster's accusation that the proposed EU action was "typical", "despicable", and an "incredible act of hostility" to the UK. See Kartal, A.G. (2021). *Coronavirus vaccine wars intensify in Europe*. Anadulu Agency (online). (30 January).

115 Deutsch and Wheaton (2021).

116 Deutsch and Wheaton (2021).

117 Deutsch and Wheaton (2021).

118 Deutsch and Wheaton (2021).

119 Deutsch and Wheaton (2021).

120 Boffey and Sabbagh (2021). See also: Boffey, D. (2021). 'EU threatens to block Covid vaccine exports amid AstraZeneca shortfall'. *Guardian*. (25 January).

121 Evenett, S. (2021). *Export controls on COVID-19 vaccines: Has the EU opened Pandora's Box?* VoxEU: Centre for Economic Policy Research (online). (11 February); Vela (2021).

122 Guarascio, F. (2021). 'EU has shipped tiny percentage of planned COVID-19 shot donations – document'. *Reuters* (online). (22 July).

123 Guarascio, F. (2021). 'Factbox: EU's COVID-19 vaccine donations so far'. *Reuters* (online). (22 July).
124 Ryan, J.M. and Nanda, S. (2023). 'Vaccines: Are we really in this together?" J.M. Ryan (Ed.) *COVID-19: Surviving A Pandemic*. London and New York: Routledge, p. 173. See also: Ryan, J.M. and Nanda, S. (2022). *COVID-19: Social Inequalities and Human Possibilities*. London and New York: Routledge.
125 This is a classic case of how competition (whether this be interstate competition or inter-capitalist competition), though rational for the *individual* competitor (whether nation-state or business corporation) must generate irrational outcomes for the *systems* of competition.
126 Pilkington, V., Keestra, S.M., and Hill, A. (2022). 'Global COVID-19 Vaccine Inequity: Failures in the First Year of Distribution and Potential Solutions for the Future'. *Frontiers in Public Health*, 10 (821117), pp. 1–8.
127 Pilkington *et al.* (2022), p. 1.
128 The UK government, for example, reportedly was on track to stockpile 210 million doses of vaccines by the end of 2021. See Allegretti, A. (2021). 'UK set to hoard up to 210 million doses of Covid vaccine, research suggests'. *Guardian*. (9 August). By 21 April 2021, the UK government had ordered 457 million of several vaccines – including 100 million each of AstraZeneca and Valneva. The volume of these procurements was 8.5 times higher than the UK's adult population of around 54 million and was (towards the end of December 2020) sufficient to put a jab in the arm of each and every person four times. See Baker, S. (2020). 'Rich countries buying most of the world's vaccine supply has left the rest scrambling for supplies, campaigners say'. *Insider*. (25 December); Stewart, C. (2021). *Number of COVID-19 vaccine doses ordered by the United Kingdom 2021*. Statista (online). (19 April).
As for the US government, by mid-March 2021, this had placed orders for 750 million vaccine doses, to cater for an adult population of 250 million. See Winfield, P. (2021). 'The Health 202: The U.S. bought enough coronavirus vaccines for three times its adult population'. *Washington Post*. (11 March). By mid-June, the US government had ordered a further 200 million jabs from Moderna, raising the total of its vaccine supply to 950 million doses. See Reuters (2021). 'U.S. buys 200 mln more Moderna COVID-19 vaccine doses'. *Reuters* (online). (16 June).
129 This approach was arguably morally defensible (given the reality of interstate competition for vaccines) during the period when the vaccines were under development and thus theoretical rather than actual. Under those circumstances, making massive orders from a number of manufacturers provided insurance protection from the possibility that some vaccines would not come to fruition. However, governments of the rich countries have also continued to place large-scale orders for jabs with companies whose vaccines were proven. Moreover, during the development period, it was clear that the US and UK governments were at least reasonably confident that the most promising vaccines already undergoing advanced trials would be effective and ready for 2021 rollout, because presumably that was the steer they were receiving from the big pharma companies based on work-in-progress.
130 Canada, on different estimates, had procured between four and nine vaccines per head. See Baker (2020); *BBC News* (2020). 'Rich countries hoarding Covid vaccines, says People's Vaccine Alliance'. (9 December); Mullard, A. (2020). 'How COVID vaccines are being divvied up around the world'. *Nature* (online). (30 November).
131 The EU's advance purchase deals signed off in 2020 were enough to double-jab every resident of the 27 member states, for example. Other major procurements were to follow. By 22 July 2021 the EU had received 500 million doses, with a further billion due for delivery before the end of September of that year. The bloc's third contract with Pfizer/BioNTech was to deliver 1.8 billion doses between 2021 and 2023. Negotiations were ongoing with eight manufacturers to deliver more than four billion vaccines

to the bloc before the end of 2022 This was to cater for an adult population across the 27 member states of around 365 million. See Arthur, R. (2021). 'EU drafts mega order for 1.8 billion Pfizer/BioNTech COVID-19 vaccine doses'. *BioPharma Reporter* (online). (15 April); Baker (2020); European Commission (2021). *Safe COVID-19 vaccines for Europeans* (online). (18 September); Guarascio, F. (2021). 'EU has shipped tiny percentage of planned COVID-19 shot donations – document'. *Reuters*. (22 July).

132   Mullard (2020).

133   Baker (2020).

134   *BBC News* (2020). 'Rich countries hoarding Covid vaccines, says People's Vaccine Alliance'. (9 December); Dyer, O. (2020). 'Covid-19: Many poor countries will see almost no vaccine next year, aid groups warn'. *British Medical Journal*, 371 (4809), pp. 1–2.

135   The EU alone, for example, placed an order from Pfizer-BioNTech in January that would account for half of the company's total output for 2021. See Farge, E. and Blamont, M. (2021). 'WHO tells rich countries: stop cutting the vaccines queue'. *Reuters* (online). (8 January).

136   According to the Duke Global Health Innovation Center. See *BBC News* (2021). 'Coronavirus: WHO chief criticises "shocking" global vaccine divide'. (10 April). Duke researchers had earlier (in January) concluded:

> While high-income countries represent only 16% of the world's population, they currently hold 60% of the vaccines for COVID-19 that have been purchased so far … Most … high-income countries have more than 100% coverage, and some can cover their populations several times over … High-income countries currently hold a confirmed 4.2 billion doses, upper middle-income countries hold 1.1 billion doses, and lower middle-income countries hold 411 million doses, and low-middle income countries hold 270 million.

See Marcus, M.B. (2020). *Ensuring Everyone in the World Gets a COVID Vaccine*. Duke Global Health Innovation Center (online). (20 January). And so predictably the competitive scramble to buy-up vaccines had by April radicalized an already dire imbalance in their worldwide distribution.

137   Padma, T.V. (2021). 'COVID vaccines to reach poorest countries in 2023 – despite recent pledges'. *Nature*, 595 (7867), pp. 342–43.

138   Cited in: Rigby, J. (2021). 'The least vaccinated countries in the world: the charts showing the scale of inequality'. *Telegraph*. (23 July).

139   Pilkington *et al.* (2022), p. 2.

140   Malpani, R. and Maitland, A. (2021). *Dose of Reality: How rich countries and pharmaceutical corporations are breaking their vaccine promises*. The People's Vaccine Alliance (online). (21 October).

141   Malpani and Maitland (2021).

142   Oxfam (2021). *More than a million COVID deaths in 4 months since G7 leaders failed to break vaccine monopolies*. Oxfam International (online). (3 June).

143   Cited in: Martin, S. and Arawi, T. (2021). 'Ensure Palestinians have access to COVID-19 vaccines'. *Lancet*, 397 (10276), pp. 791–92.

144   Human Rights Watch (2021). *Israel's Discriminatory Vaccine Push Underscores Need for Action*. Press Statement. HRW (online). (19 March).

145   *Al-Jazeera* (2021). 'Palestinian Authority calls off vaccine exchange with Israel'. (18 June).

146   Malpani and Maitland (2021). Pfizer reported profits of $3.5 billion for the first three months of 2021, of which almost 25 percent were from its COVID-19 vaccine. This made the vaccine the company's most profitable ever drug, netting at least $900 million over that short period. See Goodman, P.S. and Robbins, R. (2021). 'Pfizer Reaps Hundreds of Millions in Profits From Covid Vaccine'. *New York Times*. (5 April).

These profits were set to grow rapidly thereafter, carried by estimated sales worth $26 billion for the rest of the year, which were later projected upwards to $33.5 billion. As for AstraZeneca, the company's vaccine sales netted $1.2 billion in profits in the first six months of 2021 alone. This was during a period in which the company had claimed it was selling its vaccine "at cost". Moderna has also made a fortune from the pandemic. The company's second-quarterly report of 2021 estimated $19.2 billion worth of sales from its vaccines, and share values that were increased by seven-fold (Pilkington *et al.* 2022, p. 4). But things could only get better. "When the Biden Administration announced its booster plan in mid-August, Moderna's 2022 revenue forecast temporarily jumped 35 percent, with an expectation of $13 billion in profit from its COVID-19 vaccine sales" (Malpani and Maitland, 2021). See also: Egan M. (2021). 'Pfizer and Moderna Could Make $32 Billion Off Covid-19 Vaccines Next Year Alone'. *CNN: Business* (online). (4 November); Hart, R. (2021). 'AstraZeneca Will Now Profit From Covid Vaccine After Pledge To Sell At Cost During Pandemic'. *Forbes* (online). (12 November); Philippidis, A. (2021). 'Top 8 Best-Selling COVID-19 Vaccines and Drugs of Q1 2021'. *Genetic Engineering and Biotechnology News* (online). (24 May).

147 Oxfam International (2021).
148 Malpani and Maitland (2021).
149 Beaumont, P. (2021). 'Vaccine inequality exposed by dire situation in world's poorest nations'. *Guardian*. (30 May).
150 *BBC News* (10 April).
151 Hart, R. (2021). 'WHO Chief Implores Rich Nations – Like The U.S. – To Not Vaccinate Children And Teens Against Covid And Donate Doses For Poorer Countries'. *Forbes* (online). (14 May).
152 Allegretti (9 August 2021).
153 Goldhill, O. (2021). '"Naively ambitious": How COVAX failed on its promise to vaccinate the world'. *STAT* (online). (8 October).
154 Pilkington *et al.* (2022).
155 Pilkington *et al.* (2022), p. 2.
156 Pilkington *et al.* (2022).
157 WHO (2022). *Accelerating COVID-19 Vaccine Deployment: Removing obstacles to increase coverage levels and protect those at high risk.* G20 Indonesia (online). (20 April).
158 WHO (2022), p. 4.
159 Based on *Our World in Data* statistics presented in the *Guardian* newspaper. See Kelly, P., Kirk. A. and Ahmed. K. (2022). 'Covid vaccine figures lay bare global inequality as global target missed'. *Guardian*. (21 July).
160 Yamey, G. *et al.* (2022). 'It is not too late to achieve global covid-19 vaccine equity'. *British Medical Journal*, 376 (70650), pp. 1–6.
161 Lazarus, J.F. *et al.* (2023). 'Vaccine inequity and hesitancy persist – we must tackle both'. *British Medical Journal*, 380 (8367), pp. 1–2.
162 UN Data Futures (2023). *Global Dashboard for Vaccine Equity* (online). Accessed: 23 April 2023.
163 WHO (2023). *COVID-19 vaccination is rising in many vulnerable African communities thanks to EU-funded, WHO-led project* (online). (7 March). The participating countries were and are (the project has two more months to run): Burundi, Cameroon, Central African Republic, Chad, Democratic Republic of the Congo, Guinea, Liberia, Madagascar, Mali, Mozambique, Niger, Nigeria, Somalia, South Sudan, Sudan, and Tanzania.
164 Kelly *et al.* (2022).
165 Pilkington *et al.* (2022), pp. 3, 4.
166 Pilkington *et al.* (2022), p. 4.
167 Yamey *et al.* (2022), p. 2.

168   UN Data Futures (2023). Accessed: 24 April 2023.
169   Sung, M. *et al.* (2021). 'Pharmaceutical industry's engagement in the global equitable distribution of covid-19 vaccines: corporate social responsibility of EUL vaccine developers'. *Vaccines*, 9 (1183), pp. 1–22.
170   Pilkington *et al.* (2022).
171   Creaven (2024), Ch.1.
172   Cutler, D.M. and Summers, L.H. (2020). 'The COVID-19 pandemic and the $16 trillion virus'. *JAMA*, 324 (15), pp. 1495–96.
173   Creaven (2024), pp. 287–88.
174   WHO (2020). *Global Equitable Access to COVID-19 Vaccines Estimated to Generate Economic Benefits of At Least US$ 153 Billion in 2020–21, US$ 466 Billion by (2025) in 10 Major Economies, According to New Report by the Eurasia Group.* (December). WHO International News (online).
175   Çakmaklı, C. *et al.* (2022). *The economic case for global vaccinations: An epidemiological model with international production networks.* National Bureau of Economic Research. (November). Working paper series: Report no. 28395.
176   Cited in Rigby (23 July, 2021).
177   Cited in: Newey, S. (2021). '"Glacial" pace of global Covid vaccine rollout will cost $2.3 trillion in lost GDP, report warns'. *Telegraph.* (25 August).
178   WHO (2021). *About WHO* (online). Accessed: 30 April 2021.
179   WHO (2014). *Basic Documents.* 48th edition (online), p. 2.
180   Buranyi, S. (2020). 'The WHO versus coronavirus: why it can't handle the pandemic'. *Guardian.* (10 April).
181   The WHO's budget for 2020/21 was just $7.2 billion. The organization is wholly dependent on voluntary contributions from national governments and private donations – the bulk of which are from Western providers. See WHO (2021). *Financing of General Programme of Work 2020–2023* (online).
182   See Hanrieder, T. (2020). *Priorities, Partners, Politics: The WHO's Mandate beyond the Crisis.* Brill Publishers (online). (23 November). This paper is due for publication in Lyon, A.J. (Eds.) (2022). *Global Governance: A Review of Multilateralism and International Organizations.* Leiden: Brill.
183   Borger, W. (2020). 'White House demands WHO reforms but is vague on details, diplomats say'. *Guardian.* (17 April); Borger, W.. (2020). 'Caught in a superpower struggle: the inside story of the WHO's response to coronavirus'. *Guardian.* (18 April).
184   Nebehay, S. and Mason, J. (2020). 'WHO regrets Trump funding halt as global coronavirus cases top 2 million'. *Reuters* (online). (15 April).
185   Igoe, M. (2020). 'Why WHO doesn't like travel bans'. *Devex* (online). (1 May); Schlein, L. (2020). 'WHO Chief Urges Countries Not to Close Borders to Foreigners From China'. *Voice of America* (online). (3 February); WHO (2020). *Updated WHO recommendations for international traffic in relation to COVID-19 outbreak* (online). (29 February).
186   Guarascio, F. and Blenkinsop, P. (2020). EU fails to persuade France, Germany to lift coronavirus health gear controls'. *Reuters* (online). (6 March).
187   Clark, P. *et al.* (2020). 'Britain's open borders make it a global outlier in coronavirus fight'. *Financial Times.* (16 April).
188   *BBC News* (2021). 'Coronavirus: WHO criticises EU over vaccine export controls'. (30 January).
189   Pilkington *et al.* (2022), p. 2.
190   Yamey *et al.* (2022), p. 2.
191   Pilkington *et al.* (2022), p. 2.
192   *Al-Jazeera* (2021). 'WHO chief urges rich nations not to undermine COVAX scheme'. (22 February); *BBC News* (2021). 'Rich countries hoarding Covid vaccines, says People's Vaccine Alliance'. (9 December); *BBC News* (10 April, 2021); Dyer (2021); Ducharme, J. (2021). 'COVAX Was a Great Idea, But Is Now 500 Million Doses Short

of Its Vaccine Distribution Goals. What Exactly Went Wrong?' *Time*. (9 September); Goldhill (2021); Hart (2021); Farge and Blamont (2021).

193 Hanrieder (2020).

194 Beaumont, P. (2020). 'Scheme to get Covid vaccine to poorer countries at "high risk' of failure"'. *Guardian*. (16 December); Mullard (2021).

195 Pilkington *et al.* (2022), p. 1.

196 Kimball, S. and Mendez, R. (2021). 'WHO chief urges world to follow US lead and support waiving Covid vaccine patent protections' *CNBC News* (online). (7 May).

197 Safi, M. (2021). 'Most poor nations "will take until 2024 to achieve mass Covid-19 immunisation"'. *Guardian*. (27 January).

198 Goldhill (2021).

199 Cascini, F. *et al.* (2021). 'Attitudes, acceptance and hesitancy among the general population worldwide to receive the COVID-19 vaccines and their contributing factors: A systematic review'. *EclinicalMedicine*, 40 (101113), pp. 1–14; Mallapaty, S. (2022). 'Researchers fear growing COVID vaccine hesitancy in developing nations'. *Nature*, 601 (7892), pp. 174–75; Mutombo, P.N. *et al.* (2022). 'COVID-19 vaccine hesitancy in Africa: a call to action'. *Lancet Global Health*, 10 (3), pp. 320–21.

200 Cited in: Kelly *et al.* (2022).

201 Mutombo *et al.* (2022), p. 321.

202 Goldhill, O., Furneaux, R. and Davies, M. (2021). 'Naively ambitious': How COVAX failed on its promise to vaccinate the world'. *Stat* (online). (8 October).

203 Cited in: Kelly *et al.* (2022).

204 Goldhill (2021).

205 Malpani and Maitland (2021).

206 Malpani and Maitland (2021).

207 Adow, M. and Essop, T. (2021). 'On vaccine equality, the UK has failed to show the leadership the world needs'. *Guardian*. (16 July).

208 Malpani and Maitland (2021); Merrick, R. (2021). 'G7 rejects pleas to fund Covid jabs for poor countries pledge'. *Independent*. (11 June).

209 Wintour, P. (2021). 'Delayed Covid vaccines for poor countries "will leave Europe vulnerable for years"'. *Guardian*. (23 December).

210 Malpani and Maitland (2021).

211 According to Gordon Brown. See Elliott, L. (2021). 'West will kill thousands if it keeps on hoarding vaccines, says Gordon Brown'. *Guardian*. (9 September); Brown, G. (2021). 'The west has more vaccine doses than it needs – and no excuse not to share them'. *Guardian*. (9 September).

212 Airfinity research cited in: Gregory, A. (2021). 'Gordon Brown calls for urgent action to avert "Covid vaccine waste disaster"'. *Guardian*. (19 September).

213 Affinity cited in: Anon (2021). 'As a rich-world covid-vaccine glut looms, poor countries miss out'. *Economist*. (4 September).

214 Malpani and Maitland (2021).

215 *Economist* (4 September, 2021).

216 Brown (2021).

217 Schreiber, M. (2021). 'US throws out millions of doses of Covid vaccine as world goes wanting'. *Guardian*. (16 October).

218 Malpani and Maitland (2021).

219 *Economist* (4 September, 2021).

220 Eaton, J. (2022). 'The US has wasted over 82 million Covid vaccination doses'. *NBC News*. (6 June).

221 Yamey *et al.* (2022), p. 4.

222 Yamey *et al.* (2022), p. 4.

223 Anon (2021). 'The WHO is right to call a temporary halt to COVID vaccine boosters'. *Nature* (editorial), 596 (19 August), p. 1.

224 Cited in Kelly *et al.* (2022).

225 Pilkington *et al.* (2022), p. 2.
226 Worldometer (2023a). *COVID-19 CORONAVIRUS PANDEMIC: Total deaths* (online). Accessed: 18 January 2023.
227 Cited in Kelly *et al.* (2022).
228 Pilkington *et al.* (2022), p. 2.
229 Hanrieder (2020).
230 Malpani and Maitland (2021).
231 Malpani and Maitland (2021).
232 Pilkington *et al.* (2022), pp. 2–3.
233 Adow and Essop (2021); London School of Economics (2021). *Waive intellectual property protection for COVID vaccines and related technologies urge over 100 IP academic experts.* LSE (online). (13 July); Shaffer, J. (2021). 'Biden should use emergency powers to license Covid-19 vaccine technologies to the WHO for global access'. *STAT* (online). (25 March). As noted earlier, Joseph Biden, Trump's successor as US president, in the end offered the US's support to suspending IPRs (in the face of opposition from the Pharmaceutical Research and Manufacturers of America), but the EU and UK continued to block the move (Kimball and Mendez, 2021).
234 *Carbis Declaration* (Cabinet Office, 2021).
235 *Carbis Communique* (Cabinet Office, 2021).
236 CBI (2021). *CBI responds to G7 Communique* (online). (13 June).
237 *Carbis Communique* (Cabinet Office, 2021), pp. 1, 9–10.
238 *Carbis Communique*, pp. 1, 8.
239 *Carbis Communique*, p. 2.
240 *Carbis Communique*, p. 8.
241 *Carbis Communique*, pp. 1–2.
242 *Carbis Communique*, p. 3.
243 Worldometer (2023a). Accessed: 28 April 2023.
244 Creaven (2023), pp. 187–217.
245 Worldometer (2023b). *United Kingdom: Total Coronavirus Deaths* (online). Accessed: 26 April 2023.
246 *Carbis Communique*, p. 1.
247 *Carbis Communique*, pp. 1, 3.
248 Cited in: Meredith, S. (2021). '"The selfie summit": Why some economists and activists are disappointed with the G-7'. *CNBC* News (online). (14 June).
249 Creaven (2024), pp. 114–16
250 Cabinet Office (2021). *G7 leaders to agree landmark global health declaration: 12 June 2021.* Press Release. GOV.UK (online). (12 June).

3 Decivilization and society

A crucial line of defence of public health and public safety faced with the global novel coronavirus pandemic is of course non-pharmacological interventions (or NPIs). Indeed, NPIs were the only line of public health protection from COVID-19 until corporate science delivered its pharmacological fix at the tail end of 2020. Moreover, to this day, these remain the primary means of public self-defence for countries outside the developed world owing to the global asymmetries of the vaccine rollout that have radically compromised it from the start. My argument presented in this chapter and the next is that these defences were seriously compromised. This was not simply owing to failings of government policy internationally in response to the crisis (though these failings were commonplace, and in countries such as the UK and US, radical). Rather, this was also owing to weaknesses in the public or popular response to the NPIs. These weaknesses, I propose, may be attributed in part to decivilizing processes at work in contemporary modern societies. Before elaborating on this argument, however, it would be beneficial to address decivilization by considering it in relation to Norbert Elias's influential account of modernization as a civilizing process.[1]

Civilization and decivilization

According to Elias, the civilizing process is especially associated with modernization, though a civilizing dynamic would likely be evident wherever a centralized state establishes secure control of sovereignty over a territory. This is because, for him, the dynamic of civilizing is especially carried by urbanization, industrialization, and marketization under the auspices of the nation-state system. Processes of urbanization, industrialization, and marketization generate wider and deeper interconnections and interdependencies between people, fostering cooperation between individuals rather than competition between groups. At the same time, the consolidation of the centralized nation-state establishes state monopoly control over authoritative resources – that is, law, criminal justice, and the juridically sanctioned means of coercion and violence (police and armed forces) – within the territory that it governs. This means that societal communities are rendered as relatively pacified citizenries under the normative regulation of the state.[2]

Inter-societal or inter-community violence (or violent conflict in everyday life) is de-legitimized by virtue of the state's monopoly on authorization, including on

DOI: 10.4324/9781003437208-4

the means of violence, just as it is de-incentivized by the growing interdependencies of everyday social life. Violent inter-group competition and interpersonal aggression within society then fade away with the civilizing process as people for the most part internalize the rule of law and the legitimacy of state authority – including the legitimacy of the state's exclusive right to exercise powers of coercion and the lawful deployment of violence.[3]

> Violence was increasingly "confined to barracks", legitimately practiced only by members of the armed forces and the police, or within specific, controlled contexts such as sporting competitions. People became more sensitive with respect to witnessing or perpetrating impulsive violence, while at the same time an increase in the planned use of physical force occurred. This disposition became incorporated within the personality structure in the form of a specific kind of conscience formation, generating heightened guilt and repugnance feelings surrounding violent actions.[4]

At the same time, interdependencies and opportunities for self-advancement generated by the division of labour and role specialization allow people to imagine themselves as sovereign individuals. A new inner world of the self is generated whereby people are motivated to own and control their own interests, behaviour, and emotions. This is just as the tighter normative controls exercised over daily conduct by the sovereign state foster in people the capacities and desires to self-discipline and self-order within the bounds of a more universalized (if also more complex) framework of conduct rules.[5]

The result, as Elias sees it, is a shift away from social constraint and social steering of conduct and towards self-restraint and self-steered behaviour. This sustains a veritable barrage of etiquette or "manners" norms (along with associated technologies) with regard to every aspect of everyday life. This also leads to the emergence of a common or society-wide standard of behaviour and affectuality that universalizes and routinizes self-restraint and enlarges the potential for expanding inter-group relations.[6] With greater justice, if not greater consistency, however, the civilizing process, on Elias's account, would appear to be one in which external social constraint and social steering are internalized by the self and thereby experienced as self-restraint and self-volition. This happens as these social forces become elements of the personality system. This is an important point to make for reasons that will later become clear.

Elias also drew attention to decivilization. However, this was simply interpreted as interruptions and reversals of the civilizing process. Decivilization was simply a regression from modern civilization – a throwback "to the savagery and barbarism of earlier ages".[7] Elias thus did not provide a theory of decivilization, nor understand it as a social process that was also embedded as deeply in modern conditions as his civilizing dynamic. Rather, decivilization was referred to as occasional upsurges or spurts of "barbarism", conceived as regressions to pre-modern incivilities, which occurred where civilization had suffered major or calamitous breakdowns. The classical case of "re-barbarization" for him was the Nazi conquest of state power in Germany and the deployment of state power to murder six million Jews.[8]

But this really will not do, because, as Zygmunt Bauman has shown, the Holocaust was continuous with modern society and was not at all a departure from it. Modern social forms – centralized state authority (including and especially its monopoly on the means of violence), legal-rational bureaucracy, nationalism, industrial technology, etc. – were its essential conditions and facilitators. Without these modern institutions and forms of culture, the Holocaust could not even have been imagined let alone delivered.[9]

Not only that, alongside much of Elias's civilizing process has been the tendency for inter-state violence to grow, just as violence within national borders has generally declined (notwithstanding stand-out events such as the Nazi genocide). As a result, death tolls worldwide from modern industrial warfare have increased century by century, with the twentieth century being the bloodiest of all to date.[10] Elias published *The Civilizing Process* on the cusp of World War Two. This was having himself witnessed the terrible destruction of World War One. The remainder of the century would witness as many deaths from state violence and inter-state conflict as occurred during the latter.[11] This indicates that decivilizing dynamics have been as integral to modern societies as civilizing ones. These arguably reside in exactly the same sociopolitical and socioeconomic systems of competition (inter-state system and world capitalist economy) that have been examined in the previous chapters.

Even though Elias did not develop a theory of decivilizing processes, his own theory of civilizing processes would logically support one. This would conceptualize decivilizing as basically a reversal of three key aspects of civilizing. Instead of a shift from social restraint to self-restraint, for example, there would be a shift from self-restraint to social restraint. Instead of a movement towards the development of a common or universal standard of behaviour and affectuality that would support generalized self-restraint, for example, there would be a movement away. This would render self-restraint less stable, more unevenly distributed and constituted, and fractured or splintered along group lines. Instead of enlargement of the bonds of mutuality between or across individuals and groups that make up a society (or which extend across societies), for example, there would instead be retrenchment or diminution so that intra-group and inter-group cooperation or cohesion is weakened or undermined.

Jonathan Fletcher surmises that these elements of decivilization "would be likely to occur in societies in which there was a decrease in the (state) control of the monopoly of violence, breaking social ties and shorter chains of commercial, emotional and cognitive interdependence". Such societies would, he says, be

characterized by: a rise in the levels of fear, insecurity, danger and incalculability; the re-emergence of violence into the public sphere; growing inequality or heightening of tensions in the balance of power between constituent groups; ... [and] a freer expression of aggressiveness and an increase in cruelty.[12]

The main problem with this, of course, is that much of this may occur (and has occurred) without any decrease in a state's control of the monopoly of violence or by any shortening of the chains of commercial interdependence. This is certainly true of rising levels of fear, insecurity, and perceptions of danger in contemporary society. Such may be enhanced as well by the nature of the political authority exercised by the state (where this is wielded for the benefit of elites rather than the commonfolk and is non-inclusive of minorities) and by the extension of commercial chains (where these generate massive asymmetries in access to allocative resources). This is of course exactly what has occurred in many countries during the neoliberal era.

Such conditions may also cause self-restraint to be diminished in favour of social restraint, or of common standards of self-restraint to be undermined. Or these may bring about a decline of inter-group cooperation or cohesion. There is evidence from the public response to the pandemic that these factors of decivilization are real in those countries where state authority is quite stable and where commercial relations are most developed, as I will show. As for growing social inequality between groups, this certainly is a source of decivilization, since this would increase feelings of injustice among those at the wrong end of these divides as well as those of insecurity owing to the sense of marginalization or precarity they experience. This would also explain the phenomenon of mistrust for and alienation from the political authority of the state that is especially to be found among large numbers of people in low-income neighbourhoods and from marginalized minority communities in developed countries such as the UK and US. Such would also feed into higher incidences of inter-group hostility and interpersonal aggression.

Social inequalities internationally and within most countries have increased in the neoliberal era of untrammelled "commercial chains", as I will demonstrate in this chapter. Research has also shown that higher levels of interpersonal violence and aggression are associated with higher rates of socioeconomic inequality, just as higher rates of property crime generally are associated with higher levels of economic deprivation or income-poverty.[13] This confirms that decivilization is not simply a story of *exceptionalism* – of the "breakdown" of modernity or of a temporary "fall-back" or "regression" to a more uncivil premodernity, as Elias contends – but is rather part of the story of capitalist modernization itself.

The civilizing process is, I contend, simultaneously a process of decivilizing. As I will elaborate, decivilization is the consequence of the damages inflicted on the social bond by the impacts of the free enterprise economy, by a narrow individuated consumer-oriented rights culture, and by the undermining of public and community life in favour of the exorbitation of private commercial interests by the neoliberal state. These arguments will be pursued in the next chapter. The task of this chapter is to establish the key forces or drivers of decivilization. The first of these is simply injustice – especially but not exclusively by social class – as a hardening trend of recent decades. Such is integral to the neoliberal project, as I will show.

Decivilization as injustice under neoliberalism

Neoliberalism as an ideology is thoroughly permeated by neo-classical economics and classical liberal social theory. According to these, only private ownership of the means of production and the operation of unrestricted markets in goods and services and labour-power can deliver economic efficiency and material prosperity. This is because these not only release individuals to pursue their rational self-interest as buyers and sellers (hence allowing economic freedom to flourish) but also foster in them self-reliance, by compelling them to take responsibility for their own welfare. In the absence of the incentives generated by private ownership and market rewards, and protected from its deficits by generous welfare states that are intended to abolish social injustice (that is, lack of consumer opportunities for some owing to unemployment or low-paid work), individuals would be deflected from the work ethic, from economic enterprise, and from self-reliance Moreover, private ownership and the market mechanism, according to economic liberalism, also safeguards individual liberty, by acting as a bulwark against the encroachments of state power on civil society and on the rational pursuit of self-advantage. To wit, these also have the virtue of imposing cost-efficiency on the functions of public administration.[14]

Neoliberalism as political governance may be identified with a specific set of policies that were intended to deliver on the prescriptions of neoliberalism as ideology. Pioneered by right-wing governments in the UK and the US in the 1980s, neoliberalism was internationalized in the 1990s and 2000s, just as corporate free-trade capitalism became globally consolidated with the crisis and subsequent demise of "communism" or "state socialism".[15] Neoliberalism as state policy sought to reinvigorate national economic competitiveness by placing itself unambiguously and enthusiastically in the service of mega-capital and corporate enterprise. This has committed ruling parties to a form of class warfare from above whereby the political process is converted into a mechanism to squeeze welfare systems, emasculate the trade unions, promote labour market flexibility, liberalize finance and trade, empower MNCs, privatize public goods and services, reduce taxation on business and wealth, and "modernize" (that is, financialize and commodify) society and the state.[16] Ultimately, the secret of capitalist renewal, from the neoliberal perspective, is to bring about an anti-egalitarian redistribution of allocative resources. This is away from labour or from income from wages and the "social wage" (that is, welfare benefits) towards capital. This is out of public hands and into private ones.

Now, the paradox of the neoliberal world is that international capitalism has, in recent times, appeared as unassailable, even though it has piled misery upon a vast swathe of the global population, and its success even in its own strictly economic terms of reference is limited.[17] Neoliberalism was forged from the collapse of the long postwar economic boom (1948–73), and from the dismantling of the Keynesian model of state-regulated welfare capitalism that was its political driver in the advanced economies. But it has not ushered in a new era of universal prosperity. Neoliberal policies, even though these are globalized, have gone furthest among the developed countries in the UK and the US, where these have been accompanied since the 1980s by increasing income and wealth inequality between rich and poor (that is, a hardening of class polarization) and seemingly intractable problems of unemployment, precarity, economic marginalization, and social exclusion.[18] However, they are rendered universal policies (and problems), albeit unevenly distributed across the face of the world, in the context of combined but unequal development, under the endless ratchet of international capitalist competition.[19]

Inequality and injustice under neoliberalism in the UK

Consider the UK example. Here increases in wealth inequality have been radical. Wealth disparities narrowed in the postwar period prior to the neoliberal era. "By 1979 the share of the top 1 per cent, which had been around three-quarters, was closer to one-fifth. The share of the top 0.1 per cent, which had been a third, was by 1979 around 7 per cent", whereas the share of the top ten percent remained stable.[20] Between 1936–38, the richest one percent of the population owned 56 percent of the national wealth, whereas the richest five percent owned 88 percent of it. The lower 90 percent of the population, during this period, owned only 12 percent of total wealth. By 1971, however, the share owned by the richest one percent had fallen to 31 percent, whereas the share owned by the richest five percent had fallen to 65 percent, just as the share going to the bottom 90 percent increased to 35 percent.[21] Since the mid-1970s these trends have been reversed. Between 1976 and 1999, the share of national wealth going to the top ten percent of households increased from 57 percent to 71 percent (excluding the value of dwellings). Simultaneously, the share going to the bottom 50 percent declined from 12 percent to just three percent. This was according to data presented by *Social Trends*.[22]

Since the turn of the century, it has become more difficult to track the trend of wealth inequality in the UK, because there has not been continuity in the way the data is gathered, and it appears that the rich are increasingly adept at masking the full extent of their riches, as well as having greater opportunities to do so. Nonetheless, the evidence appears to support the continuation of the trend of hardening wealth disparities since 2000. On this timescale, the richest ten percent of households increased their pickings, from 48 percent to 52 percent of national wealth,[23] whereas the share going to the bottom 50 percent, according to the ONS, dropped back to nine percent from 12 percent.[24] This was in the period up to 2010. Since 2010, however, the process has levelled off owing to the temporary damage inflicted on share price values and bonuses by the great crash and recession. Between 2010 and 2018, the top ten percent increased their share, but only fractionally, from 43.56 percent to 44.59 percent of the total, whereas the bottom 50 percent saw their share decrease, also fractionally, from 9.61 percent to 8.48 percent.[25] These figures are inclusive of the value of dwellings. Nonetheless, the super-rich, the top 0.1 percent, the corporate elite, escaped the 2007/09 financial crisis and subsequent long depression virtually unscathed, doubling their share of national wealth between 1984 and 2013.[26]

Turning now to trends in income inequality and poverty in the UK during the neoliberal era. Here the evidence of growing disparities and of worsening poverty over the long *durée* is clear.

Prior to this, in the first few decades of the postwar period, the share of national income of the top ten percent of households fell from 33.2 percent to 26.1 percent, whereas the share of the next 60 percent increased from 54.1 percent to 63.5 percent. However, over this period, the bottom 30 percent were not the beneficiaries of the income redistribution that took place. Between 1954 and 1974, their share did not increase at all, though nor did it fall, fluctuating between 10.8 percent and 12.1.[27] By contrast, in the period from 1979 to 1997, the top 20 percent of earners saw their income grow by 2.5 percent per annum compared to 1.1 percent for those in the third quintile of earners and 0.8 percent for those in the lowest quintile. This trend was interrupted under the New Labour years, though it was not reversed. Between 1997 and 2010, the top 20 percent of earners increased their annual income by 1.7 percent, whereas the bottom 20 percent increased theirs by the same amount.[28]

Over the same period, the number of people living below the official poverty line (as defined as disposing of an income of less than 60 percent of average earnings) rose from four million to 14 million between 1979 and 1997, whereas the proportion of households on below-average earnings increased from 59 percent to 63 percent. This was just as average income increased.[29] As the New Economics Foundation reported in 2014,

> the UK saw a dramatic rise in levels of economic inequality during the 1980s; it has continued to rise since, although at a slower pace. Recent data shows that the richest one per cent of households in the UK now earn around 150 times more than the poorest one per cent of households. Wealth inequality has also risen considerably, with the top 1 per cent now having more wealth than the bottom 50 per cent put together.[30]

Between 1981 and 1992, the proportion of people living in households of less than 60 percent of average income increased from 15 percent to 25 percent, just as average income increased.[31] Between 1981 and 1993, the poorest 10 percent of the population experienced a 4.1 percent decline in income, and the poorest 50 percent a 2.9 percent decline in income, whereas the richest 10 percent increased their level of income by nearly five percent.[32] According to *Social Trends*, these trends toward increasing income differentials between rich and poor continued, albeit at a lesser pace, between 1994 and 2001.[33] Research by Brewer *et al.* confirmed this, indicating increasing income inequality from 1997 to 2000 (under the first New Labour government).

By the late 2000s, still under New Labour's watch, income inequality had "reached levels last seen in the 1920s". This was "driven by a growing share of income going to the richest, in particular the top one per cent". During the period from 1975 to 2008, "income inequality among working-age people has risen faster in the UK than in any other OECD nation … such that the UK now ranks as one of the most unequal countries in the OECD".

The UK has a net income inequality index of 0.341, and is only exceeded by Portugal (0.344), Israel (0.376), USA (0.378), Turkey (0.411), Mexico (0.466) and Chile (0.501) ... The average annual income in the UK for the top 10 per cent of the population in 2008 was roughly £55,000; for the bottom 10 per cent, it was just £4,700 – a ratio of 12:1. This is up from a ratio of 8:1 in 1985, and significantly higher than the average income gap in developed nations of 9:1.[34]

At the same time, according to Department of Work and Pension (DWP) statistics, between 1979 and 2000, the number of people in poverty increased from 7.1 million (or 13 percent of the population) to 13.3 million (or 23 percent of the population).[35] However, between 2000 and 2005, the latter increase was offset, owing to the impact of New Labour's modest reforms of the benefits and taxation systems.[36] Thus, according to the Joseph Rowntree Foundation, the proportion of people in poverty declined marginally under New Labour, from 23 percent to 20 percent between 2000 and 2005. This was a temporary respite though. These modest gains were dissolved by another upward spike in poverty rates between 2005 and 2007 that restored the level to 22 percent of the population, and still climbing.[37] Overall, in the period between 1979 and 2008, under the impact of the three main planks of neoliberal reforms – financial liberalization, social security tightening, and labour market deregulation – "the number of people living in poverty ... almost doubled, from 7.3 million people in 1979 to 13.5 million in 2008".[38]

In the aftermath of the Great Financial Crash of 2007/09, the process of growing inequality levelled off. But this was due to a more rapid depreciation of income from wages than of income from welfare benefits owing to the recession. This was possible because the poorest of the poor derive a much greater proportion of their income than others from welfare.[39] The poorer became poorer but so did many average income earners. Since 2007 the proportion of the population in poverty has been static, with minor fluctuations either way. This was still 22 percent in 2018/19, just as it was in 2007/08.[40] Indeed, as analysis by the Social Metrics Commission has shown, "over the course of the last two decades, the overall rate of poverty in the UK ... has sat stubbornly between 21% and 25% of the UK population".[41] But, in terms of raw numbers, there are more people living below the official poverty line today (14.3 million according to the Social Metrics Commission) than at any other time in the postwar period.[42]

Inequality and injustice under neoliberalism in the US

What about trends in inequality and poverty in the US over the same period? Here some of the patterns are even more severe than in the UK. In the pre-neoliberal postwar period, between 1947 and 1977, rates of income inequality were stable, with minor fluctuations. The bottom 40 percent of earners marginally increased their share of national income, whereas the top 10 percent saw their share marginally decrease.[43] Between 1977 and 1997, by contrast, the top five percent of American households increased their annual income after taxes by 43 percent, the top one percent by 115 percent, while the bottom 60 percent saw no improvement in real income at all, despite a sharp increase in the number of dual-earning families. Moreover, the bottom 20 percent witnessed an absolute decline of around nine percent over the same period.[44] In the mid-1970s, the share of national income going to the top fifth of American households was 45 percent, whereas by 2018 this had increased to 52 percent. The median income of the top-tier households increased by 64 percent from 1970 to 2018, whereas the income of the lowest-tier households *fell* by one percent over the same timeframe.[45] "Between 1979 and 2007 the share of income of the bottom 80 percent of the population fell by between 10 and 30 percent, while that of the top 1 percent increased by 130 percent".[46]

Thomas Piketty's exhaustive research concluded that over the course of three decades (1994–2014), the income growth of the poorest 50 percent of the population was virtually zero compared to a 300 percent rise for the wealthiest one percent.[47] Between 1980 and 2016, just as the share of national income accruing to the top one percent of householders increased from ten percent to 20 percent, the share accruing to the bottom half declined from 20 percent to 13 percent.[48] On a longer timescale, from 1971 to 2016, the incomes of the top tenth of households grew 80 percent more than those of middle-income households and 120 percent more than the bottom half of households.[49] Between 1989 and 2016 the share of pre-tax national income going to the top ten percent of earners increased from 43 percent to 50 percent, whereas the share going to middle-earners declined from 42 percent to 37 percent and the share going to low earners (who make up half of all earners) fell from 15 percent to 13 percent.[50]

Wealth disparities in the US are even wider than disparities of income and have shown the same tendency to increase in the neoliberal era. Again, the pattern before the consolidation of neoliberalism was for wealth disparities to reduce rather than increase. From the mid-1920s through to the end of the 1970s, the share of national wealth owned by the super-rich, the top 0.1 percent of the population, fell from 25 percent to eight percent of the total. Since the early 1980s, however, this trend has been reversed, as the share of national wealth owned by this propertied elite has risen inexorably, reaching 22 percent of the total by 2013.[51]

In 1989, the United States had 66 billionaires and 31.5 million people living below the official poverty line. A decade later, the United States had 268 billionaires and 34.5 million people living below the official poverty line.[52]

In 1989 as well the richest five percent of American households enjoyed a share of national wealth that was 114 times above the median, whereas by 2016 their share was 248 times higher.[53] At the tail end of the 1980s, the top tenth of families owned 67 percent of total wealth, whereas the bottom half owned just three percent. By 2016, however, the top tenth of families had increased their share to 77 percent, whereas the share owned by the bottom half of families had declined to only one percent.[54]

Research conducted by Saez and Zucman showed that "almost all of this increase is due to the rise of the share of wealth owned by the 0.1% richest families, from 7% in 1978 to 22% in 2012, a level comparable to that of the early twentieth century". Moreover, according to Saez and Zucman, "over the 1986–2012 period",

> the average real growth rate of wealth per family has been 1.9%, but this average masks considerable heterogeneity: for the bottom 90%, wealth has not grown at all, while it has risen 5.3% per year for the top 0.1%, so that almost half of aggregate wealth accumulation has been due to the top 0.1% alone.[55]

America's richest householders "are also the only ones whose wealth increased in the years after the start of the Great Recession".

> From 2007 to 2016, the median net worth of the top 20% increased 13%, to $1.2 million. For the top 5%, it increased by 4%, to $4.8 million. In contrast, the median net worth of families in lower tiers of wealth decreased by at least 20%. Families in the second-lowest fifth experienced a 39% loss (from $32,100 in 2007 to $19,500 in 2016).[56]

The outcome of all of this, as Barbara Ehrenreich notes, is widespread hardship alongside unprecedented riches in the wealthiest country on the planet:

> The Economic Policy Institute recently reviewed dozens of studies of what constitutes a "living wage" and came up with an average figure of $30,000 a year for a family of one adult and two children, which amounts to a wage of $14 an hour. This is not the very minimum such a family could live on; the budget includes health insurance, a telephone, and child care at a licensed center, for example, which are well beyond the reach of millions. But it does not include restaurant meals, video rentals, internet access, wine and liquor, cigarettes and lottery tickets, or even very much meat. The shocking thing is that the majority of American workers, about 60 percent, earn less than $14 an hour.[57]

The official poverty measure (OPM) in the US unfortunately offers very little purchase on the reality or extent of the hardship faced by America's working poor. This is because it is based on an absolute baseline rather than on a culturally sensitive one, which drastically undersells poverty. US poverty is calculated by comparing a person's income to a fixed threshold. This threshold is the amount of income needed to cover the most basic of needs. The threshold was set in the 1960s and has not since been changed. This was pegged at three-times the cost of a minimum food diet adjusted for family size and inflation (that is, of food prices).[58] The rationale for this was that back then (in the early 1960s), one-third of family income was typically spent on food. But this is no longer the case. The proportion of income an average American family spends on food has since shrunk to just 15 percent because the prices of non-food consumptive items have increased much faster than food items so that the OPM has become arbitrary.[59]

Such a measure does not accommodate income from subsidies or benefits (e.g. housing or nutritional assistance, tax credits, etc.). Nor does it incorporate a host of everyday elementary living expenses (transport, medical bills, medical insurance, childcare support, taxes, etc.) – the cost of most of which have increased much faster than food prices. And, of course, there is no place for exceedingly basic cultural or leisure needs (e.g. the occasional vacation, day trip, or cinema outing). Nor is this threshold linked to national median income or to increases in general living standards as a culturally relative measure of poverty would be. Consequently, whereas the OPM in the 1960s set the poverty line at roughly 50 percent of median income, today it is setting official poverty at under just 28 percent of median income.[60] This effectively renders invisible tens of millions of Americans who, on a reasonable and culturally relevant definition of poverty, are very poor indeed, and who would have been recognized as poor in the 1960s. Ehrenreich's working poor are effectively airbrushed out of the picture.

Given that the OPM has since the 1960s become outmoded and invalidated, ever more so with each passing decade, massively under-representing real deprivation, and with the undersell also increasing with each passing decade, the persistence and magnitude of poverty in the US that it reveals on its own terms is remarkable. The long postwar boom that coincided with the Keynesian-welfarist model of capitalism saw the official poverty rate as defined by the OPM halve from 22 percent in 1960 to 11 percent by 1973.[61] Since then, in the neoliberal era, progress has stalled over the long *durée*, as the poverty rate has fluctuated with the ups and downs of the economy, failing to maintain the steady downward trajectory of the earlier era. OPM rates climbed back up to above 15 percent owing to the recessions of the early 1980s and 1990s, receding in the periods in between, though without falling back to the level of the early 1970s.

> The poverty rate wavered between 11 and 12 percent for the rest of the decade [after 1973] and then rose rapidly to 15.3 percent by 1983. It gradually fell to 12.8 percent by 1989, then climbed back over 15 percent by 1993. The 1996 poverty rate was 13.7 percent.[62]

The 1990s boom left one in eight Americans below the poverty line, whereas the percentage of Americans living in absolute poverty (that is, on less than 40 percent of median earnings) rose from 4.9 percent in 1989 to 5.1 percent in 1998.[63] Poverty then climbed continually from 1999 to 2010, again topping 15 percent by the end of the period. The Great Recession increased the number of those living below the official poverty line by four million to 44 million, or 14.3 percent of the population, the highest it had been for 15 years. This also brought about a 4.2 percent drop in median household income.[64] Most recently, though, poverty has ebbed again, dipping from 14.8 percent in 2014 to 10.5 percent in 2019, resulting from a mini-boom. Hence, after more than 45 years (and most of those under neoliberal governance) "official" (that is, state-misrecognized) poverty marginally bettered the 1973 rate.[65] The reality, of course, is that poverty in America has increased *substantially* since the 1980s. Even on the official count, in 2018, the officially acknowledged American poor numbered more than 38 million, or one in seven Americans.[66] In 1973 they numbered 23 million.[67]

Neoliberalism and the workers

The neoliberal era has also witnessed a general process of redistribution of income for or from wages to income for or from capital. Across the OECD, for example, just as neoliberal reforms started getting phased in, capital-growth began to outstrip wage growth. This was from the 1980s onwards. "For the Group of Seven (G7) major industrial economies, the OECD estimates that the 'share of capital income' grew from 31.9 percent in 1975–9 to 33.9 percent in 1990".[68] This is indeed an international trend:

> The labor share of income in 35 advanced economies fell from around 54 percent in 1980 to 50.5 percent in 2014 ... Developing economies have also experienced the same phenomenon, albeit to a lesser extent. Available studies suggest that the labor share of income fell from 39 percent in 1993 to 37.4 percent in 2014, a drop of about 4 percent.[69]

In the US, on a longer timescale, workers have been especially hard hit, suffering a decline of the median wage of eight percent between 1973 and 1998, despite recording productivity gains of 46.5 percent for employers over the same period. This was even though the US economy enjoyed a 1990s growth boom that ought to have boosted wage growth.[70] According to Joseph Galbraith, four-fifths of American families witnessed an absolute fall in their income of five percent during the recession-ravaged 1980s.[71] Robert Brenner estimated that between 1979 and 1990 hourly real wages in the US economy fell by an average of one percent a year.[72] On Robert Heilbronner's calculation, the real weekly income of an American worker in 1990 was 19.1 percent below the level reached in 1973.[73] As a result, "the average real income of families was only a few percentage points higher in 1993 than in 1973, and that largely because so many more spouses were working".[74]

The American boom of the 1990s did nothing to reverse these trends, benefitting only the top third of families. This was noted even by the IMF: "One strong development of the current expansion has been the steady decline in labour's share of national income".[75] Average wages for American non-supervisory employees working in all industries and services, other than government and agriculture, were less in 1997 (at the peak of the US boom) than they were in 1973.[76] By 2000, the poorest tenth of American workers was still earning just 91 percent of the earnings they used to enjoy three decades earlier.[77]

Alongside these trends has also been a tendency for average working hours of waged or salaried workers to increase so that incomes have declined relative to the expenditure of labour time. The average working week in the US increased by

20 percent (or from 40.6 hours to 48.4 hours) between 1973 and 1985.[78] Employees were on average by then working the equivalent of more than a month extra (an additional 164 hours per year) in 1996 compared to 1976.[79]

> Between 1970 and 1990, the share of employed-for-pay U.S. men who worked more than 48 hours in the Census reference week rose from 15.4 to 23.3 percent. Between the 1980 Census and 2005 American Community Survey, the share usually working more than 48 hours per week rose from 16.6 to 24.3 percent. We find that increases in long work hours were greatest in detailed occupations (and industries) with (a) rising residual wage inequality and (b) slowly growing real compensation at "standard" (40) hours.[80]

This trend exists for female workers as well as male workers, and for lower-income as well as higher-income workers:

> The average worker worked 1,868 hours in 2007, an increase of 181 hours from the 1979 work year of 1,687 hours. This represents an increase of 10.7 percent – the equivalent of every worker working 4.5 additional weeks per year ... Annual work hours grew more among women (20.3 percent) than among men (4.4 percent) from 1979 to 2007, primarily because women increased their weeks per year in the paid workforce.[81]

Workers at the lower end of the pay scale have experienced the highest increases in annual working hours between 1979 and 2007, whereas those in the middle have experienced the next highest increase. The bottom fifth saw an increase of 22 percent over this period, the next fifth saw an increase of 15.2 percent, and the middle fifth saw an increase of 10.9 percent. By contrast, the top 80–95 percent of earners experienced an increase in annual working hours of 4.3 percent, whereas the top five percent experienced an increase of 7.6 percent over this period.[82] This trend has been accompanied by workplace speedup or intensification of work (along with increasing levels of stress and fatigue), with survey data reporting employees experiencing a significant increase in the tempo of work between 1977 and 2006.[83]

The trend towards diminishing income returns from work for ordinary workers has continued into the 2000s. Whereas "average real after-tax household income for the one percent of the population with the highest income grew by 275 percent between 1979 and 2007 ... the inflation-adjusted median income for working-age households declined by over $2000 between 2000 and 2007".[84] Hence labour's share of national income (that is, the share that is composed of wages) *vis-à-vis* capital's (the share that goes to profits) has declined at a faster rate than has happened internationally:

> The decline in labor share of income in the United States since the turn of the millennium has been particularly marked. Official data from the Bureau of Labor Statistics (BLS) suggest that, while the labor share had already started to decrease in the 1960s, three-fourths of the entire post-1947 decline

occurred between 2000 and 2016. The steepest part of the decline – from 63.3 percent in 2000 to 56.7 percent in 2016 – followed a moderate downward drift in the 1980s and early 1990s, and a slight recovery in the late 1990s.[85]

The declining share of income accruing to labour and the increasing share accruing to capital in the US is partly a story of boardroom excess. Thus: "In 1980 the top managers of the 300 biggest US corporations had incomes 29 times larger than the average manufacturing worker – by 1990 they were 93 times larger".[86] By 2018, though, the incomes of typical American CEOs were 278 times larger than those of ordinary wage earners.[87]

The same downward pressures on workers' living standards have been experienced in the UK, albeit with less draconian results than in the US. Average earnings from wages in the 1970s and 1980s grew 2.9 percent annually, but these slowed to 1.5 percent in the 1990s and just 1.2 percent in the 2000s.[88] This occurred as workers recorded average productivity gains for their employers of 4.9 percent between 1982 and 1990, and 2.3 percent between 1997 and 2007, compared to 1.9 percent between 1973 and 1979.[89] This is suggestive of greater intensification of work. And so it has been. In 1997, 23 percent of employees reported working at very high speeds for most of the time, whereas by 2001 this had increased to 38 percent, and by 2010 to 40 percent.[90] Workplace intensification continued to rise between 2012 and 2017. "Most notably, the proportion of workers in jobs where it was required to work at *very high speed* for most or all of the time rose by 4 percentage points to 31 percent in 2017".[91] This trend is especially pronounced among public sector workers, since by 2012, 53 percent of them, compared to 30 percent of them in 1992, reported higher work intensities.[92]

> Teachers and nurses are two professional groups that have experienced especially high levels of required work intensification. By 2017, a remarkable 92 percent of teachers strongly agreed that their job requires them to work very hard, up from 82 percent in 2012. Nine out of ten teachers, and nearly three quarters of nurses report that they often or always come home from work exhausted.[93]

Intensification of work has gone alongside the stalling of the postwar tendency for annual average working hours to decline, according to a report by the New Economics Foundation. The average full-time week fell from 46 hours in 1946 to 40 hours by 1979. This was owing to a "combination of increased pay and productivity, strong collective bargaining and increased labour market regulation from government". Since 1980, however, "this trend faltered following labour market deregulation, reduced collective bargaining and slower earnings growth for low income workers" so that "the average full-time week fell by just 2.5 hours to an average of 37.5 hours by 2016".

Indeed, the average working week in the UK for full-time workers has been virtually static from the 1990s right up until the cusp of the coronavirus crisis: in

1992, it was 38.1 hours; in 2019, it was 37.4 hours.[94] Between 1983 and 1995, the average working week even increased by an hour,[95] and so has since reduced only marginally, by less than an hour. This was despite continued productivity growth that outstripped pay rises up until the financial crisis of 2007/09. If trends of the first three decades of the postwar period had continued, the UK would have been on target to reach a 30-hour week by 2040.[96] "If the pre-1980 trend had continued, workers would now be working half a day less than they do today, roughly in line with annual working hours in Germany".[97]

From 2008 to 2014, in the context of the global financial crisis and its aftermath, real median weekly wages in the UK dropped by ten percent, whereas the real median hourly wage dropped by eight percent.[98] By April 2011, "average real hourly wages were 4 percent lower than they were at the start of the recession", with 70 percent of workers adversely affected, with 21 percent of workers seeing their wages cut absolutely, and 12 percent seeing their wages frozen.[99] Based on the TUC's analysis of International Labour Office (ILO) data, UK workers saw income from wages decline by an average of one percent a year from 2008 to 2015.[100] Similarly, according to the New Economics Foundation,

> In the seven years following the crash, the UK ... suffered the longest sustained decline in real wages since records began. This decline hasn't been shared equally across the income spectrum ... annual data up to the end of 2013 shows real earnings for the top 10% increasing by 3.9%, and a 2.4% fall for the remaining 90%. Households are once again piling on risky personal debt at a rate of almost £1 billion a year.[101]

This was as inflation rose faster than pay. This placed the country in 101st place internationally for wages growth and compared poorly with higher-income EU states such as France and Germany which experienced increases in real pay over the period.[102] The pay drop was owing not simply to a combination of wage freezes and wage cuts imposed by employers but, in rarer cases, an increase in casualization, as employers switched full-time workers to part-time contracts or even zero-hours contracts with lower salaries.[103]

The period of most precipitous decline was from 2010 to 2013 when real average wages fell by 2.2 percent annually.[104] This was remarkable insofar as the assault on wages was sustained even though the UK economy managed to maintain high employment and low unemployment after the initial shock of the crash.[105] By 2018/19, even though the great recession had ended, average wages showed little sign of recovery from the squeeze of the earlier period, as employer gains were consolidated in the context of slow productivity growth. Consequently, real earnings for workers were "still 3% below where they were in 2008 and ... 13% (or £3,500 per year) below where we might reasonably have expected based on rates of growth in the years prior to the crisis (of around 1.4% per year)".[106]

Inequality and poverty worldwide under neoliberalism

The past few decades have witnessed not only the radicalization of wealth and income inequalities within most national borders and across the globe but also the obdurate persistence of brutal subsistence poverty for billions on the wrong side of the North–South divide.[107] Opinions differ on the question of whether or to what extent subsistence poverty has reduced internationally under neoliberal "globalization". Under the World Bank's definitions and measures, there is a case for saying that it has, and majorly so, from around 1.9 billion in 1990 to 741 million by 2017, or from 37 percent of the world population to under ten percent.[108] However, the World Bank's timeframe for poverty trends leaves the 1980s out of the equation – which is where neoliberal "globalization" gets started. World poverty increased in the 1980s, even under the Bank's own metrics, despite the fact that there were substantial falls in China where a large proportion of the poor (20 percent) were to be found.[109] The World Bank's definition and measure of poverty is also deeply problematic, based as it is on an arbitrary dollar value. Moreover, it instructs about trends only at the absolute basement of the poverty range rather than illuminating trends across the whole poverty spectrum, for which different measures are needed.

Now, poverty, if this is understood in *absolute* terms – as the World Bank understands it, as having an income below a fixed sum that is necessary for bare subsistence – ought to diminish wherever there is economic development or "modernization" of whatever shape or hue. Employers are, after all, compelled to pay their workers at least enough to live on and be capable of working or else they would have no one to employ. Thus, poverty reduction, under these terms, ought not to be portrayed (as it is by apologists of capitalism and neoliberalism) as a dizzying triumph of a benign economic system abounding in "freedom of opportunity". On the contrary, it would be miraculous if there was not poverty reduction in the context of world economic development and de-colonization. Nor, reasonably, can poverty reduction be made a gift of "globalization", or of trade liberalization (that is, neoliberalism), or even of capitalism *per se*, though it is presented as such by the World Bank, by neoliberal politicians, by the corporate media, and by free-trade economists. Rather, this is the result simply of the global spread of the industrial mode of economic development.

The World Bank informs us that today there are around 689 million people living in conditions of *extreme* poverty, or approximately nine percent of the world's population.[110] The organization's current measure of absolute poverty, since 2015, is an income of $1.90 per day, up from $1.25 in 2008, $1.08 in 1993, and from $1.02 in 1985. But this is an inadequate baseline because hardly anyone anywhere could possibly have even their basic needs met on this level of income. Moreover, the upward adjustments in the base dollar rate have not kept up with increases in the cost of living virtually anywhere in the world.

These are reasons to call into question the validity of the World Bank's grandiose claims that even severe subsistence poverty has been *drastically* cut in the era of "globalization". This measure is also static in as much as any meaningful definition of subsistence poverty anywhere in the world ought to relate this to median income levels in the countries in question and by making cross-national comparisons of GDP capacity. This is because poverty is also relational and contextual. Poverty ought to mean having access to a level of income that is insufficient to participate in the economic and cultural life of a society that is available to the "typical" or "average" person in that society. This is not how the World Bank estimates poverty.

Another reason to dispute the World Bank's claim, according to critical economists, is major problems with their counting methods.[111] How did the World Bank settle on its own measure of absolute poverty? Well, first they found out the official national poverty lines of a sample of low-income and middle-income countries. Second, they worked out the average poverty line from across the sample and converted the figure into its equivalent in US currency. Third and finally, they gathered data from general household surveys of the countries in the sample on the percentages of people who were below the local national poverty lines.[112] By this method, back in 1985, the World Bank determined that the correct measure of poverty was living on less than $1.02 per day, whereas in 1993 they raised this to $1.08 per day, then to $1.25 in 2008, and most recently to $1.90 in 2015.

Fair enough, it could be said – the World Bank ought to adjust the poverty line upwards over time to account for things like price inflation. So they should. But the trouble is that they do not seem to adjust it often enough or generously enough. So, arguably, they are short-changing the world's poor. It just does not seem plausible, for example, that a rise of just 23 cents in the poverty baseline over a period of more than 20 years (from 1985 to 2008) could be sufficient to keep up with general price inflation anywhere in the world. This may mean that the World Bank's "evidence" for declining global poverty is literally senseless, for the simple reason that the real value of $1.90 of spending power today is quite possibly less than the real value of $1 of spending power 35 years ago.

But there are other problems with how the World Bank defines and measures poverty. Firstly, it relies on the adequacy of the local, national definitions of poverty lines. The World Bank takes as given all the local, national poverty lines that are used by all the countries in its surveys. For all sorts of reasons, these tend to be stringent, under-estimating the level of income needed to avoid destitution. So, there is right at the start of the counting and calculating process, a pressure to deflate the international poverty line that emerges as its outcome.

Secondly, it relies also on the adequacy of the local general household surveys from which data is collected on the numbers of people below the various national poverty lines – and these are often inadequate. These often do not follow a standard template and are of variable quality. They often are methodologically flawed. For example, often the questions addressed to householders neglect certain poverty indicators, which skew the data. Householders are also sometimes reluctant to admit they are facing destitution, since in many entrepreneurial societies and cultures (for example in East Asia and in India) there is a strong stigma attached to poverty. And, of course, there is also the problem that many of the poorest are not actually householders at all. Vagrants and the homeless are not included in the household surveys. There is also the problem that those governments that administer the surveys have an interest in minimizing poverty because high poverty rates may reflect badly on them by revealing inadequacies of their own economic or social policies. With that in mind, a tendency has been noticed for the recall times of the surveys to be abbreviated, from 30 days to just 7 days. This may be because shorter recalls tend to give a more favourable result. These result in people reporting higher levels of household expenditure than is the case for longer recall periods.[113]

Thirdly, the data sets from which the World Bank calculates poverty have big gaps in them. Two countries – China and India – are the most difficult of all to extract reliable data from. Chinese governments have not co-operated at all with the World Bank. This is by refusing to participate in international surveys that would allow a comparison of living costs or household expenditures in China with other countries in the sample. The Indian government, on the other hand, has co-operated only partially, by selective involvement. The Chinese data is further weakened by the fact that urban populations have not been included in calculations of the overall poverty rate.[114] Yet millions of the poor have flooded into the cities in search of work, and it is plausible to think that a lot of them remain very poor. There are good reasons for thinking that breakneck hyper-urbanization has generated masses of working poor.

For some critics, these inadequacies of methods of data collection and analysis (and other issues) are such that, at least from the 1990s through to the early 2000s, it was simply not possible to be certain whether real poverty was going up or down. All that could be said with confidence was that there was an awful lot of it and that this was devastating to the lives of the poor.[115] This is especially important because China was responsible for around 90 percent of the supposed decline in extreme poverty from the start of the 1980s up until the 2000s.[116] Indeed, on some estimates, in as much as there were poverty reductions in the 1980s and 1990s, these were almost entirely attributable to developments in China and India.[117] Even taking the World Bank's poverty data at face value, it is clear that poverty reduction is not a genuinely global trend but has been and remains localized and regionalized, reflecting the combined but uneven development of the capitalist world economy. Large parts of the world (in sub-Saharan Africa, the Middle East, Central Asia, and Latin America) have not progressed in terms of human development.

These issues impact negatively not only on the accuracy of the official poverty trends but also on estimates of trends in global inequality. These counts have been shown to be based on methods of data collection and analysis that are most conducive to generating the desired (that is, positive) results. These do not, for example, measure relative income differentials between top earners and bottom earners, both within and across national borders.[118] In any case, putting China out of the equation, there has been for a long time scarcely any improvement for the life chances of the world's poorest in the era of capitalist internationalization. This was from the 1980s up to the start of the new century,[119] although there has been progress since, which is now under threat owing to the COVID-19 crisis.[120] But China's poverty achievements (whatever they are) have little to do with neoliberal free-market policies or capitalist "globalization". These were achieved by state-capitalist methods:

massive public investments in infrastructure and housing and industry; partial (at least) state ownerships of the biggest companies; epic investments and subsidies in economic target areas under the five-year plans; plus virtually self-enclosed consumer markets and selective doses of trade protectionism.[121]

The World Bank estimated that in 2008 there were 1.4 billion people living below its then poverty line of $1.25 daily.[122] That was roughly 20 percent of the world population. They also estimated that 2.6 billion people were then living on an income of under $2 a day, more than one-third of the total.[123] In the early 1970s, by comparison, the International Labour Organization (ILO) estimated that the total number of very poor people in the world was 700 million, whereas the World Bank put the number at 800 million.[124] Now, half of the global population (around 3.6 billion people) was thought by the World Bank to live on an income of less than $2.50 per day in 2008.[125] This was the equivalent of $2.50 purchasing power in the US market, not local marketplaces. The OPM in the US was at the time, by comparison, an income of below $10 per day, whereas today the US Federal Poverty Level (FPL) – which is the cut-off threshold for a range of welfare benefits – is $35 a day.[126] Now, roughly 97 percent of the population of the developing world had an income of less than $10 per day in the mid-2000s.[127] Today around 80 percent of the world's population does,[128] whereas almost half of the world's population has to get by on less than $5.50 a day.[129]

The figure of $5.50 per day is an interesting one. This is because the World Bank itself somewhat let the cat out of the bag when it admitted that half of the world's population (that is, that portion of it earning less than this amount) suffers as it puts it from "severe hardship".[130] So, even on a highly conservative estimate of subsistence poverty (that is, an income of less than $2.50 per day at 2008 prices or of $5.50 a day at 2015 prices), which itself would scarcely be sufficient to secure the necessities of life for most people in most places, at least half of the world's population has been living under such a condition, and probably considerably more.

Even though the World Bank sees free-market capitalism's victory over poverty as imminent, if economic growth continues (a rather big "if"), the lie is also revealed by the realities that the term "hardship" denotes. These are just a few of them. One in three people worldwide do not have safely managed access to clean drinking water (2.2 billion) and half (4.2 billion) do not have access to safely managed sanitation services.[131] One-third of children worldwide under five years of age are under-nourished and half lack essential vitamins and nutrients.[132] So, we have what ought to be (from the World Bank's perspective) the incomprehensible phenomenon of widespread child "food poverty", despite the fact that (according to them) there is nowhere near as much *actual* child poverty.

Addressing wealth and income trends in the world economy now – what are we to make of these? Even though there is at least a case for seeing extreme poverty as having been reduced in the neoliberal era (though not for imagining that poverty levels are less than astronomical), this is certainly not true of inequality. Indeed, for the most part, the World Bank and pro-globalization economists concede the case but represent growing inequality as the necessary price to be paid for eliminating global poverty. This is the infamous "trickle-down" theory writ large. Today, more than 80 percent of the world's population lives in countries where earnings-differentials have been widening during the age of untrammelled capitalist internationalization.[133] Thus, inequalities *within* most countries have grown. The OECD reports: "In the 1980s, the richest 10% of the population in OECD countries earned seven times more than the poorest 10%. They now earn nearly ten times more".[134]

Inequalities *across* borders have also increased. At the close of the 1960s, "the gap between the richest and poorest fifths of the world's population stood at 30 to one, in 1990 at 60 to one, and in 1998 at 74 to one".[135] As Gabriel Zucman's recent review of a range of wealth surveys shows:

> Evidence points toward a rise in global wealth concentration: For China, Europe, and the United States combined, the top 1% wealth share has increased from 28% in 1980 to 33% today, while the bottom 75% share hovered around 10%. Recent studies, however, may underestimate the level and rise of inequality, as financial globalization makes it increasingly hard to measure wealth at the top.[136]

The wealthiest ten percent of the global population today monopolize 86 percent of global wealth, and the top one percent possess 46 percent, whereas the lower 50 percent have access to less than one percent of the total.[137] The richest 20 percent of the world's population today enjoy 75 percent of total income, whereas the lower 40 percent have to get by on just five percent.[138]

A major international survey published in 2011 investigating trends in income distribution right across the OECD over several decades – *Divided We Stand: Why Inequality Keeps Rising* – found that, since the mid-1980s, in a vast majority of OECD countries, "the household incomes of the richest 10% grew faster than those of the poorest 10%".

> The Gini coefficient, a standard measure of income inequality that ranges from 0 (when everybody has identical incomes) to 1 (when all income goes to only one person), stood at an average of 0.29 in OECD countries in the mid-1980s. By the late 2000s, however, it had increased by almost 10% to 0.316. Significantly, it rose in 17 of the 22 OECD countries for which long-term data series are available, climbing by more than 4 percentage points in Finland, Germany, Israel, Luxembourg, New Zealand, Sweden, and the United States. Only Turkey, Greece, France, Hungary, and Belgium recorded no increase or small declines in their Gini coefficients. However, the ratio varies widely from one country to another. It is much lower than the OECD average in the Nordic and many continental European countries, but reaches 10 to 1 in Italy, Japan, Korea, and the United Kingdom; around 14 to 1 in Israel, Turkey, and the United States; and 27 to 1 in Mexico and Chile.[139]

The survey noted that first-world income inequality first began to widen in the UK and US (the two neoliberal pioneers of the developed world) in the late 1970s and early 1980s, but thereafter the trend was internationalized.

The latest trends in the 2000s showed a widening gap between rich and poor not only in some of the already high inequality countries like Israel and the United States, but also – for the first time – in traditionally low-inequality countries, such as Germany, Denmark, and Sweden (and other Nordic countries), where inequality grew more than anywhere else in the 2000s.[140]

A fundamental aspect of the inequality gap, as revealed by another recent OECD study, is the growing disparity between income from median wages and from typical corporate-executive salaries. Typical pay for CEOs across the OECD is now almost 300 times higher than median wages, whereas 20 years earlier it was 20–30 times higher.[141] This OECD study also found that growth in global inequalities within and between the 34 member countries was interrupted by the financial crisis of 2007/09, but that these have since resumed their upward climb so that the average earnings gap between the top ten percent and the bottom ten percent is now at a record postwar high of almost tenfold. Emblematic of these developments, in the decade since the financial crisis, the number of billionaires in the world doubled. From 2016 to 2018, the number of billionaires owning as much wealth as the poorest half of the global population dropped from 61 to just 26. Moreover, the world's richest increased their riches by 12 percent just as the poorest half of the world's population saw their wealth fall by 11 percent over this same period. By 2015 a new landmark in world inequality was reached: the wealthiest one percent of the world's population acquired for the first time more wealth than everyone else put together.[142]

Now, radicalizing or hardening inequality together with the privations of economic marginalization and attendant social exclusion may be considered key elements of decivilization. This is because these trends are associated with status-frustration, or feelings of injustice over blocked opportunities,[143] along with a lively sense of class-conscious grievances and antagonisms.[144] These trends also correspond to popular disenchantment with political authorities that preside over them (and so can be regarded as being indifferent towards or even as supportive of them).[145] These elements (plus others – such as the pressure of economic necessity to prioritize self and family over a generalized other) are decivilizing because they corrode "public" society, communal solidarity, and the social bond.

These decivilizing drivers, I will argue, explain in part the non-compliance or lesser-compliance of many people with those NPIs and PIs (physical distancing norms mandated by the government plus the biomedical fix promised by the vaccination rollout) that were intended to protect the public from COVID-19. Those people least likely to comply in whole or in part with the NPIs and to consent to get vaccinated were disproportionately drawn from the deprivileged side of the social class and racialized class divides, as I will show in the next chapter.

Modes of individualism and decivilization

As for individualization, this is simultaneously a force of civilization and of decivilization. As a force of decivilization, individualization also allows public non-compliance with NPIs to be explained sociologically. Such an explanation would attribute the phenomenon of non-compliance, or at least the potential for it, as residing to some degree at least in the basic cultural structures of a modern society. This is in the sense that these may plausibly be regarded as enabling or even facilitating acts of deviation while also partially neutralizing the normative or moral inhibitors that would deflect people from them. Such cultural forms have become, in the "global" age, generic, since "globalization" has been a story of the international diffusion of modern ideologies and lifestyles.[146] As such they would provide part of the explanation for non-conforming behaviour everywhere, not simply here and there.

Individualized or individualistic cultures are made by modern social conditions generally. They are the effects of post-Enlightenment societies. An individualistic culture may be defined as one that orders social life in such a way that the individual is prioritized over the group or collective or community. Individualistic or individualized cultures are focused on the self rather than on the group, inasmuch as the purpose of society or community is seen as facilitating or enabling personal freedom, independence, expression, accomplishments, and development rather than furthering collective goals or interests. Individualistic cultures, in short, emphasize personal interests rather than group interests.[147] And in these cultures, individuals are encouraged to sustain social ties with other people beyond close family and indeed allegiance to societal norms or institutions less on the basis of moral obligation or duty, or general altruism, or under the impress of social authority, and more informed by strategic judgements over the pros and cons of doing so in relation to their own self-interest or that of close kin.[148]

Individualization as a fundamental dynamic of modern civilization has its genesis in the great revolutions (industrial, commercial, urban, scientific) of the eighteenth and nineteenth centuries that brought into being the first simple modern capitalist societies in Northwest Europe and North America. Since World War Two, however, individualization has been internationalized. On this timescale, modern societies across the face of the globe have consolidated, with few exceptions, albeit to greater or lesser degrees, individualized cultures. This occurred initially under the spur of the long postwar boom. This established a world market dominated by US capitalism and ushered in the de-colonization of the Global South with the dismantling of European imperialism.[149] Latterly, this was boosted by the collapse of "communism" or "state socialism" in Eastern Europe and the developing and underdeveloped world in the 1980s, which removed "collectivist" societies and cultures from the game so that liberal polity and capitalist economy were granted the opportunity to hegemonize internationally. This not only allowed the global diffusion of citizenship but also opened up every corner of the globe for commercial exploitation, allowing the full capitalization and corporatization of the world economy in the present neoliberal era.[150]

The history of so-called globalization from the second half of the twentieth century is, for this reason, as much a history of progressive individualization of social and cultural life as it is of institutional modernization. Indeed, for many contemporary social theorists, postwar modernization in all of its aspects is a story of individualization.[151] Individualization may be defined, following Emile Durkheim's example, as the process by which the power of collective cultures to build social solidarity across social groups and the conformity of individuals to social order, in effect by binding people to the same set of shared norms and values, is diminished or undermined. This is because the decline of culture as a force that binds and unites a society through the imposition of uniform moral obligations is one that opens new opportunities for people to differ from one another.[152] In effect, then, individualization results when the prescriptive force of culture to solidarize a community's or society's members through the imposition of homogenous, universally binding, normative, and moral standards is forestalled or undone since this grants people latitude to constitute themselves as autonomous beings, as bearers of distinct subjectivities or self-identities, as personally unique selves capable of exercising their own judgements of how to live their lives.

I have said that individualization is simultaneously a force of civilization and of decivilization. But, to grasp why this, is it is necessary to distinguish between modes of individualism. There are, of course, multiple drivers of individualization under modern conditions so that, rather than individualization *per se*, there are various modes of it. All of these, however, have in common the effect of diminishing the capacity of culture to impose prescriptive forms of behaviour on a society's members so that socialization and enculturation function less to bind individuals to social conformity through shared norms and values and by force of moral obligation. Yet some of these modes are heavily implicated in decivilization processes, whereas others are much less so. Indeed, certain modes would provide a potential redoubt against decivilization. Decivilization is a concept that offers an explanation of many people's non-compliance with NPIs, not individualization *per se*. The modes of individualism that will be considered in the discussion that follows are *associational individualism*, *economic individualism*, *consumerist individualism*, and *reflexive individualism*.

Associational individualism

Emile Durkheim was the first to theorize modern individualism, seeing this as emerging from the specialized social division of labour characteristic of modern industrialism.[153] Although unfashionable, owing to the close association of his work with structural functionalism in social theory, his analysis retains much of its force and relevance today. Durkheim's primary interest was with what he saw as the emergence of *moral individualism* – which was an aspect of what may be termed as *associational individualism*. Role specialization, he argued, dissolved the self-sufficiency of the traditional household-based subsistence economy, replacing this with the interdependencies of roles and functions of a market-based industrial economy. Work was made into a separate branch or sphere of social life split off from intimate relations within the domestic sphere. Yet, for Durkheim, this evolving division of labour, though originating in the economic context of capitalist industrialization, was much more than an economic phenomenon. Rather, role specialization and role differentiation were extended into all aspects of society, in order to increase the functional utility of social forms. In short, the division of labour under conditions of modern industrialism was the *social* division of labour in the fullest sense.[154]

Politics and education, like work or economic activity, thus became detached from kinship relations, and these were subsequently transformed into highly specialized departments of social activity. Culture and science too became progressively differentiated and specialized. Instead of "science", there were sciences, each a separate branch of expert knowledge with its own investigatory practice. Instead of "culture", there were different cultures, which each corresponded to the distinct spheres of social life in the social division of labour. Alongside societal role specialization, formal political and economic liberalization came to govern the steering institutions of industrial society. Hence individualism as political theory and ideology animated the political, legal, and economic spheres. A politico-judicial "rights culture" corresponding to the "contract society" was consolidated which reconstructed people as the bearers of a range of individual entitlements (legal, political, economic). This in effect transformed them from subjects (of community or sovereign or divine authority) into citizens.

According to Durkheim, the process of the social division of labour, as this came to characterize the dynamic of industrial modernity, shifted society from one dominant mode of social regulation of the behaviour of its constituent members to another – from *mechanical solidarity* to *organic solidarity*. By organic solidarity, Durkheim was referring to a form of solidarity that was created by the expanding diversity of roles in modern society wrought by the social division of labour. For him, the social division of labour based on role specialization was exactly the dynamic force that historically allowed people to be made into individuals. Such made possible the liberal "rights culture" that established political and economic individualism as a matter of legal entitlement.

This was because role diversity provided a flexible opportunity structure by which subjects may exercise freedom of choice over which roles they will take up in society. In order for a society's members to be made into more than merely communal beings beholden to collective norms, Durkheim affirmed, a choice of social roles was necessary. By virtue of exercising personal choice over which social roles to make their own, people were granted capacities to individualize themselves, since there can be no individuality unless people have freedom to choose how they will live their lives. Without freedom of choice, human beings must always be creatures of a uniform or undifferentiated culture rooted in tradition and collective obligation.[155]

Durkheim was well aware that the individualization generated by the industrial division of labour was potentially a negative as well as positive force. It was positive not simply because a society that allows personal freedom to flourish was morally preferable to one that did not, but also because such a society would dispense its functions and roles with far greater efficiency of utility for the benefit of all than one where the division of labour was rudimentary and there was little role specialization. But the danger of the individualism promoted by role differentiation and attendant political liberalism, Durkheim opined, was that this could, under certain circumstances, potentially degenerate into the egoistic pursuit of private self-interest as people compete with each other as individuals for access to the higher rewards (in terms of money and prestige) in the division of labour, placing personal or familial desires above community or societal needs. Such would threaten the dissolution of social solidarity and the community bond as society fragments and splinters into Hobbesian monads.

This negative potential existed, Durkheim thought, largely due to the fact that the economy of industrial society was based on laissez-faire capitalism. This is not a merely historical issue since in recent decades under neoliberal governance, laissez-faire capitalism has been reimposed on the world economy. In any case, for Durkheim, this was a mode of capitalism that operated wholly on the terrain of formal contracts between individuals as buyers and sellers of various kinds of commodities without much formal regulatory normative control (that is, beyond the enforcement of contracts) by community or civic organizations or the state to ensure that these contracts were fair. For Durkheim, nineteenth-century capitalism, based on free trade and unregulated markets, generated a host of social problems for industrial society.

The primary one was that this form of capitalism encouraged wholly self-interested behaviour by rendering status success dependent on the acquisition of material rewards (hence legitimizing a materialistic outlook on life – the anomie of "insatiable appetites"). Others included unjust inequalities between employer and employee; blocked opportunities for upward social mobility for those at the lower end of the class structure; periodic commercial crises; and industrial conflict that threatened to spill over into class war (especially during periods of economic crisis). Durkheim classed these problems as those of the "abnormal forms" of the social division of labour – the anomic division of labour (generated by the lack of regulatory rules to civilize capitalist markets)[156] and the forced division of labour (generated by arbitrary rules that restrict access to certain trades or professions or which defend hereditary privileges)[157] – which he regarded as obstructing progress towards organic solidarity.

Nonetheless, Durkheim thought that modern industrial society would resolve these problems. Indeed, he was optimistic that modern industrialism made possible a higher, better form of social solidarity than had gone before. This is why he classed organic solidarity as the natural or typical form of the social division of labour under industrial modernity to be contrasted with the deviant or "abnormal forms". As he put it: "Human beings cannot live together without acknowledging and, consequently, making mutual sacrifices … Every society is a moral society. In certain respects, this character is even more pronounced in organised societies".[158] The reason for his optimism was that for him modern individualization was rooted not simply in social differentiation in the division of labour but also in the functional interdependence of roles. The highly specialized division of labour, Durkheim observed, not only fragmented a societal community into separate micro-systems of social action but also ensured that a society's members were made dependent on each other for their livelihood. The car-worker, for example, cannot live off the products of his or her own labour; rather, he or she must exchange them with those of other goods-providers in order to acquire the things he or she needs.

So, for Durkheim, differentiation of roles was also inevitably interdependence of roles, whereas interdependence of roles has the potential to rein in egoism. With greater choice and diversity of roles, people are made individuals, rather than just members of one big group or homogeneous community. But, at the same time, the modern division of labour potentially allowed individuals to recognize alongside their own needs and interests those of others, plus also the need to cater for those other needs and interests. This makes possible the building of bonds of solidarity rooted in a sense of *mutual moral obligations*. Under modern conditions of role specialization, where individuals cannot cater for their own needs by drawing exclusively on their own resources, they are thereby bound together by ties of mutual dependence. Owing to the functional interdependence of roles, social cooperation is enforced on a society's members. This was Durkheim's definition of organic solidarity – that is, solidarity through differentiation and interdependence, or solidarity by means of *complementary differences* in the social division of labour – which he believed modern industrial society was gravitating towards.[159]

This was to be contrasted with mechanical solidarity, which Durkheim regarded as the type of community bond that characterized traditional pre-industrial societies. Mechanical solidarity, he affirmed, was the dominant mode by which people's behaviour was regulated in the pre-modern world. This was a form of solidarity emergent from societies in which the division of labour was static and rudimentary. In traditional society, families were the basic units of economic life; family members worked together in household enterprises, with tasks divided up on the basis of a simple sexual division of labour between husbands and fathers and male dependents on the one hand, and wives and mothers and female dependents on the other.

The domestic or familial unit that made up the household-based economy was self-subsistent or self-sufficient, catering for all of the subsistence needs of its members so that exchanges of goods or services beyond community borders were negligible. The household economy was mostly based on the land in agricultural subsistence production, where from generation to generation family members performed the same basic work roles. Community life was the stuff of extended kin or clan relations (so that community members were always personally known to each other) and of collective rituals that drew together the different families into a shared culture of norms and values and beliefs.[160]

The lack of specialized or diverse roles in the division of labour meant that virtually everyone shared the same basic interests and experiences. Moreover, because virtually everyone shared the same basic interests and experiences, this ensured that they also shared the same basic perspectives on life. Community life was also insular in the sense of being radically parochial, since confined to the village, with limited geographical mobility, the villagers rarely if at all strayed outside community borders, whereas visitors from outside were few and far between. Hence cultural horizons defining the rights and wrongs of social behaviour and moral sensibility were totalizing (in the sense of being culturally fixed or bound by community tradition and largely insulated from external influence). They were also homogenizing inasmuch as culture enforced cohesion of social life by imposing uniformity of attitudes and beliefs on community members, installing a sense of the fundamental sameness or likeness of moral sentiments that bound them together. This meant that in traditional societies, for Durkheim, there was a narrow and powerfully restrictive, indeed powerfully prescriptive group consensus on what people should or should not think or feel, on what they should or should not believe, and on how they should or should not conduct themselves.

Thus, for Durkheim, mechanical solidarity was, in short, a solidarity of sameness or of group-oneness (not of diversity and interdependence). This was a sameness of roles, identities, perspectives, and values. Social solidarity of the community or group was safeguarded simply by the fact that its members tended to think and act in very similar ways and to conform to a single cultural template. Based on a radically undeveloped division of labour, mechanical solidarity was characterized by a collectively endorsed community bond, a totalizing moral code (invariably religious in nature) that instructed community members on how to live their lives and which insisted that they do so in fundamentally the same ways.[161]

But how might the prescriptive or binding power of the collective over the individual be explained under conditions of mechanical solidarity? Durkheim's answer was that, in traditional society, based on mechanical solidarity, the collective moral sentiments that bound a community's members together tended to be high in volume, intensity, rigidity, and content. This was the opposite of the state of affairs under modern organic solidarity where collective norms and values were weak under each of these categories.

They were high in volume because the minds of individuals were almost completely suffused with the cultural standards that defined a community's way of life so that there was little scope for independent thought outside those parameters. They were high in intensity because the community members had a high degree of emotional and moral attachment to the cultural standards of their society so that deviation from these was seen as abrogation of a sacred duty. They were high in rigidity inasmuch as the cultural standards governing right from wrong action and attitude were sharply delineated so that there were starkly marked out do's and don'ts, with little room for ambivalence. Finally, they were also content-rich in a spiritual sense inasmuch as the cultural standards were represented as belonging to the order of the sacred rather than of the secular. The moral sentiments of the community or group to which the individual belonged were typically sanctioned by religion, Durkheim affirmed, so that an individual's sense of social duty was fused with a sense of religious duty.[162]

The logic of Durkheim's theory would support the perspective that in traditional societies based on mechanical solidarity there would tend to be less deviance than in modern societies based on organic solidarity. This does appear to be Durkheim's view, though he was not terribly explicit about it.[163] The reason for this would be that owing to the sameness of roles, and hence the sameness of socialization into near-identical norms and values, the scope for deviation from community-level obligations was much reduced. Where there is little scope for individualization, the capacity of individuals to do other than defer and submit to the group is considerably curtailed. Lacking a developed sense of personal identity or uniqueness, people are less able to formulate a sense of private interests that stand in clear opposition to collective ones. Yet this is necessary if deviation is to become a major part of the life of a society.

Rather, in traditional society, the collective interest is more likely to be interpreted by the group member as his or her personal interest. Thus, deviation from group norms is more difficult in communities where the purpose of the individual is to serve the community or some aspect of it. Moreover, deviation from group norms under mechanical solidarity functions to isolate and atomize the rule-breaker, because this literally places him or her outside the moral compass of the social universe he or she inhabits. The rule-breaker is individualized in a society that places no value on individualization. For this reason, the moral pressure exerted by group solidarity on the individual to avoid deviant behaviour is typically experienced as prohibitive.

Since diversity and differentiation of social roles under industrial modernity have allowed individualization to flourish (that is, an individualization based on the freedom to choose one's roles and hence identities), it is, therefore, no surprise that where this is lacking (that is, in pre-modern society), the opposite effect has been generated. Individualization by its nature must diminish the prescriptive force of community-level regulation of individual lives, since freedom to choose roles is also greater freedom to disregard social norms where these are seen to obstruct or forestall the satisfaction of personal wants. Therefore, because we have been turned into individuals by the huge variety of roles in the division of labour and by attendant rights of citizenship, which renders freedom of choice and differentiation meaningful, this also means we have more freedom to deviate. This means that there will inevitably be more deviance in modern societies than in traditional societies, whether for good or for ill. Since there is more individualism and less mechanical conformity to community values, there is far more rule-breaking. Indeed, rule-breaking becomes normalized as an aspect of everyday society.

Role specialization fragments collective cultures so that pluralized cultures replace unitary ones, and individuals may then benefit from the opening up of new vantage points from which they may formulate personal interests in opposition to collective ones. Just as individuals can pick and choose and judge between social roles, precisely because different options are available, so can they choose between if or when to follow moral or normative rules. The volume of collective sentiments, as these impact the individual consciousness, diminishes. Individualization released by the organic division of labour also empties a community's collective sentiments of their religiously prescribed status of sacredness so that the abrogation of cultural normative standards cannot incur the same intensity or energy of moral censure or punitive response as previously. Deviance is secularized, inasmuch as it is no longer sinfulness against divinity so that a key normative constraint that would deflect people from rule-breaking (fear of other-worldly as well as worldly sanctions) is undermined. Consequently, the power of collective culture to build and enforce consent also declines by virtue of the diminution of the intensity, rigidity and prescriptive moral content of its normative elements.

But, in modern industrial societies, according to Durkheim, not only does the specialized social division of labour mean there is far greater scope for people to be made into individuals, but this also makes possible a more flexible and subtle system of moral and legal rules based on citizenship. This is a system of rules that balances the need for people to exercise individual freedoms of various types with their obligations to everyone else as members of society. In modern societies, law and morality have to be ambivalent enough to allow very different groups (with different beliefs) to coexist and cooperate in the social division of labour. Law and public morality must recognize social differentiation and individual rights as well as the need to protect the community.[164]

Since the singular totalizing moral order of traditional society is replaced by "a patchwork of differentiated moral domains", and since conformity to social order is secured by mutual obligations in the division of labour rather than by prescriptive religious norms, this renders the solidarity-building normative elements that arise in industrial modernity as

> not strict codes of shared morality but what one might term "moral ground rules" – framework values such as freedom, humanism, individuality, reason and security – which form the bedrock of agreement upon which the diversity and pluralism of modern society can be built.[165]

There is also, as was noted by Michel Foucault, a relative shift away from largely retributive and coercive punitive sanctions in the classical age of sovereign power and towards those that are more hemmed in by the need of judicial authorities to accommodate the fact that community members are no longer merely subjects, that is, objects of communal service and control, but are the repositories of rights of citizenship.[166] Durkheim himself identified this shift as being from the dominance of wholly repressive law in traditional society (which he regarded as religiously sanctioned) to its partial supplanting or supplementing by restitutive law in modern society. He classified the whole of criminal or penal law in modern society as repressive, just as he did the whole of criminal law in traditional societies. But, with the development of modernity, Durkheim drew attention to the rise of parallel legal forms ("civil law, commercial law, procedural law, administrative and constitutional law"),[167] which were of the restitutive kind.

For Durkheim, the emergence of restitutive law (which requires the wrongdoer to compensate the victim for breach of contract) alongside criminal law (which punishes retributively the wrongdoer for offending against the normative order) was an indicator of the transition from mechanical to organic society.[168] Whatever the rights or wrongs of this perspective, the rise of modern citizenship is certainly associated with a transformation of criminal justice in the early modern period. The old judicial methods, typically arbitrary and excessive, based on physical punishment (torture or destruction of the body) were phased out in the eighteenth and nineteenth centuries in favour of those that were more tolerant, less severe or intense, or those which were more nuanced and differentiated, based on the suspension of liberty – or which were, as Foucault puts it, governed by the "carceral imperative".[169]

For Durkheim, the prison was the quintessentially modern method of punishment, since this was he thought consistent with the demands of moral individualism and of citizenship, which forbade harsh or excessive or cruel judicial sanctions.[170] In more recent times, of course, the carceral imperative of modern criminal justice has been conjoined with a new emphasis on reform or rehabilitation (normalization) of the wrongdoer.[171] Thus, since the moral and legal elements are more flexible and complex than in traditional societies, by virtue of which they possess less prescriptive moral force than before, and since the judicial methods are based on "softer" restitutive (disciplinary) forms of power, this means that individuals under modern conditions have greater latitude to question and dispute legal norms. By the same token, they also have the latitude to voluntarily abide by them on the basis of moral endorsement.

Economic (egoistic) individualism

As we have seen, Durkheim also recognized the emergence of *economic individualism*, which he associated with the Industrial Revolution that ushered in laissez-faire capitalism. This may be simply referred to as *capitalistic* individualism. Arguably, though, Durkheim did not give this mode of individualism its proper due, despite the dangers to the social fabric and community life that he thought it posed. This was because, as I noted earlier, he thought that, with the consolidation of organic solidarity and its associational (and moral) individualism, its negative impacts could be neutralized.

At this point, it is worth briefly revisiting Durkheim's concept of anomie. This is because anomie is the concept that Durkheim uses to explain how organic solidarity may founder, hence tipping society or some part of it into a disordered or "pathological" state. By anomie, Durkheim, meant a situation where there is a precipitous decline in the power of regulatory norms to solidarize a society's members so that these are no longer effective in deflecting people from deviant behaviour. Anomie is therefore indicative of decivilization. Thus, rapidly escalating rates and volumes of crime and disorder are suggestive that society or a sphere of society is entering an anomic state. An anomic society or sphere of society would be one where a failure of controlling norms threatens (through escalating lawlessness and social conflict) its own reproduction.

For Durkheim, anomie became a major problem in Europe starting from the period of modernization that brought industrial societies into being, owing to the destruction of traditional communal society by rapid processes of urbanization and industrialization. This was because the rapidity of the changes undermined the modes of solidarity that had previously given meaning and unity to community life and individual lives. Industrialization and urbanization dissolved mechanical solidarity, by virtue of undermining traditional society, but without establishing in its place a new inclusive regulatory moral and normative framework that would reintegrate society, re-establish social bonds, and place social order on a secure foundation. As Durkheim put it: "The scale is upset; but a new scale cannot be immediately improvised. Time is required for the public conscience to reclassify men [sic] and things".[172]

Swept along by industrialization, people were flung into towns and cities as a collection of strangers without clear guidelines about their duties or obligations to each other and without access to resources beyond those they must generate from their own private labours. The securities of small-scale village society – based on stable traditional work, the reciprocal obligations of landlord and tenant, and the old system of parish "outdoor" relief to support community members when harvests were poor – were swept away, to be replaced by the new insecurities of the cash nexus, the logic of hire and fire governed by the impersonal laws of market supply and demand. In the absence of moral regulation, a culture of egoism emerged from the daily competitive struggle to prosper or survive in the new urban centres. In short, mechanical solidarity was undone but without organic solidarity yet being established, so in the period of industrialization, people lost a sense of moral purpose and communal responsibility for each other, just as society was wracked by major group conflicts for access to the new bounties of material resources that industrial production had generated.

But Durkheim also argued that the threat of anomie was not confined to the birth of industrial society but would be one that continued to haunt it in its developed form. This is because industrial modernity is ephemeral, in constant flux and change, so the ever-evolving social division of labour and attendant production of new role-based subgroups may outstrip existent regulatory frameworks which forever are playing catch-up.[173] Yet, as we have seen, Durkheim seems clear enough that a major cause of the anomic state of society during the Industrial Revolution and thereafter, if not the major cause of it, was the specific mode of economy (free-market capitalism) that was associated with industrialization. Indeed, according to Durkheim, this mode of economy was a major obstacle to society achieving for itself a state of organic solidarity. This was because this was a type of capitalism (based on free trade, unregulated labour markets, and unjust employer–employee contracts) that was especially promotive of the egoism of materialism and was prone to all manner of disequilibria stemming from its emancipation from all forms of collective regulation in the service of social justice.[174]

Capitalism, opined Durkheim, if it was not regulated by the state and civic organizations, would not be capable of inculcating in people a sense of the mutual obligations that the "organic" interdependence of their roles in industrial society made possible. Rather, in the absence of collective normative regulatory control, individuals would lack the resources to resist seeing economic life as a kind of war of all against all. This was for the simple reason that free-market capitalism is based on unbridled economic competition for purely material rewards and also represents the division of labour as a wholly economic benefit and commercial private self-interest as the source of economic success.[175] Under "pure" (private free-market) capitalism, therefore, it is not simply that participation of people in the "rat race" (competition between individuals in the service of their own narrow self-interest or those of their kin) is ideologized as functionally indispensable to rational economic order. Rather, it is also that this is thrust upon them by their daily experience of market-mediated competition, whether this competition be motivated by the pressure to maintain or enhance social status measured in material terms or to merely "make ends meet".

According to Durkheim, therefore, the anomies threatened by laissez-faire capitalism stemmed from the failure of its agents (buyers and sellers of various kinds of commodities) to recognize the system's own normative and moral foundations in the mutual obligations generated by the interdependence of roles in the modern industrial division of labour. This made it (capitalism) a force that obstructed or undermined rather than facilitated the moral and normative regulation of society. Since, in Durkheim's view, the problem of modern society was that the sources of organic solidarity were occluded so that there was a lack of moralization of the economic sphere in particular, the solution was, therefore, to re-moralize the social division of labour.

To achieve this, Durkheim thought that major and specific institutional reforms were necessary. Firstly, democratization of the industrial sphere and state regulation of economic competition (prices, profits, and wages). Consequently, Durkheim recommended that exchange relations be situated within a normative and valuational framework supervised by the state that went beyond the merely contractual. Rather, this would be based on reciprocal agreements between the various parties on what were fair rewards or returns for the various services or functions.[176] Durkheim also argued that the economy should be overseen by elected boards formed from occupational associations.[177] These would cover each branch of industry and would be made up of representatives of consumer groups, employers, and trade unions. These boards would "regulate ... relations of employers and employees – conditions of labour, wages and salaries, relations of competitors to one another, and so on".[178]

Such would ensure that there was a balance of power between the interests of employers, employees and general citizens so that unjust contracts perpetuating the forced division of labour and industrial conflict were undone. This would also rein in egoistic individualism by overcoming the atomism of narrow occupational specialisms and by placing moral checks (rooted in social consensus on "reasonable expectations") on personal aspirations for material success.

Secondly, encourage occupational groups to turn themselves into professional associations with their own distinctive codes of ethics. That (that is, the professionalization of roles in the occupational sphere) was necessary, Durkheim opined, in order to make sure these groups served the public interest rather than simply their own private interests, hence offsetting the egoism encouraged by market-mediated work roles.[179] Thirdly, re-establish a baseline framework of societal-wide norms and values, which all groups in society would subscribe to, because they were those that fit with the needs of organic solidarity. This would distil the unity-in-difference (individuality, diversity, pluralism) that was implicit in the modern division of labour. For this to happen, it was necessary for the state to take upon itself the task of implementing a universal compulsory secular system of education by which core moral values as well as those fundamental cognitive, technical, and social skills needed for role specialization may be installed in the young.[180]

Finally, modern society needed to be meritocratized. The state must also act to ensure that there was equality of opportunity in society. This meant abolishing all forms of hereditary privilege or status advantage – including the arbitrary rules informed by "distinctions" or "prejudices" that blocked access to certain networks or elite professions, but especially inheritance of wealth or property through the family line. As Durkheim observed:

> There cannot be rich and poor at birth without there being unjust contracts ... If one class of society is obliged, in order to live, to take any price for its services, while another class can abstain from such action thanks to resources at its disposal which, however, are not necessarily due to any social superiority, the second has an unjust advantage over the first in law.[181]

If people saw their opportunities for social advancement cut off unfairly, Durkheim argued, they would withdraw their allegiance to normative order. The normative order would be undermined because it would be incompatible with collective moral sentiments. So, the abolition of "the anomie of injustice"[182] was necessary to consolidate a properly organic society.

As noted earlier, Durkheim argued that, although organic solidarity was the "normal" or "natural" state to which modern society gravitated, there were also abnormal or deviant forms of the social division of labour that may partially obstruct or deflect it from attaining its ideal state. But since he was unable to theorize how one might distinguish between normal and abnormal (pathological) states of any given type of society, this raises the question of how the supposed normalcy of organic solidarity as an integral aspect of modern civilization can be established. The problem is an acute one, for the simple reason that capitalist modernity since Durkheim's death has not transcended the range of acute social problems that he himself diagnosed and which he thought would be overcome by the consolidation of organic solidarity. Rather, these problems have since been spread far and wide by the internationalization of capitalism.

This means that organic solidarity has not been empirically validated – not if its existence is to be inferred from its (positive) effects, as Durkheim argued it ought. These supposedly residual problems of modernity were those Durkheim attributed to the abnormal forms of the division of labour – the anomic and forced types of social differentiation. These included: the acquisitive egoism encouraged by economic competition along with the discontents of secular materialism (that is, "insatiable appetites" for money and possessions that can never be fulfilled); recurrent financial and trade crises; asymmetrical bargaining power between capitalists and workers in the marketplace (hence unjust contracts); and limited opportunities for upward social mobility for those at the wrong end of the class structure (hence status-frustration for those excluded from roles or positions their talents merited).

These problems (along with many others – most notably those of oppression and disadvantage by ethnicity and gender) have proven so intractable, despite the continued development of the system, that any doubt that these are not structural must be dispelled. Since this is so, the compatibility of a capitalist society and economy with Durkheim's organic solidarity appears doubtful. Rather, the evidence is point-ing the other way. The so-called abnormal forms of the division of labour are com-monplace. For that reason, these may be seen as typical, even though doubtless the effects of these have been somewhat, to varying degrees, reduced over the past 100 years.

Of course, it could be argued that the failure of modern society to attain an organic state does not expose a failure of Durkheim's sociology of modernity but rather a historical failure of politics that was hardly inevitable. This would be the failure of state and governance in the advanced societies to introduce the range of reforms that Durkheim considered necessary to establish organicism and deci-sively see off the threat of the anomic and forced divisions of labour. That there has been a failure of politics is undeniable. This has been a historical failure of political power to confront economic power. But the failure of politics itself confirms the fundamental weakness of Durkheim's theoretical perspective on modern society since this begs the question of its cause.

Durkheim could specify no mechanism by which the "cult of the individual" (his notion that under modernity the individual is made sacred rather than the com-munity as under tradition) would necessarily commit people to reciprocal obliga-tions. Organic solidarity was not and could not, he rightly concluded, be a "given" of the modernization process. Individuals who recognize themselves as sacrosanct are not compelled to extend this recognition to others, especially in a market-mediated society where livelihoods are won or lost in competitive exchange. So, organic solidarity could only be a political project that must be won at the expense of property and capital. Bringing it into being required deploying the power of the state to substantially erode or curtail the liberties of ownership and the market. Yet the modern liberal-democratic state was never going to commit to that project. Durkheim could not see this, however, owing to his failure to recognize the class character of the state and the structural interdependence of state and capital under modern conditions.[183]

And so it came to pass. States rarely attempted the kind of close regulation of capitalist markets to ensure a fair balance between prices, wages, and profits that Durkheim wanted to see. Income policies were occasionally implemented, but to defend profits against wages, not vice versa.[184] The occupational associations and elected industrial boards never anywhere got started. Even at the height of peace-time state-corporatism and of the mixed economy in the 1950s and 1960s, these did not materialize. In countries such as the UK, public ownership assumed the corporate form, with managers recruited from the private sector (typically former owners). At best there was minority trade union representation on the boards of certain nationalized companies.[185] This was of course swept away in the neoliberal era, along with the nationalized industries, in an orgy of privatizations.

Nor was the "anomie of injustice" abolished. Hereditary inter-generational transmission of property and wealth was never challenged, since that would be an affront to free competition that had bestowed these bounties. Postwar welfare states in the developed countries succeeded in preventing the immiseration of the poor but did not particularly reduce social inequalities. This was unsurprising because income redistribution was not the intention of welfare politics in this era. Postwar economic growth together with strong labour organization and progressive taxation did a better job of reducing the income gap between the wealthy and unionized workers. But this, as we have seen, succeeded only in ameliorating inequality not substantially reducing it, whereas the lowest income earners and those people dependent on welfare benefits were left behind. These limited gains were then also reversed in the neoliberal age that saw private-corporate free-market capitalism resurgent.

Universal schooling was established, of course, but this was hardly classless, nor always and everywhere secular, nor particularly a vehicle for humanistic or cosmopolitan values. Education systems have tended to reflect if not actively reproduce the social hierarchies and class relations of the societies of which they are a part and are heavily skewed towards functioning as providers of exploitable human resources for capitalist employers.[186] The occupational structure certainly has undergone a considerable degree of professionalization, but professionalization has not always been accompanied by the kinds of ethics (of selfless or altruistic public duty) that are community-building. Often, professionalism has been deployed as a market strategy of occupational groups to artificially limit access to their own trades, restrict the supply of their services, preserve inflated material rewards and social status, or define itself instrumentally in terms of technical performativity.[187]

This forces us to confront a conclusion that Durkheim's sociology of modernity shied away from. This is that a major, if not *the* major driver of individualization, or of an especially potent form of it, is the capitalist economic system. This was the case when Durkheim was alive and it has remained so ever since. The worldwide dominance of the capitalist mode means that everywhere, economic life and material prosperity (the wealth of nations and the well-being of peoples) are governed by what Marx understood as the law of value. This is, as he puts it, "the labour-time required to produce any use-value under the conditions of production normal for a given society and with the average degree of skill and intensity of labour prevalent in that society".[188] This, in other words, is *socially necessary* labour time, the logic of competitive exchange.[189] This means that rational economic life under capitalism is subverted because the satisfaction of collective human needs is secondary or coincidental to the profit motive that drives the system. Subsistence production, production for human and community needs, and use-value as the governing principle of economic life are supplanted by commodity production, production for corporate interest and for private profit, the self-expansion of capital, or the optimization of exchange value.

The economic mode of individualism that capitalism supports is certainly a primary force of decivilization. This is because it is essentially acquisitive or egoistic, based as it is on the pursuit of self-interest. This is also decivilizing in the sense that it is pursued (and can only be pursued) for purposes other than those of community interest, since capitalism allocates resources individually (in profits or wages or other entitlements) rather than collectively, through asymmetric opportunity structures and on the basis of market competition or state rationing.[190]

Market relations and miserly rationing of public goods (such as access to welfare resources) exert pressure on wage workers to view each other as competitors for jobs, homes, healthcare, and so on. At the same, inter-capitalist competition for control of markets and to generate profits for reinvestment compels companies to reduce labour costs so that productivity gains outstrip wage increases.

Under capitalism, any coincidence of self-interest (that is, business interest) with social interest is accidental rather than intended, as this is governed by the "hidden hand" of the market. This undoubtedly provides an important part of the explanation of why modern capitalist societies generate large volumes of especially (though not exclusively) economically motivated criminality at all levels of the social structure, albeit for reasons of cause or conditioning that differ for people in accordance with their position in the class structure.[191] Thus, capitalism facilitates, in equal measure, crimes of the rich and powerful (that is, of accumulation and domination) and of the powerless and poor (that is, of subsistence and estrangement).[192]

Capitalism is individualizing and decivilizing because it transforms community or collective property into private property and renders public welfare dependent on the success of private commercial enterprise. Capitalism is individualizing and decivilizing because its key structural forms (private ownership, commodity production, and wage labour) must generate vast asymmetries in the distribution of allocative resources. These ensure that class-based inequalities will grow unless the state intervenes to hold these in check or unless the labour unions are strong and resolute enough (which they rarely are) to win for workers through industrial action wage rises that are commensurate to productivity growth. The law of value, whereby the pressure of capitalist competition for profits and markets forces each unit of capital (that is, each business enterprise) to undermine or undercut each other by seeking out methods of reducing labour costs to below the social average that prevails in any particular branch of production, is exactly the force that animates this dynamic.[193]

This is why there is underconsumption for workers and their families on the one hand (since the subordination of wages to profits ensures that these may purchase only a declining proportion of the total economic output of labour)[194] just as there is over-accumulation of capital on the other (as the prodigious surpluses grow faster than the opportunities to profitably reinvest them).[195] The result is the manufacture of artificial resource stress for the majority subordinate class alongside the alienations wrought by intra-class competition for access to scarce resources, which exacerbates the tendencies towards prioritization of atomistic self-interest and egoistic individualism over collective societal interest.[196] Capitalism is thus individualizing and decivilizing because it splits or fractures hitherto relatively homogeneous communities into a myriad of atomized competitors (whether individuals or different kinds of groups) on the terrain of various markets – those for status or income from the alienation of labour capacity, or those for access to housing or social security or health care or education resources.

Capitalism, for these reasons, is an economic way of life that is actively corrosive of the social bond, of community solidarity, of collective public morality, of Durkheim's organic solidarity. This is owing to the economic pressures, constraints and imperatives the system imposes on its agents (whether these be state actors, wageworkers, small business owners, or corporate bosses) to prioritize private interests over public interests. The relevance of this to the COVID-19 crisis and its management is obvious. This is of course in the negative sense that capitalism itself places major constraints on the prospects of success for any community-based response aimed at curbing the spread of the virus that relies on social solidarity, a sense of public duty, or on collective altruism. Yet capitalism does not and cannot undermine these things altogether. This is owing to the basic sociality of human beings as a natural kind or "species being", which ensures that basic sympathy and empathy for others is not simply dissolved.[197] Nonetheless, capitalism is certainly a force that interrupts, disrupts, and counteracts the translation of these human sentiments into actual social behaviour.

Thus, as far as the current pandemic is concerned, millions of workers worldwide (despite furlough schemes in some countries) had impelling economic motives to carry on going to work wherever opportunity allowed, even if symptomatic, because otherwise their jobs and livelihoods were under threat. They would also be incentivized by market rationality to eschew testing or disregard test results if these were the "wrong" ones. For them – many of whom would be struggling to make ends meet, especially if precarious "gig" workers – placing public interest before self-interest was a luxury they could not afford. Non-compliance to public health restrictions, where these were legally mandated, would then, wholly plausibly, be a case of Richard Quinney's "crimes of subsistence".[198]

Turning now to the capitalist employers of wage labour. They could see, during the lockdowns and all the restrictions around the lockdowns, only harm to profits and markets, so governments had to be actively lobbied to dismantle these at the first opportunity, irrespective of the public health situation. (Neoliberal governments – those faithful servants of corporate capital – were only too happy to oblige as soon as the peaks of the immediate crises were passed). This was just as these employers browbeat reluctant risk-averse employees to switch from home-working to office working or otherwise return to the fold if homeworking was not feasible. Doubtless, some smaller businesses (which were much less protected by government aid schemes than were the corporations) risked legal sanction during the lockdowns by carrying on as before, pulling employees on site. This would be in order to opportunistically encroach on the markets of competitors not open for business or simply to survive. As for the general population, many people would have been incentivized to ignore stay-at-home guidance or disregard social distancing requirements on the basis of favourable cost-benefit calculations of personal risk (and of risk to loved ones) without consideration of risks to an anonymous "public". This, after all, was culturally mandated by economic individualism.

Consumerist individualism

Neither Marx nor Durkheim lived to witness the ascendancy of consumer capitalism, of course. The capitalism that they were familiar with was a much more austere capitalism of production. However, in more recent times, the system is also individualizing in that it creates mass consumer markets that are indispensable to its own reproduction. This has given rise to *consumerist individualism.*

Even though capitalism is driven to subordinate consumption to accumulation, it must also seek out ways of expanding consumption to find markets for its goods and services so that surpluses can be valorized as profits. Capitalist "globalization" has in part been driven by the need for large-scale monopoly capital to escape dependence on restricted home markets where productive capacity has radically outstripped local demand for its outputs.[199] To survive, therefore, capitalism was compelled to expand, and to expand it had to mobilize people as consumers.[200] Indispensable to the viability of this consumer capitalism became the promulgation (by media capitalism, the advertising industries, and corporate branding) of the culture ideology of consumerism.[201] The consolidation of this ideology worldwide has opened up huge new markets that cater for people acting on the basis of what in a different context have been described as subterranean values – the pursuit of "thrills and spills", fun and games in leisure.[202]

Consumer culture since World War Two was thus built on a profusion or super-abundance of objects and attendant signs with which individuals were extolled and interpellated to form attachments.[203] In their daily lives, particularly in affluent societies but also in the urban hubs of the developing world, people had ever-growing opportunities to interact more with things than with people, or with things *instead* of people (whether objects on the supermarket shelves or the images on the TV screen), or with people *as* things (e.g. sexualized bodies, vendors of consumables, etc.).[204] The shopping mall along with the television emerged as the locus of a new leisure society, with shopping and TV-viewing becoming by far the most popular and frequent types of leisure or consumption activity in developed countries and more generally. Most recently, with the rise of the internet and cyberspace, a vast new opportunity structure for virtual consumer-oriented leisure has been opened. This has given fresh impetus to individualized and privatized entertainment and acquisition.[205]

Shopping malls became the centrepiece of "public" space and "community" life, and in so doing marked a diminution of both. This was for two main reasons. Firstly, because malls are typically corporately owned sites, exist only for commerce, and typically discourage or even forbid any other use of that space. Secondly, actors as shoppers function in these spaces as consumerist atoms or monads, as individuated agents of commerce, engaging in one-to-one transactions with anonymous commodity providers. In doing so, they participate in subject-object relations rather than interpersonal ones, in order to satisfy privatized (personal or familial) wants. As such, the consumer as shopper is a wholly privatized and atomized subject, because his or her relations with things are in effect relations with his or her own desires, albeit desires that are incited by consumer ideology. Consumerism is primarily self-centred in that its motive and object of choice is one's own, at best influenced only by those who are part of the individual's intimate network, screening out all other social or public influences.

As Jean Baudrillard explains, consumerism developed as a system of signification. This was a "system of objects", assembled in categories, with each category linked relationally to or correlated with consumerist signs that defined their life-style appeal in the eyes of those who would purchase them.[206] This system of con-sumerism, or mode of consumption, has been key in fermenting in peoples across the world the psychic motivational dispositions to wish to consume, not simply or primarily for the sake of satisfying objective material needs but for a range of other reasons: to acquire, for example, high status in the ever-proliferating style or taste hierarchies, or to differentiate themselves from others as particular (and often superior) kinds of cultural agents. Or, it was to realize through the use of lifestyle and leisure commodities purely hedonistic or libidinal pleasures, or to simply be a player where culture is no more than games so that "sporting a fixed taste and nar-rowing one's choices could be only a symptom of deprivation and retardation ... not the 'culturally correct' model of conduct ... likely to be embraced and practised by those aiming at the top".[207]

Consumerism as culture functions to refer all problems of living to the mar-ket so that these may be resolved by buying or selling remedies. Privatizing pub-lic issues and individualizing social tasks represents a further exorbitation of the individual as a sovereign artificer.[208] This is because consumerism demands that affirmation of personal identity and social status is realized not through reciprocal social interactions, or through associative work, or through participation in com-munity relations, but through the relations that atomized selves initiate with objects of desire (that is, commodities as the bearers of lifestyle images that the consumer wishes to personify).

> Neither a class in itself nor for itself, the mass now engages with consumer-ism individually, together – divided, they shop. Its members have no inter-ests, no concern for their "wellbeing", no collective beliefs, community or identity they can call their own.[209]

Therefore, this "consumer syndrome" or "consumer attitude" (as Bauman calls it),[210] this marketized way of life, aims to establish the asocial uniqueness of the individual as a matter of his or her choices of style or taste, rather than his or her substantive obligations (e.g. moral or political or interpersonal affiliations). Indeed, it aspires to establish a person's individuality through his or her styles of and tastes in largely hedonistic pursuits, sensation-seeking, and the pleasure principle, rather than through his or her personification in social roles of normative commitments (such as to a professional vocation or to a political cause or to some form of public service).

This consumerism, as Baudrillard tells, makes its appeal through seduction, as this is experienced by individuals as obscene fascination.[211] Seduction replaces meaning because the market-mediated way of life replaces being with having, whereas having reduces to ephemerality and is forever radically incomplete. This is because the having is of consumables that are no sooner acquired than used, discarded, replaced, or upgraded, along with the identities they mark out. Consumer syndrome, *homo consumus*, accommodates or reconciles its subjects to lives without meaning. This is because it educates that life has no purpose beyond sensation-seeking, that consumption will fulfil that need for sensation, and that the sense of personal incompleteness that accompanies consumption can be plugged only with more consumption.[212]

As Bauman suggests, the appeal of consumerism is that what it instructs imposes an order of structure on lives that are left increasingly in "liquid times" to fend for themselves without the securities of stable employment, community support networks, or inclusive welfare systems.[213] Since consumption is a matter of personal choice, exercised in a microsystem where an atomized subject relates to a constellation of things only as extensions of his or her desire, the individual has a sense of control over this circumscribed personal sphere where control elsewhere is lacking.[214] This is also obscenity in so far as the commodification of culture renders people's experience of it as trivial or superficial, an encounter with surfaces or appearances since commodities as things contain no hidden mysteries or deeper meanings beyond the phenomenal and sensational. This is obscene too in the sense of the voyeuristic since commodification of culture demands that the personal and taboo be rendered phenomenal and transparent so that these too may be consumable as objects of sensation.[215]

The individualization wrought by the commodification of culture as objects of consumption is one that is rooted in fetishism. The fetishism of commodities, as Marx explained, consists of the misreading of human and social relations between people as material relations between things:

> The mysterious character of the commodity-form consists therefore ... in the fact that the commodity reflects the social characteristics of men's [*sic*] own labour as objective characteristics of the products themselves, as the socio-natural properties of these things ... The commodity-form, and the value-relation of the products of labour within which it appears ... is nothing but the definite social relation between men [*sic*] themselves which assumes here, for them, the fantastic form of a relation between things.[216]

This may also be seen as the subordination of human relations to object relations, which for Marx was the key aspect of alienated labour. For Marx, "although private property appears to be the basis and cause of alienated labour, it is rather a consequence of the latter",[217] since capitalist property is made from appropriated labour time objectified as things (money, commodities, means of production). Alienated labour, as Marx put it, could not be "otherwise in a mode of production in which the labourer exists to satisfy the needs of self-expansion of existing values, instead of, on the contrary, material wealth existing to satisfy the needs of development ... of the labourer".[218]

Under consumerism, social relations between subjects are increasingly converted into the mere means of entering into relations with things, that is, the acquisition and exploitation of things as objects of consumption. Such can only degrade human relations, social solidarity, and community obligations. Indeed, the culture ideology of consumerism can only exacerbate the longstanding tendency of capitalist commodity cultures to encourage people to adopt an instrumental view of each other as well as of things (whether artefacts of nature or manufactured goods or services), as objects of utility or resources of various kinds.

For example, this may encourage a depersonalized view of people as wholly or largely objects of sexual pleasure; hence the burgeoning pornography industries, sex tourism, and the acquisition of "trophy wives" by rich Westerners. For example, this may allow people to be regarded as objects of economic exploitation: hence the far from opposite poles of "normalized" labour-subordination in "legitimate" corporate enterprises, on the one hand, and the trafficking of children and women for sweatshop enterprise or domestic servitude, on the other. For example, this may sanction the treatment of people as objects of political or ideological manipulation: hence the mobilization of populations by state authorities to serve strategic goals through misinformation, withholding of information, propagandizing, or other devices.

This sociological critique of consumerist individualism is powerful and persuasive. Yet a problem with this critical sociological reading of contemporary culture, especially in the work of Bauman and Baudrillard, is that it represents its negative impacts as almost irresistible forces so that consumerism is seen as having succeeded completely in transforming contemporary citizenries into passive agents of capitalist reproduction. This, I suggest, is a one-sided reading, which founders for two main reasons.

Firstly, because it is yet another species of sociological imperialism – the latest in a long series. To be plausible, this kind of perspective has to embrace an over-social subject, in the sense of positing an individual personality who is cultural "all the way down", a passive object of socialization or enculturation. But individuals are more than social selves. They are also beings of a natural kind, bearers of a definite species being, rooted in biological reality, which is the product of a long history of natural evolution. This human nature that links people together as a common species is not merely definable in terms of its plasticity or flexibility, as sociological imperialists would have it – and so humans are not like Durkheim's indeterminate material or Louis Althusser's *tabula rasa* until filled with social and cultural content. Rather, human nature is such that it supports behavioural, psychological, and cultural plasticity rather than being definable as such, and this is owing to its determinate structured properties.[219]

These properties include a specific range of capacities: sociality (humans are by nature communal beings who can individuate themselves only in the context of society),[220] intelligence, self-consciousness, rationality, language, and constitutive labour. These properties also include a range of objective physiological and psychological needs (for sufficient food, clothing, and shelter maintain the physical health of the organism, for love and intimate relations, for dis-alienated labour, for community and fellowship, for intellectual and emotional self-development, and for as much personal freedom as is objectively possible within material-social and nature-imposed constraints). And they also include a range of emotional of affective dispositions that support some basic behavioural norms shared by human beings in all known human societies.[221] Now, if the social theorist is to avoid explanatory tautologies when accounting for the possibility of human society and of social history, the capacities must be treated as elements of human reality rather than of specific contingent sociocultural realities. This is for the simple reason that their indispensability to society and culture is transcendentally given.

Human plasticity (of behaviour, of attitudes, of mores, of social and cultural forms) cannot be its own explanation but must be rooted in some antecedent set of conditions that make it possible. For sure, actual social and community life in an actual society or community is necessary to distil or grow human properties, but this does not make these properties products of society, not least because it is an integral part of a human being to be a social or communal being. Rather, humans have to possess certain of these properties as capacities (that is, intelligence, abstraction, self-consciousness) in order for their socialization or enculturation into the ways of their society or culture to even get started,[222] whereas others (that is, sociality and hence constitutive social labour) are exactly conditions of existence of social and cultural evolution.[223]

As for human properties as emotional or affectual dispositions, these are established as elements of human nature rather than as a gift of society by virtue of their universality. These are "cultural universals" precisely because they are not socially or culturally relative but are found wherever humans are. Cultural universals are universal because they are rooted in transcendental human emotions. Complex language, family and kin relations, marriage, incest prohibition, hygiene rules, art, music, dancing, storytelling, bodily ornament, gift-giving and gift-taking, game-playing, jokes and humour, etc. – these are integral to every known human society.[224] But, at a more elementary level, directly affectual actions have always been the bedrock of social life. Loving, sympathizing, empathizing, identifying, trusting, solidarizing, and committing (including acts of reciprocal altruism) – these are forms of behaviour that hold societies together, even societies such as ours whose organizational features and formal ideologies run counter to these affectual behaviours. This is because these are energized and motivated by basic human needs and psychological dispositions.[225]

An emotional attachment to egalitarianism and distrust of hierarchy has also been a pervasive feature of popular sentiments across the range of "civilized" (state- and class-based) societies. This has translated everywhere into norms of distributive justice, which are typically motivated by the needs of powerholders to legitimize social inequalities and unjust practices that serve their socially structured interests.[226] Of course, humans are as capable of negative emotions – hate, fear, anger, greed, selfishness, etc. – as they are of positive ones. And, of course, the emotional negativa will support equally negative acts, such as those of oppression or discrimination or interpersonal violence. But there is a sense in which for human beings the negative passions are parasitic on the positive ones.

This is because the latter arise from contingencies of society or culture (resource stress, social inequalities, group competition, ideologies legitimizing patterns of advantage and disadvantage, etc.) or from contingencies of personal life (e.g. being oppressed or victimized or abused or neglected), whereas the latter are emergent properties of the self-conscious sociality of humanity's species being. Thus, one important obstacle to the total absorption of people today in a culture of consumerism and commodification is that such a culture can never fulfil their fundamental needs – for sociality, for community, for fairness, for justice, for the exercise of creativity and imagination, for all-round self-development – since these needs are integral to humans as a natural kind.

Secondly, the impact of consumerism in shaping modern subjectivities and identities is partially offset by the fact that individuals have a rich diversity of social and other experiences to draw on other than lifestyle consumption (e.g. of relations of kinship and intimacy, of workplace and professional associations, of peer group relations, of gender relations, of class membership, of physical and practical interactions with natural-kind things, and so on). These other experiences act as mediators of personality and self and also exert directional guidance on one's self-constitution as a particular kind of social or cultural or political subject.[227] These experiences may include those of a social kind which are quite at odds with consumer freedom and media-spun hyper-realities. For example, those of unemployment, social exclusion, low-paid casualized employment, or simply restricted household budgets owing to child-rearing costs, or the burden of financially supporting elderly or infirm dependents, or the need to save funds for a mortgage – all of which curtail lifestyle consumption opportunities fairly radically. Such experiences may foster resentments over blocked opportunities for lifestyle freedoms enjoyed by others,[228] or they may inspire either a negative (reactively formed) or positive rejection of consumer values.[229]

But cultural experiences may also mitigate against the absorption of the individual by the culture ideology of consumerism, for the simple reason that not all of culture is commodified, not even in the corporate age. There are still aspects of culture that cater for cultural needs or wants other than the affirmation of individual status through lifestyle (e.g. health and education), or which mobilize resources of critique against corporatism and consumerism on the grounds of their ecological or human costs, or which appellate us as moral altruistic subjects (e.g. as opponents of injustice and champions of cosmopolitan inclusivity). Even much of leisure today cannot be said to be commodity-based or consumer-status-oriented. Walking, gardening, reading, keeping a diary, stargazing, and so on – these would not typically fall into that category. Even popular pastimes that are mediated by commodities (such as pubbing or clubbing) are not typically motivated by the desire to consume commodities (e.g. alcohol or other leisure drugs) but are more usually motivated simply by the desire to socialize or participate in some kind of group activity. Sometimes people hit the dancefloor simply because they enjoy dancing.

However, none of this means that the radical critique of capitalist-driven consumerism is misplaced. Far from it. This is a powerful, developed, defensible critique of the dehumanizing logic of this culture. The problem is not that the critique of consumerism is mistaken, but that the goals of this culture are regarded as almost wholly accomplished. This is owing to errors of social theory that themselves degrade and debase the targets and victims of consumer ideology. Consumer culture itself at the point of production is guilty as charged.

Moreover, clearly this culture does have negative impacts on those who are exposed to its enchantments and seductions, as the radical critics rightly diagnose.

Consumerism is a corrosive force – of subjectivities and communities and of inclusive socialities. It promises consumers what it cannot possibly deliver: freedom and personal fulfilment by consuming life rather than by living it. Nonetheless, people are not cultural dopes or cultural dupes. They are capable of exercising critical judgements. They have inner and outer resources to draw upon that would allow them to resist or reproach, partially or in whole, the negative impacts of this culture. And where resources of resistance exist there will always be those who will take them up, especially given the spiritual emptiness of the market-mediated consumerist way of life.

Despite this, a generally positive reading of the impact of consumer culture on people's lives and consciousness has recently become the order of the day. This has been under the auspices of postmodernist social theory, and it is a development that evidences the way in which mainstream sociology of culture (or cultural studies) has accommodated itself to cultural power. As neoliberal governance and corporate "globalization" have in recent decades consolidated their worldwide grip, and as this process has encountered little organized political resistance (though much misery on the wrong side of the class divides), it is unsurprising that a sociology that has made a fetish of the immediate and the fashionable wishes to find virtue in the cultural forms it has spawned. This is not least because the course of acquiescence is an intellectually undemanding endeavour, whereas swimming with the tide of power rather than against it is politically easier. This also has the added attraction of permitting poseurs to whoop it up on consumerism with a clear conscience since this is endorsed by cutting-edge social theory. Such entails a kind of "forgetting" of the critiques that have been made, or their dismissal as one-sided, since there is no serious attempt to engage with them.

The postmodern embrace of consumer culture focuses on the idea of commodification as a process that allows the pluralization and differentiation of consumption so that individuals have greater latitude to determine their own lifestyles. This then represents and lauds, it is claimed, freedom as a "lifestyle choice" or "lifestyle opportunity" as a strategy of life by means of which people make of themselves by way of their consumer preferences in the subjects they wish to be and situate themselves voluntarily in the groups they wish to be identified with.[230] Leisure, it is argued, is made into an end in itself, an aesthetic of existence, rather than into a means for achieving some other goal, such as relaxation and replenishment of the body's spiritual and physical energies, or self-education, or improved health and fitness.[231]

This focuses also on the idea that consumerism is in a sense inclusive and democratic because it detaches lifestyle choices from specific social groups (such as class membership, gender, ethnicity, or age) so that choices are not constrained (or are very much less constrained) by group pressures or social hierarchies than hitherto; that is, these are unconstrained or less beholden by the need to adapt to the expectations of others.[232] A further theme of this kind of work is that consumerism is as much a force that facilitates sociality as it does individuality since a person's consumer choices not only distinguish his or her lifestyle from others but also solidarize the chosen lifestyle with others who also embrace it. Consumerism is, in short, a means by which people fulfil their desire to be "part of a crowd" as well as a unique self-subsistent individual.[233]

The problems with this approach are manifold – and many of these are illuminated by the previous discussion. These will now be briefly summarized. The argument that consumerism is unreservedly a force for pluralization, differentiation and democratization of lifestyle founders on the fact that those who would consume do not have the same capacities for consumption. These capacities are profoundly structured by economic and social inequalities that show no sign of abating. Purchasing power in the cultural marketplace is thus asymmetric so that although there is something purchasable for most within the "system of objects", there is also much else that only the wealthy can afford.[234]

This is why the developed countries (which contain less than 16 percent of the world's population) account for 80 percent of total global consumption, whereas low-income countries (home to approximately 32 percent of the world's population) account for only three percent.[235] The real imbalance in consumption is even much greater than these statistics indicate because in rich countries most people are not rich, and very many are poor, so if consumption was calculated on the basis of class on a world scale, the asymmetries would be far higher, and the proportion of people at the high end the consumption spectrum would shrink dramatically, whereas the proportion of those at the low end would increase equally dramatically.

In the UK, for example, the bulk of spending by the average income household is devoted to essential consumption rather than to lifestyle consumption. Spending on transport, housing, utilities, and subsistence amounts to 45.1 percent of it. If you factor in clothing and footwear, communication, miscellaneous services (which would include childcare), health, and "other expenses", this would amount to 71.4 percent of total household expenditure. Of course, some of this would fit the category of lifestyle or leisure or identity-affirming expenditure, though more likely most would not, not for most families. By contrast, only 21.7 percent of the average UK household spending is on items that may be loosely interpreted as status- and lifestyle-affirming: recreation and culture, restaurants, and hotels.[236]

Again, these figures obscure as much as they illuminate, for if the average income household spends less than a quarter of its income on lifestyle commodities, then low-income households will spend very much less than this – and a vast majority of UK households have incomes below the current average of £35,900 per annum. The median household income in the UK is £29,600 per annum, so 50 percent of UK households make a maximum of up to that amount while 50 percent make more.[237] Data cited earlier has shown that the poorest UK households have experienced a decline in their median income of 4.3 percent between 2017 and 2019 owing to benefits cuts and freezes,[238] which is the most recent incarnation of a long-run pattern of growing inequalities of wealth and income since the 1980s. This would appear to place fairly stringent constraints on the lifestyle consumerism of many. The poorest households currently spend just seven percent of their income on restaurants and hotels (£18.20 per week), for example, whereas the richest spend 10 percent (£110.60 per week) of theirs.[239]

Addressing the class-based obstacles to lifestyle consumerism is important, because the outputs of consumer culture are commodities produced for sale, and these outputs are ranked in hierarchies of taste and style, with different "price tags" attached that reflect their differential status in the cultural pecking order. In short, some lifestyles are more expensive than others, and many are priced beyond the reach of most, even in the limited sense of being able to buy into their symbolic representations. And, contrary to the commands of postmodernists, the distinction between the authentic and the inauthentic in terms of cultural consumption remains firmly in place, with access to the authentic being the marker of superior consumption taste, whereas settling for its reproductions is indicative of a lesser lifestyle status.[240] At the bottom of the cultural pecking order, of course, are the "flawed consumers",[241] whose marginal or precarious economic position not only excludes them from work-role status but from the world of lifestyle consumption.

The argument that the consumer or commodity culture facilitates sociality as much as individuality is especially impoverished. What kind of sociality or community is established by shopping? Shopping does not establish a community or a social bond because it establishes no shared obligations or commitments around which a community or bond can be built. Any "group affiliation" based on similarity of lifestyle consumerism would exist only until the next fashion was projected by the advertisers as the "in thing" and hence would be ephemeral. The level of appearances is in any case, by definition, a superficial indicator of shared cultural sentiments that would allow a network to persist. Such would also be a strictly local affair, based in the main on known others within a small intimate network, rather than something that was community-facing or community-building. Nor is it clear why fashion preferences would alone be sufficient to draw people together into a group. This may be an aspect of group affiliation, but it would hardly be the mainstay. Lots of people prefer specific "brands" or "labels", but that does not encourage them to seek out others so inclined on social media.

I contend that consumerist individualism is, as much as economic individualism is, a force of culture that is inherently hostile to the maintenance of collective moral solidarity within a society. This means that societies where consumer culture is most developed and embedded in everyday life (that is, those of the high-income countries of the developed world) are those least likely to be able to muster community-level defences against pandemic events such as COVID-19. They are, in other words, those that are least well equipped to mobilize citizenries for safeguarding the lives and well-being of the communal Other.

This may help us explain something that would otherwise appear anomalous if not counter-intuitive. This is that disproportionately represented among the world's poorest performing countries for minimizing public health harms from the novel coronavirus so far have been those of the Global North, including and especially the West.[242] At the time of writing this chapter (midyear 2021), the developed world has for the most part done a much worse job of holding down fatalities than the semi-developed and underdeveloped worlds. This is despite enjoying the advantages of higher per capita income, superior general life expectancy, more segregated or privatized living arrangements, and better-resourced public health services. This, of course, is a situation that likely cannot hold, owing to the huge inequalities in vaccine protection coverage across the inter-state system between richer and poorer countries. But it has been a feature of the pandemic for a year and more.

Part of this may be accountable in terms of the older age demographic of the Global North. But this can hardly explain all of it, given the magnitude of North–South inequalities. The developed world can sustain a bigger elderly population than the rest of the world, true enough. But this is owing to its major economic and healthcare advantages that generally allow for better life chances across the board. As far as the pandemic is concerned, the less developed countries would appear to have many more and greater COVID vulnerabilities than the richer ones. These include substantial populations of people with radically weakened immune systems owing to poverty and malnutrition and exposure to contaminated water sources; the lack of protection for workers from the virus afforded by furlough schemes that render home quarantine feasible; the far larger numbers of workers in "material" and "manual" employment incompatible with home-working than in "immaterial" or "virtually-mediated" occupations; less popular access to medical resources; higher residential densities in the cities; and higher exposure to the risks associated with crowded and multi-generational households and dormitories.

Given these circumstances, it seems feasible that the especially poor pandemic record of countries such as the US, UK, Italy, Spain, France, etc., may have at least something to do with lower levels of voluntary public compliance with NPIs. This is in comparison with those levels of compliance in many countries in the less developed world – and especially levels of compliance in the more culturally "collectivist" countries of Southeast Asia. If so, this lesser engagement of the general population in the Global North with NPIs may be attributable to the fact that the culture ideology of consumerist individualism is, by and large, much more deeply and pervasively embedded here than in those countries where major income disparities together with relatively low per capita income basically cut off much of the population from consumer opportunities.

Yet, as is the case with economic individualism, consumer culture does not and cannot extinguish the social bond altogether, even in those countries particularly under its spell. This is for reasons I have elaborated but which I will now restate. For a start, consumerism's ideological grip on the popular mind is diminished by the social reality of economic inequality, since this places millions of people (even in the developed world) at least partially beyond its seductions. But, at a deeper level, this is because the constitution of human beings as social beings biologically wired for basic empathy and altruism for others of their own kind is not (and cannot) be simply dissolved by consumerism. The human capacity to accept moral responsibility for the Other is given by what Bauman has called our primaeval animal sociality.[243] This, I have argued elsewhere, is a personal emergent property (PEP) of our species being. It emerges from natural selection in *homo sapiens* in the direction of social cooperation and our resultant long history of "being with others".[244] It manifests as our self-conscious capacity for the positive projection of the qualities of ourselves onto other human beings.[245] This is a redoubt against the egoistic (economic and consumerist) modes of individualism.

Reflexive individualism

So too perhaps may be (or could be under certain circumstances) a form of individualism that Anthony Giddens has dubbed as "reflexive", albeit indirectly. *Reflexive individualism* for Giddens is also a gift of modernization.[246] The basis for it is rather similar to Durkheim's associational individualism. In traditional societies, says Giddens, people did not tend to self-reflect or interrogate their social world. This was because their choices of social action (roles, practices) were already mostly predetermined within a highly restrictive and insular cultural framework. This was a framework set by the customs, traditions, and habits of the local society as these were largely untouched and unaffected by social worlds beyond community borders. In pre-modern societies, Giddens acknowledges, people were also reflexive subjects. But their reflexivity was largely focused on the clarification and renewal of tradition. This meant that people's choices of action (and of beliefs) in pre-modern society were far more fixed by immediate embedded contexts – that is, by the borders and horizons of the locality – than the choices of modern people, which in the "global" age have transcended borders.

Social practices in pre-modern times, according to Giddens, may then (following Weber's example) be classed as *traditional* action.[247] This is action that is relatively fixed by local customs and precedents, and which consequently does not vary much from generation to generation. By contrast, in late-modern society, Giddens observes, people are much less beholden to the precedents set by earlier generations or by the traditions of local place. As he puts it, "we live in a world where we have to decide what values to hold, as individuals, and in a democracy, collectively – essentially through reflexive discourse".[248]

Durkheim himself spelt out many of the reasons for this. It was, he said, because law and morality are more flexible or liberal and less restrictive. It was, he said, because politics is liberalized with the consolidation of individual rights. It was, he argued, because there is more cosmopolitanism owing to migration and cross-border exchanges. It was, he proposed, because there is more occupational diversity owing to a far more complex and specialized division of labour. To these drivers may be added others. Enhanced geographical and social mobility (and with this the expansion of leisure and lifestyle pluralism) has been fuelled respectively by technological advances and the expansion of educational opportunities for all. Owing to these changes, Giddens points out that people have vastly more opportunities to exercise choice in every area of their lives than before. And by exercising these choices, they individualize themselves. By contrast, pre-modern subjects had much less scope to self-individualize. This was because their actions and beliefs were much more hemmed in by the narrowness of the social roles and cultural horizons by which or within which they lived their lives.

This self-individualizing is inherently reflexive, Giddens rightly says. Reflexive individualism, for Giddens, entails "the routine incorporation of new knowledge or information into environments of action that are thereby reconstituted or reorganised" so that subjects orient themselves towards "the strategic adoption of lifestyle options, organised in terms of the individual's projected lifespan".[249] More choices, Giddens instructs, means more reflection on available choices:

> The reflexivity of modern social life consists of the fact that social practices are constantly examined and reformed in the light of incoming information about those very practices ... In all cultures, social practices are routinely altered in the light of ongoing discoveries which feed into them. But only in the era of modernity is the revision of convention radicalized to apply in principle to all aspects of human life.[250]

But this is also because more choices mean more uncertainties and therefore greater risks attached to exercising those choices. Thus, reflexivity and risk go together in the contemporary age. This means that individual actions now require of their agents more analysis and thought (that is, more *self-reflection* and *social reflection)* than they did in the pre-modern age. Our social dependence on personally unknown others to facilitate our needs or wants (owing to the complex social division of labour and fragmentation of roles) ensures that we must simultaneously risk and trust anonymous persons and abstract social systems. We must trust them and risk them because we cannot be fully knowledgeable of how they will impact our lives. Yet we are incentivized to strive for ever higher levels of self- and societal reflexivity to minimize risk and rationalize trust. This, says Giddens, is a progressively growing demand placed on contemporary lives, for with worldwide interconnectedness under "globalization" and with ever-increasing disembedding of social systems from purely local contexts, individuals are confronted with ever-changing complexities upon which to reflect when navigating their social worlds.

Late-modern selves, therefore, are uniquely well placed historically to translate or articulate our innate species sociality and attendant primaeval sense of responsibility for each other into self-reflective political and cultural humanisms. This is where the mute herd sociality of human nature is elevated into self-conscious organic communities such as Durkheim and Marx envisaged whereby the "free development of each is the condition for the free development of all".[251] Such would dissolve the alienated and fetishized egoistic individualisms based on capitalist economism and consumerism that have so degraded the bonds of social solidarity and of the attendant ethics of collective nurture and dis-harm – and which as we shall see have seriously compromised the cause of public health in the current pandemic. This is only to identify potential that is merely abstract until energized by real political struggles, however. And these struggles would be motivated by rather more prosaic or secular concerns (for bread, shelter, recognition, and justice) than those of a universal humanism.

But, at present, reflexive individualism may allow for recognition by some of the necessity of moral and associative individualism to curb the pandemic. This is just as our instinctual empathy for those of our own kind has offered some defence against it in the face of political and economic counterforces of zombie capitalism. For these reasons, perhaps, there was sufficient voluntary public acquiescence with NPIs for them to do their job, just about, even though these (as we shall see) were undoubtedly compromised by significant levels of non-compliance. But the non-compliance, I contend, was symptomatic of powerful decivilizing processes at work in contemporary society. This will be explored in the next chapter.

17 August 2020 (updated July 2021)

Notes

1 Elias, N. (2000). *The Civilizing Process: Sociogenetic and Psychogenetic Investigations.* (Revised edition). [1939]. Oxford: Blackwell.
2 Elias (2000).
3 Elias (2000); Elias, N. (1988). 'Violence and Civilization: On the State Monopoly of Physical Violence and Its Infringements'. J. Keane (Ed.). *Civil Society and the State: New European Perspectives.* London: Verso, pp. 134–54; Elias, N. and Dunning, E. (2008). *Quest for Excitement: Sport and Leisure in the Civilising Process.* Dublin: University College Dublin Press.
4 Fletcher, J. (1995). Towards a Theory of Decivilizing Processes'. *Amsterdams Sociologisch Tijdschrift*, 22 (2) (October), pp. 283–96. See p. 284.
5 Elias, N. (1991). *The Society of Individuals.* Oxford: Basil Blackwell.
6 Elias (2000).
7 Elias's essay on *The Breakdown of Civilization* cited in Fletcher (1995), pp. 287–88.
8 Elias cited in Fletcher (1995), p. 288.
9 Bauman, Z. (1989). *Modernity and the Holocaust.* Cambridge: Polity Press.
10 See Rees, J. (1998). *The Algebra of Revolution: The Dialectic and the Classical Marxist Tradition.* London: Routledge, p. 1.
11 Rees (1998), p. 1.
12 Fletcher (1995), p. 299.
13 See for example: Adrienko, Y. (2002). 'Crime, Wealth and Inequality: Evidence from International Crime Victim Surveys'. Moscow: Economics Education and Research Consortium; De Courson, B. and Nettle, D. (2021). 'Why do inequality and deprivation produce high crime and low trust?' *Scientific Reports*, 11 (1937), pp. 1–11; Demombynes, G. and Özler, B. (2002). 'Crime and Local Inequality in South Africa'. New York: World Bank; Fajnzylber, P., Lederman, D., and Leayza, N. (1998). *Determinants of Crime Rates in Latin America and the World,* Washington DC: World Bank; Fajnzylber, P., Lederman, D., and Loayza, N. (2002). 'Inequality and violent crime', *Journal of Law and Economics*, 45 (1), pp. 1–40; Hsieh, C-C and Pugh, M. (1993). 'Poverty, income inequality, and violent crime: a meta-analysis of recent aggregate data studies'. *Criminal Justice Review*, 18 (2) (August), pp. 182–202; Jongmook, C. (2008). 'Income Inequality and Crime in the United States'. *Economics Letters*, 101 (1), pp. 31–33; Kelly, M. (2000). 'Inequality and crime'. *Review of Economics and Statistics*, 82 (4), pp. 530–39; Taylor, I. (1997). 'The political economy of crime'. M. Maguire *et al.* (Eds.), *Oxford Handbook of Criminology*, 2nd edition. Oxford: Oxford University Press.
14 Friedman, M. (1962). *Capitalism and Freedom.* Chicago: Chicago University Press; Hayek, F.A. (1949). *Individualism and Economic Order.* London: Routledge and Kegan Paul; Hayek, F.A. (1944*). The Road to Serfdom.* London: Routledge and Kegan Paul; Hayek, F.A. (1960). *The Constitution of Liberty.* London: Routledge and Kegan Paul; Seldon, A. (1967). *Taxation and Welfare.* London: Institute of Economic Affairs; Seldon, A. (1981). *Wither the Welfare State.* London: Institute of Economic Affairs.

15 See Callinicos, A. (1991). *The Revenge of History: Marxism and the East European Revolutions*. Cambridge: Polity Press, Ch 2.
16 Duménil, G. and Lévy, D. (2004). *Capital Resurgent: Roots of the Neoliberal Revolution*. Cambridge MA: Harvard University Press; Glyn, A. (2006). *Capitalism Unleashed: Finance, Globalization and Welfare*. Oxford: Oxford University Press; Harman, C. (2008). 'Theorising neoliberalism'. *International Socialism*, 117 (Winter), pp. 87–121; Harvey, D. (2005). *A Brief History of Neoliberalism*. Oxford: Oxford University Press; Saad-Filho, A. and Johnston, D. (Eds.). (2004). *Neoliberalism: A Critical Reader*. London: Pluto Press.
17 As I demonstrate in my *Contagion Capitalism* (Routledge). Forthcoming.
18 Bourquin, P., Cribb, J., Waters, T., and Xu, X. (2019). *Living Standards, Poverty and Inequality in the UK: 2019*. London: Institute for Fiscal Studies; Collins, C., Hartman, C., and Sklair, H. (1999). *Divided Decade: Economic Disparity at the Century's End*. New York: UFE; Gilbert (2007). 'Inequality and Why It Matters'. *Geography Compass*, 1 (3), pp. 422–47; Hurst, C., Gibbon, H.F., and Nurse, A. (2016). *Social Inequality: Forms, Causes and Consequences*. London and New York; Saez, E. and Zucman, G. (2014). *Wealth Inequality in the United States Since 1913: Evidence from Capitalized Income Data*. Working Paper 20625: NBER Working Paper Series. Cambridge MA: National Bureau of Economic Research; Westergaard, J. (1995). *Who Gets What? The Hardening of Class Inequality at the End of the Twentieth Century*, Cambridge: Polity Press.
19 Duménil and Lévy (2004); Harvey (2005); Hertz, N. (2002). *The Silent Takeover: Global Capitalism and the Death of Democracy*. London: Arrow; Sklair, L. (2001). 'The Transnational Capitalist Class and Global Politics: Deconstructing the Corporate: State Connection'. *International Political Science Review*, 23 (2), pp. 159–74.
20 Alvaredo, F., Atkinson, A.B., and Morelli, S. (2017). *Top wealth shares in the UK over more than a century*. Institute for New Economic Thinking. INET Oxford Working Paper No. 2017–1.
21 Westergaard, J. and Resler, H. (1976). *Class in a Capitalist Society*. Harmondsworth: Penguin, p. 112.
22 National Statistics (2002). *Social Trends, 32*. London: ONS, p. 102.
23 Alvaredo *et al.* (2017).
24 ONS (2018). *Wealth in Great Britain: 2014 to 2016*. GOV.UK (online); ONS (2016). *Wealth in Great Britain: 2010 to 2012*. GOV.UK (online).
25 ONS (2019). *Total Wealth in Great Britain: April 2016 to March 2018*. GOV.UK (online).
26 Alvaredo *et al.* (2017).
27 Atkinson, A.B. (1983). *The Economics of Inequality*. Oxford: Oxford University Press, p. 63.
28 Cribb, J., Joyce, R., and Philip, D. (2012). *Living Standards, Poverty and Inequality in the UK: 2012*. London: Institute of Fiscal Studies, p. 30.
29 Callinicos, A. (2000). *Equality*. Cambridge: Polity Press, p. 135.
30 Green, B. and Shaheen, F. (2014). *Economic Inequality and House Prices in the UK*. New Economics Foundation (online), p. 7. See also: Equality Trust (2018). *How Has Inequality Changed? Development of UK Income Inequality* (online).
31 National Statistics (2006). *Social Trends, 36*. London: ONS, p. 81.
32 Goodman, A., Johnson, P., and Webb, S. (1997). *Inequality in the UK*. Oxford: Oxford University Press, p. 22.
33 *Social Trends, 36* (2006), pp. 76–77.
34 Oxfam (2013). *The True Cost of Austerity and Inequality: UK Case Study* (online). (September). Based on: OECD (2011). *Divided We Stand: Why Inequality Keeps Rising. Country Note: United Kingdom* (online); OECD (2013). *Crisis squeezes income and puts pressure on inequality and poverty* (online).

35 DWP (2012). Households Below Average Income Statistics: First Release. (14 June). London: DWP; Howard, M., Garnham, A., Fimister, G., and Veit-Wilson, J. (2001). *Poverty: The Facts*, 4th edition. London: Child Poverty Action Group, p. 21.

36 Brewer, M., Goodman, A., Shaw, J., and Sibieta, L. (2006). *Poverty and Inequality in Britain*. London: Institute for Financial Studies.

37 Aldridge, H., Kenway, P., Macinnes, T., and Parekh, A. (2012). *Monitoring Poverty and Social Exclusion 2012*. York: Joseph Rowntree Foundation, p. 23.

38 DWP (2013). *Households Below Average Income: An analysis of the income distribution 1994/95 – 2011/12 June 2013*. GOV.UK (online). See Table 3, p.74. Cited in: Oxfam (2013). *The True Cost of Austerity and Inequality: UK Case Study* (online). (September).

39 Belfield *et al.* (2014), p. 57.

40 Joseph Rowntree Foundation (2020). *UK Poverty Statistics: Poverty Levels and Trends* (online).

41 Social Metrics Commission (2019). *Measuring Poverty 2019: A Report by the Social Metrics Commission* (online). (July), p. 20.

42 Full Fact (2019). *Poverty in the UK: a guide to the facts and figures* (online). (27 September). Full Fact's statistics are based on the Social Metrics Commission's new measures of poverty.

43 Apel, H. (2015). 'Income inequality in the U.S. from 1950 to 2010 – the neglect of the political'. *Real World Economics Review*, 72, pp. 1–145. See p. 6.

44 Collins *et al.* (1999).

45 Schaeffer, K. (2020). *Six Facts about Economic Inequality in the U.S.* Pew Research Center (online). (7 February).

46 Trudell, M. (2012). 'The occupy movement and class politics in the US'. *International Socialism*, 133. (Winter), pp. 39–53. See p. 44.

47 Piketty, T. (2014). *Capital in the Twenty-First Century*. Cambridge MA: Harvard University Press.

48 Alvaredo, F., Chancel, L., Piketty, T., Saez, E., and Zucman, G. (2018). *World Inequality Report 2018: Executive Summary*. World Inequality Lab (online).

49 Kuhn, M., Schularick, M., and Steins, U.I. (2019). *Income and Wealth Inequality in America 1949–2016*.

50 Kent, A., Rickets, L., and Boshara, R. (2019). *What Wealth and Income Inequality in America Looks Like: Key Facts and Figures*. Federal Reserve Bank of St Louis (online).

51 Saez, E. and Zucman, G. (2014). *Exploding Wealth Inequality in the United States*. Washington Center for Equitable Growth (online). (20 October).

52 Collins *et al.* (1999).

53 Schaeffer (2020).

54 Kent *et al.* (2019). Similarly, according to Saez and Zucman, the share of national wealth going to the top 10 percent of households increased from 64 percent in 1987 to 77 percent in 2012. Saez, E. and Zucman, G. (2014). *Wealth Inequality in the United States since 1913: Evidence From Capitalized Income Tax Data*. Working Paper 20625. NBER Working Paper Series. Cambridge MA: National Bureau of Economic Research, p. 56.

55 Saez and Zucman (2014), p. 1.

56 Schaeffer (2020).

57 Ehrenreich, B. (2003). *Nickel and Dimed: Undercover in Low-Wage America*. New York: Henry Holt, p. 213.

58 Institute for Research on Poverty (2020). *How Is Poverty Measured?* University of Wisconsin-Madison (online).

59 Greenberg, M. (2009). *It's Time for a Better Poverty Measure*. Center for American Progress (online). (25 August).

60 Greenberg (2009).
61 Morrill, R. (2010). '50 Years of US Poverty: 1960 to 2010'. *New Geography* (online). (19 February); Chaudry, A. *et al.* (2016). *Poverty in the United States: 50-Year Trends and Safety Net Impacts.* (March). US Department of Health and Human Services: Office of Human Services Policy (online).
62 Plotnick, R.D., Smolensky, E., Evenhouse, E., and Reilly, S. (1998). *The Twentieth Century Record of Inequality and Poverty in the United States.* Discussion Paper no. 1166–98. Institute for Research on Poverty, p. 21.
63 Collins *et al.* (1999).
64 Eckholm, E. (2010). 'Recession Raises Poverty Rate to a 15-Year High'. *New York Times.* (16 September).
65 Morrill (2010); Chaudry *et al.* (2016); Semega, J. *et al.* (2020). *Income and Poverty in the United States: 2019.* United States Census Bureau (online). (15 September).
66 Fessler, P. (2019). 'U.S. Census Bureau Reports Poverty Rate Down, But Millions Still Poor'. *NPR News* (online). (10 September).
67 Miller, R.H. (1973). *Characteristics of the Low-Income Population: 1973.* Current Population Reports. Series P.60, No. 98. US Department of Commerce and Bureau of the Census. Washington DC.
68 Harman, C. (1993). 'Where is capitalism going?' *International Socialism*, 2 (58), pp. 3–57. See p. 53 for OECD data.
69 Manyika, J., Mischke, J., Bughin, J., Woetzel, J., Krishnan, M., and Cudre, S. (2020). *A new look at the declining labor share of income in the United States.* McKinsey Global Institute (online). (22 May).
70 Collins *et al.* (1999).
71 Galbraith, J. (1993). *The Culture of Contentment.* Boston: Houghton Mifflin Harcourt.
72 Brenner, R. (2006). *The Economics of Global Turbulence: The Advanced Capitalist Economies from Long Boom to Long Downturn, 1945–2005.* London: Verso, pp. 191–92
73 Heilbronner, R. (1993). *Twenty-First Century Capitalism.* New York: W.W. Norton and Co.
74 Madrick, J. (1997). *The End of Affluence: The Causes and Consequences of America's Dilemma.* New York: Random House, p. 16–17.
75 IMF. (1999). *Why Has Inflation in the United States Remained So Low? Reassessing the Importance of Labor Costs and the Price of Imports.* Working Paper 99/149. New York, p. 5.
76 Luttwak, E.N. (1999). *Turbo Capitalism: Winners and Losers in the Global Economy.* London: Harper-Collins, pp. 95–96.
77 Collins *et al.* (1999).
78 Hunnicut, B.K. (1990). *Work Without End: Abandoning Shorter Hours for the Right to Work.* Philadelphia: Temple University Press.
79 Schor, J. (1991). *The Overworked American: The Unexpected Decline of Leisure.* New York: Basic Books, p. 26.
80 Kuhn, P. and Lozano, F. (2005). *The Expanding Work Week: Understanding Trends in Long Work Hours Among US Men, 1979–2004.* Working Paper 11895. National Bureau of Economic Research: Cambridge MA, pp. 1–2.
81 Mishel, L. (2013). *Vast majority of wage earners are working harder, and not for much more: trends in US work hours and wages over 1979–2007.* Issue Brief #348. Economic Policy Institute. (30 January), p. 2.
82 Mishel (2013), p. 3.
83 Kalleberg, A.L. (2011). *Good Jobs, Bad Jobs.* New York: Russell Sage Foundation; Maume, D.J. and Purcell, D.A. (2007). 'The "Over-Paced" American: Recent Trends in the Intensification of Work'. B.A. Rubin (Ed.) *Workplace Temporalities: Research in the Sociology of Work*, vol. 17. Bingley: Emerald Group Publishing Limited; Steiber,

N. (2014). 'Trends in Work Stress and Exhaustion in Advanced Economies'. *Social Indicators Research*, 121, pp. 215–31; Green, F., Felstead, A., Gallie, D., and Henseke, O. (2021). 'Working Still Harder'. *ILR Review*, 20 (10), pp. 1–30.

84 Congressional Budget Office. (2011). *Trends in the Distribution of Household Income Between 1979 and 2007*. CBO Publications (online). (25 October).

85 Menyika *et al.* (2019).

86 Harman, C. (1999). *A People's History of the World*. London: Bookmarks, p. 607.

87 Mishel, L. and Wolfe, J. (2019). 'CEO compensation has grown 940% since 1978: typical worker compensation has risen only 12% during that time'. Economic Policy Institute (online). (14 August).

88 Taylor, C., Jowett, A., and Hardie, M. (2014). *An Examination of Real Falling Wages*. London: Office of National Statistics, p. 3. See also: *BBC News* (2014). 'Drop in real wages longest for 50 years, says ONS'. (31 January).

89 Hardy, J. and Choonara, J. (2013). 'Neoliberalism and the British working class: A reply to Neil Davidson'. *International Socialism*, 140 (Autumn), pp. 103–30 (p. 7).

90 Felstead, A., Gallie, D., Green, F., and Inanc, H. (2013). *Work Intensification in Britain: First Findings from the Skills and Employment Survey 2012*. Economic and Social Research Council and UK Commission for Employment and Skills: University of Oxford. See also: Burchell, B. (2006). 'Work intensification in the UK'. D. Perrons *et al.* (Eds.) *Gender Divisions and Working Time in the New Economy: Changing Patterns of Work, Care and Public Policy in Europe and North America*. Cheltenham: Edward Elgar; Chartered Institute of Personnel and Development (2013). *Megatrends. Are we working harder than ever?* London: CIPD; Green, F. (2001). 'It's been a hard day's night: The concentration and intensification of work in late twentieth-century Britain'. *British Journal of Industrial Relations*, 39 (1), pp. 53–80; Green, F. (2006). *Demanding Work. The Paradox of Job Quality in the Affluent Economy*. Woodstock, UK: Princeton University Press.

91 Green, F., Felstead, A., Gallie, D., and Henseke, G. (2018). *Work Intensity in Britain: First Findings from the Skills and Employment Survey 2017*. ESRC and UKCES: University of Oxford (online).

92 Felstead *et al.* (2013).

93 Green *et al.* (2018).

94 ONS (2021). *Average actual weekly hours of work for full-time workers (seasonally adjusted)*. GOV.UK (online).

95 Harman, C. (1995). *The Economics of the Madhouse: Capitalism and the Market Today*. London: Bookmarks, p. 49.

96 New Economics Foundation (2019). *Average Weekly Hours Fell Faster Between 1946 and 1979 than Post-1980*. New Economics (online).

97 Dmitracova, D. (2019). 'UK working hours would be shorter if pre-1980 trend had not been derailed, new study says'. *Independent*. (12 September).

98 Machin, S. (2015). *Real Wage Trends*. Understanding the Great Recession: From Micro to Macro Conference. (23–24 September 2015). London: Bank of England, pp. 8–9.

99 Blundell, R., Crawford, C., and Jin, W. (2012). *What can wages and employment tell us about the UK's productivity puzzle?* London: IFS. Working Paper W13/11.

100 Osborne, H. (2015). 'UK workers' wages fell 1% a year between 2008 and 2015, TUC says'. *Guardian* (27 February).

101 Martin, A. (2014). *Why Inequality is an Economic Problem*. New Economics Foundation (online).

102 Osborne (2015).

103 Belfield, C., Cribb, J., Hood, A., and Joyce, R. (2014). *Living standards, pay and inequality in the UK: 2014*. Institute for Fiscal Studies (online). (15 July).

104 Taylor, C., Jowett, A., and Hardie, M. (2014). *An Examination of Real Falling Wages*. London: ONS, p. 3. See also: *BBC News* (2014). 'Drop in real wages longest for 50 years, says ONS'. (31 January).

105   Elliott, L. (2017). 'Missing wage rises give lie to picture of full employment'. *Guardian*. (15 February).
106   Cribb, J. and Johnson, P. (2018). *10 years on – have we recovered from the financial crisis?* IFS (online). (12 September).
107   Greig, A., Hulme, D., and Turner, M. (2006). *Challenging Global Inequality: Development Theory and Practice in the Twenty-First Century*. London: Red Globe Press; Korzeniewicz, R.P. and Moran, T.P. (2009). *Unveiling Inequality: A World-Historical Perspective*. New York: Russell Sage Foundation; Nye, H. and Reddy, S. (2003). 'Weaknesses of recent global poverty estimates: Xavier Sala-i-Martin and Surjit Bhalla'. Social Analysis (online); Pogge, T. (2007). *Freedom from Poverty as a Human Right: Who Owes What to the Very Poor?* Oxford: Oxford University Press; Pogge, T. and Reddy, S. (2009). *How not to count the poor*. Initiative for Policy Dialogue Working Papers Series (online); Reddy, S. (2006). *Counting the Poor: The Truth About World Poverty Statistics. Socialist Register*; Reddy, S. and Pogge, T. (2002). *How Not to Count the Poor: a reply to Ravallion*. Social Analysis (online); Reddy, S. and Minoiu, C. (2007). 'Has World Poverty Really Fallen? *The Review of Income and Wealth*, 53 (3), pp. 484–502; Sengupta, R. (2006). *Poverty and Inequality in the New World: Moving forward or backward? A Critique of 'Globalization, Poverty and Inequality since 1980' by David Dollar*. Network-Ideas.org (online); Vandemoortele, J. (2002). *Are we really reducing global poverty?* New York: United Nations Development Programme: Bureau for Development Policy; Wade, R.H. (2004). 'Is Globalization Reducing Poverty and Inequality?' *International Journal of Health Studies*, 34 (3), pp. 381–414; Wade, R.H. (2007). 'On the causes of increasing world poverty and inequality, or why the Matthew effect prevails'. *New Political Economy*, 9 (2), pp. 163–88; Wade, R.H. (2017). 'Global Growth, Poverty and Inequality: the globalization argument and the "political" science of economics'. J. Ravenhill (Ed.) *Global Political Economy*. Oxford: Oxford University Press, pp. 319–55; Weller, C.E. and Hirsch, A. (2004). 'The long and short of it: Global liberalization and the incomes of the poor'. *Journal of Post-Keynesian Economics*, 26 (3), pp. 471–504; Weller, C.E., Hirsch, A., and Scott, R.E. (2001). 'The unremarkable record of liberalized trade'. Briefing Paper 113. Economic Policy Institute (online). (1 October).
108   World Bank (2020), pp. 2–3.
109   Chen, S. and Ravallion, M. (2004). 'How Have the World's Poorest Fared since the Early 1980s?' *World Bank Research Observer*, 19 (2) (Autumn), pp. 141–46.
110   World Bank (2020), p. 2.
111   Nye and Reddy (2003); Pogge (2009*)*; Pogge and Reddy (2009); Reddy and Pogge (2002); Reddy and Minoiu (2007); Sengupta (2006); Weller and Hersh (2004); Vandemoortele (2002); Wade (2004, 2007).
112   Wade (2004).
113   Wade (2004).
114   Wade (2004).
115   Pogge (2009); Reddy and Minoiu (2007); Wade (2004, 2007).
116   Wade (2004, 2007). See also Wade, R.H. (2006). 'Globalisation isn't working'. *Prospect Magazine*, 124. (22 July).
117   Wade (2004, 2007); Vandemoortele (2002).
118   Weller and Hersh (2004).
119   According to the World Bank, between 1980 and 1993 world extreme poverty excluding China fell by only 6.9 percent, from 29 percent of the world's poor to 27 percent. Between 1993 and 2002 it had fallen 14.9 percent so that the proportion of the world's poor excluding China was reduced only to 23 percent from 29 percent. Since then, progress has quickened, and world poverty outside China halved between 2002 and 2015. See Roser and Ortiz-Ospina (2017). These are much less impressive results than the overall picture inclusive of China headlined by the World Bank.

120   World Bank (2020), p. 5. Their estimate was that the crisis had likely pushed 88 million below the poverty line in 2020 and would likely push a further 35 million below in 2021.

121   Cendrowski, S. (2015). 'China's Global 500 companies are bigger than ever – and mostly state-owned'. *Fortune*. (22 July); Weightman, W. (2018). 'Why China Won't Abandon Its Controversial Trade Policies: Protectionist policies play a key role in China's national strategy'. *Diplomat*. (24 May).

122   Chen, S. and Ravallion. M. (2008), 'The Developing World Is Poorer Than We Thought, but No Less Successful in the Fight Against Poverty'. Policy Research Development: Paper No. 4703. Washington DC: World Bank, pp. 31, 36.

123   Chen and Ravallion (2008). Indeed, as Chen and Ravallion noted, just as the number of people living under $1 a day declined from the 1980s through to the 2000s: "At the same time the number of people in the world living on less than $2 a day rose so that there has been a marked bunching up of people living between $1 and $2 a day". Chen, S. and Ravallion, M. (2004). How Have the World's Poorest Fared since the Early 1980s? *The World Bank Research Observer*, 19 (2) (Autumn), pp. 141–69. Again, China was at the centre of this dynamic. Breakneck industrialization and urbanization took 300 million out of severe poverty on the World Bank's numbers, but this was won by creating a new mass of the working poor hovering precariously above the $1 daily rate. More generally, perhaps the great achievement of neoliberal capitalist "globalization" is the replacement of a mass of absolutely impoverished rural farmers with a mass of slightly less impoverished urban proletarians.

124   Hayter, T. (1990). *The Creation of World Poverty*, 2nd edition. London: Pluto Press, p. 18.

125   Chen and Ravallion (2008).

126   Hayes, A. (2020). *Federal Poverty Level* (FPL). Investopedia (online). (13 October).

127   Ravallion, M., Chen, S., and Sangraula, P. (2008). 'Dollar a Day Revisited'. *World Bank Economic Review*, 23 (2), pp. 163–84.

128   Shah, A. (2013). *Poverty Facts and Stats*. Global Issues (online). (7 January).

129   World Bank (2018). *Nearly Half the World Lives on Less than $5.50 a Day*. Press release. (17 October).

130   World Bank (2018).

131   UNICEF and WHO (2019). *Progress on drinking water, sanitation and hygiene: 2000–2017: Special focus on inequalities*. New York: UNICEF and WHO.

132   UNICEF (2019). *The State of the World's Children: Children, Food and Nutrition*. UNICEF (online).

133   UNDP (2008). *Human Development Report 2007*. New York: UNDP, p. 25.

134   Keeley, B. (2015). *Income Inequality: The Gap between Rich and Poor*. Paris: OECD Publications, p. 3.

135   Harman (1999), p. 607.

136   Zucman, G. (2019). 'Global Wealth Inequality'. *Annual Review of Economics*, 11, pp. 109–38. See p. 109.

137   Credit Suisse (2013). *Global Wealth Report 2013*. Geneva and New York: CS Research Institute, pp. 21–22.

138   UNDP (2008). p. 25.

139   OECD (2011). *Divided We Stand: Why Inequality Keeps Rising* (online), p. 22.

140   OECD (2011), p. 22

141   OECD (2015). *In It Together: Why Less Inequality Benefits All* (online).

142   Oxfam (2018). *An Economy for the 99%*. Oxfam Briefing Paper. For a summary see Elliott, L. (2019). 'World's 26 richest people own as much as poorest 50%, says Oxfam'. *Guardian*. (21 January).

143   As has been demonstrated by those working within the research programme of Strain Theory in academic criminology building on the pioneering work of Robert K. Merton. See, for example, Agnew, R. (1992). 'Foundation for a general strain theory of crime

and delinquency', *Criminology*, 30 (1), pp. 47–87; Agnew, R. (2001). 'Building on the foundation of General Strain Theory: specifying the types of strain most likely to lead to crime and delinquency'. *Journal of Research in Crime and Delinquency*, 38 (4), pp. 319–61; Featherstone, R. and Deflem, D. (2003). 'Anomie and strain: context and consequences of Merton's two theories', *Sociological Inquiry*, 73 (4), pp. 471–89; Messner, S.F. and Rosenfeld, R. (2001). *Crime and the American Dream*, 2nd edition, Belmont CA: Wadsworth; Rosenfeld, R. (1989). 'Robert Merton's contributions to the sociology of deviance'. *Sociological Inquiry*, 59 (4), pp. 453–66.

144 In the UK, for example, the proportion of people who self-identify by class has not declined at all over the past 30 years. Only five percent rejected the idea that they belonged to one in the 2013 Social Attitudes survey. This was the same as in 1988. Survey data since the 1980s also evidences a radicalizing sense of class dissonance and injustice in popular attitudes in the UK during the neoliberal epoch. See Burrage, M. (2008). *Class Formation, Civil Society and the State: A Comparative Analysis of Russia, France, the US and England*. Basingstoke: Palgrave-Macmillan; Jowell, R., Witherspoon, S., and Brook, L. (1988). *British Social Attitudes 1987: The 5th Report*. Aldershot: Dartmouth; Jowell, R. *et al*. (1997). *British Social Attitudes 1996: The 14th Report*. London: Ashgate; Park, A. *et al*. (2013). *British Social Attitudes: The 30th Report*. London: National Centre for Social Research; Rose, D. and Marshall, G. (1988). 'Social Stratification'. M. Haralambos. (Ed.) *Developments in Sociology*, 4. Ormskirk: Causeway Press.

145 Park *et al*. (2013, pp. 62–66), for example, mobilize survey data to demonstrate a growing disengagement of people from the political process since 1983 in the UK. The disengagement is certainly indicative of increasing popular disenchantment with and distrust of government and politicians. Such is evidenced by: (1) a sharp rise in the number of people who think that political parties are interested only in votes and who think governments put the interests of their own party ahead of the public interest; (2) a decline in the number of people who participate in elections; (3) a decline in the number of people who think that taking part in elections is a moral duty or civic responsibility; (4) a decline in the number of people who identify with a particular political party; and (5) a decline in the number of people who identify strongly with a political party. This popular disenchantment with neoliberal democracy has been paralleled by a collapse of public confidence in key institutions of corporate power, such as the banks and the press (Park *et al*. 2013, pp. xv–xvi).

146 Beck, U. (1999). *What is Globalization?* Cambridge: Cambridge University Press; Giddens, A. (1990). *The Consequences of Modernity*. Cambridge: Polity Press; Robertson, R. (1992). *Globalization: Social Theory and Global Culture*. Thousand Oaks: Sage.

147 Hofstede, G. (2001). *Culture's Consequences*. Thousand Oaks: Sage.

148 Rothwell, J. (2010). *In the Company of Others: An Introduction to Communication*. New York: Oxford University Press.

149 Harman (1999), pp. 548–58, 566–70; Hobsbawm, E. (1994). *Age of Extremes: The Short Twentieth Century*. London: Abacus, pp. 217–22, 257–86.

150 Harman (1999), pp. 586–97; Hobsbawm (1994), pp. 403–32, 461–99, 558–85.

151 Bauman, Z. (2000). *Liquid Modernity*. Cambridge: Polity Press; Beck, U. (1992). *Risk Society: Towards a New Modernity*. London: Sage; Beck, U. (2000). *World Risk Society*. Cambridge: Polity Press; Beck, U. and Beck-Gernshein, E. (2002). *Individualization*. London: Sage; Giddens, A. (1990). *The Consequences of Modernity*. Cambridge: Polity; Giddens, A. (1991). *Modernity and Self-Identity*. Cambridge: Polity Press.

152 Durkheim, E. (1964). *The Division of Labour in Society*. New York: The Free Press.

153 Durkheim (1964).

154 Durkheim (1964), p. 41.

155 Durkheim (1964). Ch.3.

156   Durkheim (1964), pp. 353–73.
157   Durkheim (1964), pp. 304, 374–88.
158   Durkheim (1964), p. 228.
159   Durkheim (1964). Ch.3.
160   Durkheim (1964). Esp. Ch.2.
161   Durkheim (1964). Ch.2. See also pp. 129, 153–35.
162   Lee, H. and Newby, R. (1983). *The Problem of Sociology*. London: Unwin Allen, p. 217.
163   Durkheim, E. (1985). *The Rules of Sociological Method*. [1895]. New York: The Free Press, pp. 65–73; Durkheim (1964). Ch. 2 and Ch.3.
164   Durkheim, E. (1973). 'Two Laws of Penal Evolution'. S. Lukes and A. Scull. (Eds.). *Durkheim and the Law*. London: Martin Robertson.
165   Garland, D. (1999). 'Durkheim's sociology of punishment and punishment today'. M.S. Cladis (Ed.). *Durkheim and Foucault: Perspectives on Education and Punishment*. Oxford: Durkheim Press.
166   Foucault, M. (1995). *Discipline and Punish: The Birth of the Prison*. [1975]. New York: Vintage.
167   Durkheim (1964), p. 69.
168   Durkheim (1964), pp. 64–75.
169   Foucault (1995), pp. 73–103; Durkheim (1973).
170   Durkheim (1973).
171   Foucault (1995), esp. pp. 170–292.
172   Durkheim, E. (2015). 'Suicide'. L.D. Edles and S. Applerouth (Eds.). *Sociological Theory in the Classical Era*. Thousand Oaks: Sage, p. 139.
173   Durkheim (2015), pp. 136–40; Durkheim (1964), pp. 229–31.
174   Pearce, F. (1989). *The Radical Durkheim*. London: Pluto Press.
175   Durkheim (1964, p. 204) criticized the utilitarian economists of his day for claiming exactly that the rational self-interested actor, *homo economicus*, was the foundation of modern economic and social order so that public virtue would flow from egoistic utility. "There is nothing less constant than interest. Today it unites me to you; tomorrow it will make me your enemy. Such a cause can give rise only to transient relations and passing associations".
176   Durkheim (1964).
177   Durkheim, E. (1957). *Professional Ethics and Civic Morals*. London: Routledge and Kegan Paul.
178   Durkheim (1957), p. 166.
179   Durkheim (1957).
180   Durkheim, E. (1961). *Moral Education:* A Study in the Theory and Application of the Sociology of Education [1925]. Glencoe Ill: The Free Press.
181   Durkheim (1964), p. 384.
182   Merton, R. (1964). 'Anomie, Anomia and Social Interaction – contexts of deviant behaviour. M Clinard (Ed.) *Anomie and Deviant Behaviour*. Glencoe Ill: The Free Press.
183   Harman, C. (1991). 'The state and capitalism today'. *International Socialism*, 2 (51), pp. 3–54.
184   For example in the US and UK. See Purdy, D. (2006). *The Wages of Militancy: Incomes Policy, Hegemony and the Decline of the British Left*. Scientific Literature Digital Library (online); Walker, W.N. (2011). *Forty Years After The Freeze*. Word Press (online).
185   Cliff, T. and Gluckstein, D. (1996). *The Labour Party: A Marxist History*. 2nd edition. London: Bookmarks, pp. 218–23.
186   Apple, M.W. (1988). 'Review: Standing on the Shoulders of Bowles and Gintis: Class Formation and Capitalist Schools'. *History of Education Quarterly*, 28, pp. 231–241; Boliver, V. (2010). *Maximally Maintained Inequality and Effectively Maintained Inequality in Education: Operationalising the Expansion-Inequality Relationship*.

Department of Sociology Working Paper: University of Oxford, Working Paper no. 2010–05; Boudon, R. (1974). *Education, Opportunity and Social Inequality.* New York: Wiley; Bourdieu, P. (1977). 'Cultural Reproduction and Social Reproduction'. J. Karabel and A.H. Halsey (Eds.) *Power and Ideology in Education.* Oxford: Oxford University Press; Bourdieu, P. and Passerson, J-C. (1977). *Reproduction in Education, Society and Culture.* London: Sage; Bourne, M. (2015). *Social-Class Inequality in Educational Attainment and Participation in England.* School of Social Sciences: University of Manchester; Bowles, S. and Gintis, H. (2011). *Schooling in Capitalist America: Educational Reform and the Contradictions of Economic Life.* [1976]. Chicago: Haymarket Books; Bowles, S. and Gintis, H. (2002). 'Schooling in Capitalist America Revisited'. *Sociology of Education,* 75 (1) (January), pp. 1–18; Bowles, S. and Gintis, H. (2002). 'The Inheritance of Inequality'. *Journal of Economic Perspectives,* 16 (3), pp. 3–30; Greaves, N., Hill, D., and Maisuria, A. (2007). 'Embourgeoisement, Immiseration, Commodification – Marxism Revisited: a Critique of Education in Capitalist Systems'. *Journal for Critical Education Policy Studies* (online), 5 (1); Heath, A. and Clifford, P. (1990). 'Class Inequalities in Education in the Twentieth Century'. *Journal of the Royal Statistical Society,* Series A (153), pp. 1–16; Jackson, M. (2013) 'How is Inequality of Educational Opportunity Generated? The Case for Primary and Secondary Effects'. M. Jackson (Ed.) *Determined to Succeed? Performance versus Choice in Educational Attainment.* Palo Alto CA: Stanford University Press; Kumar, R. (Ed.) (2012). *Education and the Reproduction of Capital: Neoliberal Knowledge and Counterstrategies.* Basingstoke: Palgrave-Macmillan; Prandy, K. (1998). 'Class and Continuity in Social Reproduction'. *Sociological Review,* 46 (2), pp. 340–64.

187 Abbott, P. and Meerabeu, L. (Eds.) (1998). *The Sociology of the Caring Professions.* London: Routledge; Be-David, J. (1964). 'Professions in the Class System in Present Day Societies'. *Current Sociology,* 12 (3), pp. 247–98; Ben-David, B. (1990). *Professions in the class system of present-day societies: a trend report and bibliography.* Boston: De Gruyter Mouton; Elliot, P. (1972). *The Sociology of Professions.* London: Macmillan; Griffith, J.A.G. (1977). *The Politics of the Judiciary.* Oxford: Harper-Collins; Illich, I. (1973). 'The Professions as a Form of Imperialism'. *New Society,* 13 (September), pp. 633–35; Johnson, T.J. (1972). *Professions and Power.* London: Macmillan; Macdonald, K. (1998). *The Sociology of the Professions.* London: Sage; Millerson, G. (1964). *The Qualifying Associations.* London: Routledge and Kegan Paul.

188 Marx, K. (1976). *Capital,* vol. 1. Harmondsworth: Penguin, p. 129.

189 Marx, K. (1976), pp. 129–31, 165–66, 171–75, 739–42; Marx, K. (1972). *Theories of Surplus Value,* vol. 3, pp. 129–31, 138.

190 Bonger, W. (1969). *Crime and Economic Conditions* [1916]. Bloomington: Indiana University Press.

191 Chambliss, W. (1976). 'Functional and conflict theories of crime'. W. Chambliss and M. Mankoff (Eds.) *Whose Law? What Order?* New York: John Wiley; Chambliss, W. (1978). *On the Take: From Presidents to Petty Crooks.* Bloomington: Indiana University Press; Gordon, D. (1976). 'Class and the economics of crime'. Chambliss and Mankoff (Eds.).

192 Quinney, R. (1977). *Class, State and Crime.* New York: McKay.

193 Marx diagnosed no "iron law of wages" by which the workers under capitalism would experience objective immiseration from an absolute decline in wages owing to competition. But his analysis showed that relative impoverishment of the class would result from their declining share of the value they produce as labour-saving technology pushes up labour productivity faster than the increase in wages. Mandel, E. (1970). *Marxist Economic Theory.* New York: Pathfinder Press, pp. 211–15; Mandel, E. (1983). 'Economics'. D. McLellan (Ed.). *Marx: The First 100 Years.* London: Fontana, pp. 204–08.

194 Baran, P. and Sweezy, P. (1968). *Monopoly Capital*. Harmondsworth: Penguin; Wright, E.O. (1978). *Class, Crisis and the State*. London: Verso.
195 Brenner (2006); Harman, C. (1984). *Explaining the Crisis: A Marxist Reappraisal*. London: Bookmarks.
196 Bonger (1969); Chambliss (1976); Gordon (1976).
197 Creaven, S. (2000). *Marxism and Realism: A Materialistic Application of Realism in the Social Sciences*. London and New York, pp. 48–58, 71–136.
198 Quinney (1977).
199 Callinicos, A. (1991). *The Revenge of History: Marxism and the East European Revolutions*. Cambridge: Polity Press. See ch. 5.
200 Baudrillard, J. (1996). *The System of Objects* [1968]. London: Verso; Baudrillard, J. (1998). *The Consumer Society: Myths and Structures* [1970]. London: Sage.
201 Sklair, L. (1995). *Sociology of the Global System*. London: Harvester Wheatsheaf; Sklair, L. (1997). 'Social Movements for Global Capitalism: the Transnational Capitalist Class in Action'. *Review of International Political Economy*, 4 (3), pp. 514–38; Sklair, L. (2000). 'Media Imperialism'. J. Beynon and D. Dunkerley (Eds.) *Globalisation: The Reader*. London: Athlone Press; Sklair, L. (2002). *Globalization: Capitalism and its Alternatives*. Oxford: Oxford University Press.
202 Matza, D. (1961). 'Subterranean traditions of youth'. *Annals of the American Academy of Political and Social Science*, 338, pp. 102–18; Matza, D. and Sykes, G. (1961). 'Juvenile delinquency and subterranean values'. *American Sociological Review*, 22, pp. 712–19.
203 Baudrillard (1996, 1998).
204 As Bauman notes, consumerism is an aspect and force of universal strangerhood. See Bauman, Z. (1990). *Thinking Sociologically*. Oxford: Blackwell.
205 Lury, C. (2011). *Consumer Culture*. 2nd edition. Cambridge: Polity Press.
206 Baudrillard (1996); Baudrillard (1998).
        Baudrillard (1996); Baudrillard, J. (1973). *The Mirror of Production*. St Louis: Telos Press.
207 Rojek, C. (2004). 'The Consumerist Syndrome in Contemporary Society: An Interview with Zygmunt Bauman'. *Journal of Consumer Culture*, 4 (3), pp. 291–312 (p. 303).
208 Bauman (1990), p. 204.
209 Blackshaw, T. (2004). 'Bauman on Consumerism: Living the Market-Mediated Life'. M.H. Jacobsen and P. Poder (Eds.) *The Sociology of Zygmunt Bauman: Challenges and Critique*. Aldershot: Ashgate.
210 Rojek (2004).
211 Baudrillard, J. (1979). *On Seduction*. Basingstoke: Macmillan.
212 Žižek, S. (1989). *The Sublime Object of Ideology*, London: Verso; Žižek, S. (1993). *Tarrying with the Negative*, Durham: Duke University Press.
213 Bauman, Z. (2000). *Liquid Modernity*. Cambridge: Polity Press.
214 As Bauman (1990, p. 204) puts it, the consumer attitude "dissolves the problem of control over the wider setting of life (something most people will never achieve) in the multitude of small shopping acts that are – at least in principle – within your reach". The constraints on the exercise of consumer freedom are lessened by the abundance of "consumer credit" – so that individuals can for a time at least participate in consumerism beyond their material means.
215 Baudrillard (1979).
216 Marx (1976), pp. 164–65.
217 Marx, K. (1962). *Early Writings*. T. Bottomore. (Ed.). Harmondsworth: Penguin, p. 132.
218 Marx (1976), p. 582.
219 Creaven (2000), pp. 71–89.
220 Marx, K. (1973). *Grundrisse*. Harmondsworth: Penguin, p. 84.

221   Creaven (2000), pp. 75–87.
222   Creaven (2000), pp. 188–92.
223   Creaven (2000), pp. 84–85.
224   Giddens, A. (1990). *Sociology*. Cambridge: Polity Press, pp. 39–40. Giddens notes the conclusion drawn from the anthropological record. But he does not draw out the anthropological consequences because he too is fully committed to the over-social self. See Giddens (1991) for his account of self-identity. See Creaven (2000, pp. 126–36) for a critique.
225   Creaven (2000), pp. 89–104.
226   Creaven (2000), pp. 108–09.
227   Creaven (2000), pp. 155–201.
228   This may be illuminated with the application of Merton's strain theory. See Merton, R. (1938). 'Anomie and social structure'. *American Sociological Review*, 3, pp. 672–82; Merton (1964) in Clinard (Ed.). Blocked cultural opportunities would result from blocked economic opportunities. And from blocked cultural opportunities for consumer participation may emerge innovation (embrace of illegitimate means in order to acquire either the material resources to force consumer access or to simply acquire the consumer access directly). Or blocked cultural opportunities may facilitate retreatist or rebellious adaptations to consumerism – either by individuals simply abandoning it and accepting lesser status as culturally flawed or incomplete beings or by wholesale rejection of consumerism in favour of a different and for them better cultural way of life.
229   Similar to Albert Cohen's lower-class gang members. See Cohen, A. (1955). *Delinquent Boys: The Culture of the Gang*. Chicago: Free Press.
230   Crook, S., Pakulski, J., and Waters, M. (1992). *Postmodernization: Changes in Advanced Society*. London: Sage.
231   Rojek, C. (1995). *Decentring Leisure: Rethinking Leisure Theory*. Sage: London.
232   Crook *et al.* (1992); Rojek (1995).
233   Katz, J. and Sugiyama, S. (2005). 'Mobile phones as fashion statements: the co-creation of mobile communication's public meaning'. R. Ling and P. Pederson (Eds.) *Mobile Communications: The Renegotiation of the Social Sphere*. London: Springer; Ling, R. (2000). 'It's "in". It doesn't matter if you need it or not, just you have to have it: Fashion and Domestication of the Mobile Phone among Teens in Norway'. Working Paper: Telenor Research. Telenor: Norway; Ling, R. (2003). 'Fashion and vulgarity in the adoption of the mobile telephone among teens in Norway'. L. Fortunati, Katz, J.E., and Riccini, R. (Eds.) *Mediating the Human Body: Technology, Communication and Fashion*. London and New York: Routledge; Scraton, S. and Brahman, P. (1995). 'Leisure and postmodernity'. Haralambos, M. (Ed.). *Developments in Sociology*, vol. 11. Ormskirk: Causeway Press.
234   Strinati, D. (1995). *An introduction to Theories of Popular Culture*. London: Routledge.
235   Casara, A. (2007). *How Much of the World's Consumption Occurs in Rich Countries?* Global Policy Forum (online).
236   ONS (2019). *Family spending in the UK: April 2017 to March 2018*. GOV.UK (online).
237   ONS (2020). *Average household income, UK: financial year ending 2019*. GOV.UK (online).
238   Romei, V. (2020). 'Income inequality increases in the UK'. *Financial Times*. (5 March).
239   ONS (2019).
240   Strinati (1995).
241   Bauman, Z. (1998). *Work, Consumerism, and the New Poor*. Cambridge: Polity Press.
242   By mid-July 2021, six of the top ten countries for COVID-19 deaths were among the most economically developed in the world, and all of these were in the Global North. This was according to Worldometer (2021). *COVID-19 Coronavirus Pandemic: Reported Cases and Deaths by Country or Territory* (online). Accessed: 18 July 2021.
243   Bauman (1989), Ch.7.

244   As Bauman (1989, p. 182) puts it. See Bauman, Z. (1989). *Modernity and the Holocaust*. Cambridge: Polity Press.
245   Creaven (2000), pp. 48–58, 71–136, 154–81.
246   Giddens (1990). See also: Giddens (1991); Giddens, A. (1994). 'Living in a Post-Traditional Society". U. Beck, A. Giddens, and S. Lasch (Eds.) *Reflexive Modernisation*. Cambridge: Polity Press; Giddens, A. and Pierson, C. (1998). *Conversations with Anthony Giddens: Making Sense of Modernity*. Cambridge: Polity Press.
247   Weber, M. (1968). *Economy and Society*, vol. 2. New York: Bedminster Press.
248   Giddens and Pierson (1998), p. 219.
249   Giddens (1991), p. 243.
250   Giddens (1990), p. 38.
251   Marx, K. and Engels, F. (1975). *Collected Works*, vol. 6. London: Lawrence and Wishart, p. 506.

4 Decivilization and the pandemic

Non-pharmaceutical interventions (NPIs), at the centre of which are physical distancing practices, are established by a large body of research as effective measures for controlling pandemics. This was the case long before the present one.[1] However, the COVID-19 crisis has incentivized a massive expansion of research into the effectiveness of NPIs, which has basically confirmed their efficacy, indeed indispensability, for pandemic management.[2] These studies demonstrate that each of the different NPIs has yielded major benefits worldwide in reducing transmission rates and saving lives, albeit variably, with some having greater efficacy than others.

These studies have also shown that the best public health outcomes result from deploying the NPIs together. "Previous simulations and current reports affirm that a combination of all strategies has the greatest success rates in containing the disease".[3] As summarized by N'Konzi et al.,[4] NPIs, if applied consistently, "result in a substantial decrease in the peak prevalence" of epidemic waves, considerably reducing infection curves. Yet strictness or stringency as well as consistency of NPIs is key to their success. "The ultimate conclusion … is that the higher the stringency of NPIs, the more effective disease control is".[5]

But the success or otherwise of NPIs (self-isolation, self-testing, reporting positive test results, avoiding social gatherings, respecting physical distancing, regular hand-washing, public mask donning, etc.) in bringing the current pandemic under control has obviously depended on the degree of public compliance with these practices. The stringency of NPIs will be effective only if enough people acquiesce to the stringency of controls. Before vaccination, NPIs were the only line of defence for people against the virus. Given the tardiness and unevenness of the vaccine rollout internationally, these will have to remain the primary defence mode for many people and governments for some time yet. However, as I will argue, the NPIs have been rather less successful in curbing the pandemic than they have usually been made out to be. This is because their stringency has been compromised by significant levels of non-compliant behaviour.

This chapter will explore the limitations of the various NPIs (physical distancing of various kinds, mask-wearing, and self-hygiene), also of test-and-trace (which I consider separately), as well as the phenomenon of vaccine resistance. The argument that is outlined in the account that follows is that these limitations (which are exactly those generated by public non-compliance with NPIs and vaccination

DOI: 10.4324/9781003437208-5

scepticism to various degrees) may be explained to some degree as consequences of decivilization. There are of course other explanations, which I will address. But the impact of decivilization should be counted among them and indeed may illuminate if not contextualize other explanations.

Trajectories of compliance with NPIs

There is extensive research literature exploring those factors that appear to account for or predict public compliance with NPIs faced with epidemiological crises. This literature predates the current pandemic but has been substantially enlarged by it. Those factors more commonly associated with conforming public behaviour include: (1) having higher education level or status;[6] (2) certain demographic characteristics (being an older person, of female gender);[7] (3) possession of social, cultural and civic capital;[8] (4) access to spacious residential conditions and green leisure opportunities;[9] (5) employment or labour market situation and status (having secure full-time employment, as well as capacity and opportunity for virtual or lone working);[10] (6) pro-social attitudes (including of empathy and altruistic concern for others);[11] and (7) personality traits (including conscientiousness, risk-aversion, and introversion) and subjective states (personal life satisfaction).[12]

Conversely, then, higher levels of non-compliance, at the empirical level, are linked to the opposites of these factors. That is, to young people; to males; to lack of social, cultural, or civic capital; to residential overcrowding and lack of access to green space; to unemployment, economic hardship, labour market precarity, and work that cannot be performed virtually or apart from others; to socially indifferent attitudes; to personality traits including extroversion, impulsiveness, and egoism; and personal life dissatisfaction. I will address compliance and non-compliance in the analysis ahead, including these "factors". But in advance of that, I will address levels and trends of public compliance with NPIs during the COVID-19 pandemic to date.

The pandemic and NPIs in Britain

In the UK, media commentators, politicians and the government's scientific advisers have for the most part suggested that public engagement with the various pandemic restrictions during the first lockdown in the spring of 2020 was generally very good. As the Cabinet Office put it: "The overwhelming majority of the British public have complied with the regulations and guidance". Similarly, the Independent SAGE Group commended the "impressively sustained high levels of adherence to lockdown the public has achieved".[13]

But, of course, such evaluative judgements are hardly objective. This is because these are in relation to expectations that have tended towards pessimism owing to the fact that they are accommodated to a liberal notion of people as egoistic monads and as acting in pursuance of wholly individuated rights. This accounts, for example, for dubious notions of "behavioural fatigue" which justified the decision of the Swedish government to avoid legally mandated NPIs and which legitimated the politics of delayed lockdown in the UK.[14] (In the UK, the necessity to evade pandemic "tiredness" was trotted out by ministers and by the UK government's chief medical officer Chris Whitty to head off pressures for a more proactive policy response to the pandemic).[15] This is also because the benchmark of what would count as a strong community response is (since there are not precedents) arbitrary. The rose-tinted view of the success of lockdown policies in the UK as conveyed by dizzying levels of public support for NPIs has also been supported by British insularity and parochialism. A comparison of the UK's performance on NPIs with that of higher-performing countries may have led to more sober appraisals.

There is, however, some evidence in favour of the rose-tinted viewpoint inasmuch as the lockdowns did cause caseloads to tumble (which would not have happened unless most people stuck to the rules) and in that even before the British government brought in the first lockdown people were "jumping the gun" by taking their own precautions and withdrawing from or reducing their own social interactions with others. The British case was not of course an anomalous one, however. Lockdowns everywhere caused caseloads to tumble and this was because enough people supported the restrictions to allow disruption of the virus's capacity to reproduce itself.

This is confirmed by a major international survey of public responses to NPIs to control the pandemic in the runup to or during the first lockdowns of 2020 conducted in 58 countries involving more than 100,000 participants. This was during a period in which 92 percent of known COVID-19 cases were in these countries. The survey found that

> 91% of respondents reported that they did not attend any social gatherings in the past week; 89% washed their hands more frequently than a month earlier; 93% say that they would have immediately informed people around them if they had experienced COVID-19 symptoms; 69% reported keeping a distance of at least 2 meters to other people; and 78% said that they stayed home in the past week. People also plan to maintain these behaviors in the future; for example, while 42% of respondents report that they will leave their home in the next 5 days to buy food, only 19% say that they will go to work, and 45% of respondents say that they will not leave their home for any reason in the next 5 days. Thus, respondents report closely adhering to protective behaviors.[16]

In the UK, a panel survey of ten cities in the aftermath of the first national lockdown covering the period from 24 March to 21 April 2020 revealed the following "high" rates of compliance (compared to expectations) with the new restrictions: 86 percent of respondents reported that they had never since lockdown socialized with persons outside their household; 87 percent reported that they had never since lockdown travelled for non-essential or non-permissible purposes; and 62 percent reported that they had never since lockdown gone outside their homes for purposes of recreation and leisure rather than exercise.[17] Similar but better results for the UK are to be gleaned from other studies. For example, Ganslmeier, Van Parys, and Vlandas, basing themselves on YouGov self-report data derived from a sample of

105,000 people, found that almost 97 percent of respondents were complying with the range of lockdown restrictions, at least initially – or at least they said that they were.[18]

There was also for a period in the UK the once-weekly Thursday-evening ritual (apparently well supported by the public) of the doorstep handclap in recognition of National Health Service (NHS) frontliners.[19] This was suggestive that conformity to lockdown restrictions for many people in Britain may have been intended to a degree at least to ease pressures on the NHS as well as for whatever other motives they had for it. This would demonstrate the resonance in the public mind of Public Health England's slogan of "stay home, save lives, protect the NHS" – which was intended to connect to people as community members, as elements of a collective, as a citizenry "all in it together" and as "all for one and one for all" faced with the crisis. The survey referred to above found evidence that this was indeed a motivating factor. This led the authors of the "ten cities" survey to make the bold claim that "the belief that 'we're all in it together' is more important than other factors in explaining why the UK public has complied with lockdown measures".[20] This explanation of NPI compliance has persisted beyond the first lockdown. A poll conducted by Ipsos MORI in October 2020 concluded that social responsibility (for the vulnerable) and defending the NHS were the main drivers of compliance.[21]

This kind of public response would perhaps be no surprise to the philosopher Slavoj Žižek. This is because for him the pandemic has turned people without realizing it into socialists or "communists". His meaning of "communist" is in the sense that people have been motivated by the pandemic to imagine a new kind of society based on "new forms of local and global solidarity" that may even transcend reliance on "market mechanisms" to deal with social problems. These are, opines Žižek, the unintended benefits of lockdowns and furloughs (that is, of the unexpected resurgence of the socially and economically interventionist welfare state in order to ward off economic collapse) and of the citizenry being drawn into a collective effort to look out for the welfare of each other.[22]

This is, of course, a remarkably if not heroically optimistic perspective. Žižek could not draw on any survey evidence that people regarded the "lockdown state" as anything other than a temporary aberration or as anything more than a necessary evil. Nor, arguably, is the lockdown state a particularly robust model for the "caring" society. Not when agents of that state in Britain were at one point taking actions that decimated society's most vulnerable members. I refer to the appalling decision of Matt Hancock's Department of Health and Social Care (DHSC) to release thousands of COVID-untested people from hospitals into care homes.[23] Moreover, public conformity to burdensome NPIs may be more or as much motivated by self-interest than by communal solidarity or support for public health services and workers. This would be fear of possible harm to oneself and to one's immediate intimates (or of harm to one's own interests) rather than of being expressive of a new collective spirit of care for unknown community others. I will return to this matter later.

The positive results for the UK revealed by the "ten cities" survey of public conformity to physical distancing have not generally been duplicated by others.

Even Ganslmeier *et al.*'s study reveals a steady decline in compliance rates (or a steady increase in the number of non-compliers) almost from the start of the first UK lockdown on 24 March 2020. The decline was gradual and modest for the rest of March, but accelerated in April, and rose quite steeply from the start of May. By mid-May 2020, non-compliance with distancing restrictions was running at almost 13 percent of the adult population, according to the YouGov self-report data of respondents upon which Ganslmeier *et al.*'s study drew.[24]

Even the "ten cities" survey conducted in the context of the first British lockdown revealed that plenty of people were from the start not at all consistent distancers (or who were "somewhat" distancers), with a small percentage core (though sizeable in actual numbers) who were radical non-compliers, despite this being legally prohibited. Of course, *real non-compliance would have likely been significantly higher*. This is owing to the fact that compliance rates would be exaggerated by research based on self-report data, as most of the research into public adherence to the NPIs has been, owing to over-reporting.[25]

If people think that following the rules is the morally right or socially expected thing to be doing, which is obviously most likely when the rules have formal legal status, those of them who are not doing so (in whole or in part) are incentivized not to admit this to pollsters or researchers. They also have motives not to admit non-compliance even if they do not regard rule-following as either morally correct or socially approved simply because this would be an admission of unlawful action. Interestingly, though unsurprisingly, respondents of pandemic surveys who report high levels of *self*-compliance to the COVID-19 restrictions tend to report much higher incidences of non-compliant behaviour by *others*.[26]

A London-based study that was inclusive of the whole period of the first UK lockdown from March 2020 and thereafter right up until the end of May 2021 reported that

> the vast majority of participants (92.8%; 632) did not adhere to all SD rules. Similarly, 90.7% (618) of participants were unable to always maintain two metres distance from others when they went out for permitted reasons indicating significant overlap between non-adherence of all rules and unintentional non-adherence. Slightly less than half (48.6%; 331) of participants intentionally did not adhere to SD rules. The more common intentional violation was unpermitted leaving of the house, which a third (227) of participants did not adhere to. Less frequent were unpermitted meeting of others with 28.8% (196) of participants not adhering to this rule.[27]

This study found that intentional non-compliance was associated with "lower intention to SD, which was associated with a lower sense of social responsibility, a higher sense of self-interest and lower normative pressure from family and friends".[28] The non-vulnerable were three-and-a-half times more likely to deliberately disregard physical distancing than the vulnerable and were on average ten years younger than those who were compliers. As one of the researchers, Yolanda Eraso, concluded:

Nearly half of the individuals in our sample deliberately broke the rules by meeting with others from outside their households or going out for unpermitted reasons. Such behaviours seem to indicate that acting for the common or the social good have dwindled in favour of a greater sense of self-interest. Clearer public health messages, maintaining a consistent sense of collective responsibility, and deterrence policies as seen in policing practices in France and Italy, could play a more relevant role in improving adherence to the guidance.[29]

But, as well as growing numbers of the simply or serially non-compliant, many other people reported in surveys that they were "bending" lockdown rules "on occasion". Such has been described as acts of "creative non-compliance". This behaviour was rationalized by these "occasional" non-compliers as violations only of the "letter" of the law that would protect public health rather than of its "spirit" (to which they claimed commitment).[30] Such decisions may be interpreted as being informed by moral judgement. But, perhaps more plausibly, they may be counted as examples of David Matza's and Gresham Sykes' techniques of neutralization.[31] Techniques of neutralization, on Matza's and Sykes' definition, are preconceived justifications that allow the setting aside of those norms that would prohibit acts that are seen as injurious to self-interest and to pleasurable or rewarding experiences, whether one's own or those of members of one's intimate circle.

A major Office for National Statistics (ONS) study conducted from 23 December 2020 to 22 January 2021, which includes a period encompassing part of the third national lockdown, casts light on self-reported non-compliance with NPIs. The qualitative aspects of the research certainly illuminate what may plausibly be interpreted as people mobilizing techniques that neutralize pandemic restrictions to legitimize rule-breaking. Popular neutralizations, especially by young adults, tended to invoke mental well-being concerns as imperatives to set aside physical distancing rules for the protection of self and intimate others. This was on the grounds that temporary barriers to socializing were not only sources of unhappiness owing to boredom or isolation but were radically and potentially permanently injurious to self or loved ones, harbingers or promulgators of mental illnesses. More mundanely, other rule-breakers justified this as resulting from confusion over rule complexity or rule changes.[32] In other cases, whether for occasional or frequent rule-breakers, neutralizations of lockdown norms functioned as blame-shifting. Some self-reported non-compliers rationalized non-compliance with certain NPIs on the grounds that proximate others in certain settings they could not avoid were disregarding them, which demotivated their own compliance under these circumstances.[33]

Less dramatically than was the case for those invoking mental health concerns, some rule-"benders" (that is, selective rule-breakers) during the first lockdown rationalized their non-compliance with certain NPIs by claiming these were counteracted by their acts of compliance with other (and in their judgement more important) NPIs.[34] Others, during the third lockdown, rationalized rule-breaking by claiming that they were taking precautions to minimize the health risks associated with their own non-complying behaviour.[35] Such included scrupulous adherence to home sanitization by themselves as visitors or hosts and of guests when participating in illegal indoor gatherings of friends and kin, or respecting distancing from strangers while relaxing distancing with known "trustworthy" others.[36]

This type of reasoning was, according to the ONS survey, especially associated with high-income professionals who were knowledgeable of the rules they were legally required to follow. Such chimes with research conducted by Liam Wright and Daisy Fancourt, namely their analysis of predictors of non-compliance to COVID-19 restrictions in the UK during the first five months of the pandemic.[37] According to this,

> individuals with higher incomes had higher initial compliance but faster decreases over time. It is possible that these individuals were able to maintain a strict compliance initially due to not facing any financial barriers such as an inability to pay bills that may have driven to rules being broken in a search for work. However, as the pandemic continued, it may be that greater wealth and a sense of privilege or a lack of financial fear over fines may have driven a more relaxed approach to compliance.[38]

The suggestive "may be" here was not idle speculation. The later ONS survey cited one high-income participant who self-reported rule-"bending" on the grounds that "the house was safe and clean, friends were not touching handles, I'm happy to take a chance with a fine".

The international picture

Beyond the UK, a substantial body of international research into public compliance with NPIs more generally (that is, not simply physical distancing) also paints a much less rosy picture than the "ten cities" survey does for the UK. This reveals a highly variable picture, with levels of compliance as high as 90 percent among some populations, but as low as 67 percent among others, by mid-April 2020.[39] At the start of the pandemic, as the first wave grew, initial public compliance with lockdown policies was uniformly strong worldwide. This has been demonstrated by a range of national-level studies – including those conducted in France,[40] in Portugal,[41] in Hungary,[42] in China,[43] in India,[44] in Israel,[45] and of course in the UK, to cite just a few. However, virtually as soon as lockdowns were brought in, public compliance began to slip. I will highlight a range of studies that establish the point. There have been plenty to date.

A study of compliance and non-compliance focusing especially on government-mandated 1.5-metre distancing in the Netherlands found that

> even though people complied with the social distancing directives prior to and immediately after these were first implemented, compliance started to decline gradually in the following weeks. This decline occurred despite repeated calls from government officials to continue keeping distance.[46]

This study was based on mass non-participatory video observations rather than self-report data – a more reliable method of gauging people's behaviour. As the researchers noted: "The observed pattern of declining compliance to social distancing directives is in line with findings from other studies on the COVID-19 pandemic and mirrors patterns observed in studies on medical adherence outside the pandemic context, which found that rapid declines in compliance occurred even in the first five to ten days of treatment ". The study found that incidents of non-compliance increased even though pandemic death tolls were rising in the Netherlands at the same time. This was suggestive "that people's willingness to comply is not as strongly driven by fear and anxiety related to the virus as has been suggested in survey research".[47] Nor, apparently, was this motivated by concerns for the protection of community others.

The Netherlands study also found that non-compliance with physical distancing rules was associated with non-compliance with stay-at-home guidance.

It appears that when people do not comply with stay-at-home directives, they also do not comply with 1.5-meter distancing directives. This means that the physical distancing violations are likely to increase as soon as the government relaxes the preventive measures and allows for schools, restaurants, and similar venues to reopen. It also means that policy makers cannot rely on people keeping the 1.5-meter distance from others in public while allowing for relaxation of stay-at-home directives.[48]

Who, then, were the doubly non-compliant? The researchers draw attention to other research which "suggests that individuals who perceived one type of protective behavior to be effective (e.g., wearing facemasks, home disinfection) are more likely to engage in other types of protective behaviors".[49] Conversely, non-compliers with physical distancing did not seem to be those who believed that measures other than 1.5-metre distancing were more effective in protecting themselves and others and who were instead following these other alternatives. Rather, non-compliers were simply those who were generally non-compliant.

Particularly high levels of non-compliance with specific NPIs (namely, personal hygiene practices and physical distancing rules) have been revealed by a study in Germany conducted between 13 and 27 March 2020.[50] This research, like the Netherlands study, was obviously at an early stage of the development of the pandemic, so "pandemic fatigue" could not be a factor explaining non-compliance. The study found that only 25 percent of respondents self-reported as "high compliers" (committing themselves to protective personal hygiene practices and distancing measures), whereas 24 percent self-reported as "low compliers" (expressing low commitment to both practices). The rest (51 percent) were classified as "public compliers", in that they self-reported their intention to adhere to distancing in public places but not to protective personal hygiene practices (that is, frequent handwashing, avoidance of face contact, tissue disposal, frequent ventilation). The low compliers were predominantly young and male.

Rather better rates of compliance with NPIs have been reported for Greece, however. A study by Kamenidou, Stavrianea, and Liava found much smaller numbers of the radically or serially non-compliant than in other European countries over a longer time span (1 March–20 May 2020).[51] Less than five percent (4.6 percent) of respondents fitted the definition, according to their results, which the research-ers classed rather aptly as belonging to the "unconcerned citizens" group. These were people who completely eschewed all NPIs. The largest group of respond-ents in their sample (making up 48.6 percent of it) were the "meticulous proac-tive citizens", who self-reported as consistently compliant with all of the required NPIs. But another sizeable group (making up 10.1 percent of respondents) were the "occasionally cautious citizens". These were people who self-reported as some-times compliant with the NPIs but as often if not most often not. So, in Greece, as in other European countries, compliance with NPIs was variable, with a large num-ber of people (14.5 percent approximately) who were either totally disengaged or somewhat disengaged from them almost from the start of the pandemic. Consistent with the findings of other studies, the least compliant people were disproportion-ately younger adults, of the male sex.

Substantial degrees of non-compliance with NPIs have been revealed not only by "people" research (that is, studies or surveys of people's observed behaviour or self-reported behaviour) but also by surveys of media reporting on the issue across a range of countries. As summarized by Ölcer, Yilmaz-Aslan, and Brzoska,[52]

> protective precautions such as self-isolation, the rules on social distancing, and the closure of all entertainment venues in the public sphere have received mixed reactions, particularly from young individuals, many of which do not comply with current advice. For instance, beaches, hiking trails, and parks in California and Florida were swarmed with crowds over the weekends thus defying the bans and recommendations of authorities on social distanc-ing. In France, Belgium, England, the USA, Germany, and New Zealand, an increase in parties has been reported by the media, particularly after the closure of schools and universities … The videos and pictures illustrating non-compliance with social distancing recommendations and regulations, which [have] occupied social media … have been accompanied by many discussions. Governments' methods of coping with SARS-CoV-2, particu-larly imposing social distancing and self-isolation regulation, have led to a divide between people: the rule followers and the risk-takers.[53]

Media reports of non-compliance became commonplace in the UK, for example, during the piecemeal de-escalation of the first national lockdown and during the second and third national lockdowns. These included those that drew attention to mass commutes that filled beaches, parks, and resorts during various public holi-days, especially in the spring and summer of 2020, and those that highlighted ille-gal raves and parties on New Year's Eve at the end of the pandemic's first year.[54]

These above-cited studies were based on data gathered in the earlier period of the pandemic where compliance rates would be expected to be higher than at later times owing to the effects of attrition. Yet levels of non-compliance were already significant. Later studies that gather data relevant to compliance and non-compliance beyond the spring of 2020 and continuing into 2021 report similar results. For illustrative purposes, I will consider just two more, from many others that could be considered.

Hengartner *et al.*'s Swiss survey, which was based on data gathered between 11 December 2020 and 5 January 2021, reported high or strong compliance with NPIs for only 75 percent of the adult population.[55] As for the rest, 20 percent were classified as somewhat or moderate compliers, whereas five percent were classed as "remarkably non-compliant".

> The highest non-compliance was found with respect to avoiding public transportation (22.7% were rather or definitely noncompliant) and making a SARS-CoV-2 test when having (cold) symptoms (29.9% were rather or definitely noncompliant).[56]

Again, in accordance with the findings of a number of other studies,[57] the "remarkably non-compliant" were mostly of young age and male sex. These were also those who reported "low appraisal of negative consequences" of catching COVID-19, "less fear and worries" about the pandemic, "not obtaining regular information from health authorities", and "not trusting in medical experts".[58]

A particularly interesting study of compliance and non-compliance with NPIs (for reasons that will become apparent) was conducted by Kaine, Greenhalgh, and Wright.[59] This was in Auckland, New Zealand, and was based on data gathered between 7 and 22 September 2020. This revealed a considerable degree of public ambivalence and scepticism towards the pandemic and NPIs in a country where one might least expect it. A number of distinct categories of respondents were identified. These included the "Covid-19 ambivalents", 15 percent of the respondents, "who were unsure about what to believe about Covid-19", and the "Covid-19 sceptics", 10 percent of the respondents, who "believed, variously, that Covid-19 was a hoax, was no worse than the seasonal flu, and that fears about Covid-19 are exaggerated".[60] Other categories of respondents with regard to the NPIs included "elimination sceptics" (10 percent), "mask ambivalents" (27 percent), "mask sceptics" (seven percent), "self-isolation doubtfuls" (11 percent), "testing selectives" (12 percent), and "testing doubters" (18 percent).[61] As the researchers found,

> a substantial minority of respondents exhibited low-to-mild involvement with wearing face masks and getting tested for Covid-19. This result suggests a minority of Auckland residents may inadvertently fail to comply with government measures intended to prevent the spread of Covid-19 in the community … These results [also] … suggest a small minority of Auckland residents would deliberately choose not to comply with government measures intended to prevent the spread of Covid-19 in the community.[62]

Now, what was remarkable about these results was that they were derived from the public of one of the few high-income countries that was then making a decent fist of suppressing COVID-19. The government was pursuing a strategy of "elimination" of the virus from New Zealand until a vaccination "fix" was feasible. This was not in the sense of eliminating COVID-19 altogether, once and for all, but by substantially cutting importations from overseas, and undermining transmission chains in the community, by nipping these in the bud.

Border closure (except for returning citizens and permanent residents) alongside a four-tier alert system that sanctioned a range of controls that would be tightened or eased based on the alert level was actually succeeding (at the time of this study and beforehand) in curbing the virus in the pre-vaccination era so that rates of hospitalizations and deaths were also being suppressed. In accordance with this policy, mandated NPIs were relaxed only following a period in which zero new cases were reported.[63] Yet a substantial minority doubted the efficacy of the NPIs that were delivering that result, whereas a smaller but significant number rejected the idea that they should be bound by them. This was perhaps because the success of the "elimination" strategy undermined fear of the virus, which in turn threatened to undermine the "elimination" strategy.

Initial compliance with NPIs

Despite the sobering findings of studies such as these, as YouGov data sets show, in all parts of the world, public compliance with a number of NPIs (avoiding crowded public places, working from home, washing hands regularly, using hand sanitizer, and avoiding direct contact with physical objects and surfaces outside the home) did increase dramatically at the start of the pandemic, albeit at different rates and magnitudes. This was not the case for all NPIs, but it was for most. Notably, public mask-wearing was slow to get started in most countries of the North Atlantic region on this timescale, in stark contrast with other places. The exceptions were in Italy (up to 75 percent compliant toward the end of March) and Spain (up to 45 percent compliant by the start of April).[64] Rapidly increasing public compliance with the other NPIs was, however, the international norm during the period from the latter part of February and throughout March (2020). During this period, initial compliance, if not high everywhere, was certainly at its highest, albeit with major (and disquieting) regional and national variations.

In the US, the percentage of people who self-reported avoiding crowded public places rose from 24 percent at the start of March to 77 percent by the close of March. Over roughly the same period, the percentage of people who self-reported working from home increased from three percent to 29 percent, peaking at 32 percent in the second week of April. Similarly, the percentage of people who self-reported improved personal hygiene in response to the pandemic (regular hand-washing and sanitizer usage) peaked at 72 percent by the end of March, whereas those who self-reported avoiding direct hand-touching of physical objects or surfaces (door handles, etc.) in public places rose to 59 percent by the end of March, peaking at 60 percent a couple of weeks later.[65]

In the UK, initial compliance with these same NPIs increased faster than in the US and reached higher levels. Here the percentage of people who self-reported avoiding crowded public places rose from 14 percent in the first week of March, peaking at 80 percent in the last week of March and in the first week of April. On the same timescale, more or less, the number of people who self-reported working from home increased from one percent to 38 percent, peaking at 39 percent at the start of April. As for the number of people self-reporting improved personal hygiene in response to the pandemic, this rose from 35 percent at the start of March to 77 percent by the beginning of April, whereas the number of people self-reporting avoiding hand contact with physical objects or surfaces in public places over the same period rose from 14 percent to 56 percent, peaking at 59 percent by mid-April.[66]

Across the EU, over the same timescale (early March up to the start of April 2020), the same pattern holds as for the US and UK, albeit in most cases at somewhat higher levels. Here are some case examples to illustrate the general trend.

In France, self-reported public crowd avoidance increased from 39 percent and peaked at 82 percent, on this timescale. In Germany, over the same period, this rose from 38 percent and peaked at 80 percent. So too in Spain, where this rose from 47 percent and peaked at 85 percent. In Italy, facing the earliest upsurge of the European pandemic, self-reported public crowd avoidance was already close to its peak before the end of the second week of March (at 87 percent), and this peaked (at 90 percent) a couple of weeks later. In Sweden, this rose from 42 percent to 72 percent, though peaking rather later than in the other EU countries (at 75 percent) in the last week of April.[67]

In France, self-reported home-staying and home-working over the same period rose from five percent to its peak of 41 percent. In Germany, on the same timescale, this rose from three percent to its peak of 29 percent. In Spain, this rose from eight percent to its peak of 51 percent, during this same period. In Italy, this rose from 27 percent to its peak of 49 percent, again on the same broad timescale. In Sweden, over this period, it rose from 10 percent to 30 percent, peaking much later than in other EU countries (32 percent) at the start of May.

As for self-reported compliance with improved personal hygiene and avoidance of touching physical objects outside the home, the period witnessed the same big upswings. In France, this peaked at 76 percent (2 April) for personal hygiene improvements and at 64 percent (also 2 April) for public touching avoidance. In Germany, this peaked at 72 percent (23 March) for personal hygiene improvements and at 54 percent (12 April) for public touching avoidance. In Spain, this peaked at 86 percent (19 March) for personal hygiene enhancements and at 67 percent (7 April) for touching avoidance. In Italy, this peaked at 82 percent (11 March) for improved personal hygiene and 63 percent (2 April) for touching avoidance. And, in Sweden, this peaked at 72 percent (11 April) for enhanced hygiene and 61 percent (25 April) for touching avoidance.[68]

However, rates and volumes of public compliance with these NPIs over the same basic timescale (from March up to April 2020), indeed from an earlier date in the development of the pandemic, were at their highest level by some distance in the Asia-Pacific region, and these were maintained over a much longer period. This was especially the case in most of the countries of Southeast Asia. These countries were at the vanguard of public mask-wearing, which by contrast grew slowly and fitfully in the West and in the Global North. This may be evidenced by YouGov data from several case examples: Malaysia, the Philippines, Thailand, Hong Kong, Vietnam, Singapore, and Taiwan.

In Malaysia, by early March, 55 percent of people self-reported public mask-wearing, which increased to 82 percent by the start of April, and which peaked at 92 percent in mid-October. In the Philippines, at the start of March, 59 percent of people self-reported public mask-wearing, which increased to 84 percent by early April, and which peaked at 88 percent by mid-October. In Thailand, 73 percent of people were self-reporting wearing masks in public places before February's end, rising to 89 percent by the end of March, and peaking at 90 percent by mid-April.

In Hong Kong, towards the end of February, self-reported public mask-wearing was already running at 90 percent, which twice more attained this level (in mid-April and early June) during the first wave, and which did not peak (at 92 percent) until mid-March the following year (2021). In Vietnam, this rose from 59 percent towards the end of March to 85 percent in the first week of April and peaked at 87 percent in the last week of April. In Singapore, a regionally low threshold of mask-wearing compliance (of 21 percent in mid-March) thereafter grew at an astronomical rate, reaching 90 percent towards the end of April. This did not peak (at 93 percent) until mid-June 2021. As for Taiwan, at the start of March, already 84 percent of people were self-reported maskers, which rose to a peak of 89 percent in early April.[69]

As for compliance with the other cited NPIs in these countries during the first pandemic wave, these too were much ahead of and in advance of those in the North Atlantic region (North America and Europe). Public crowd avoidance in Malaysia, according to self-report data, rose from 40 percent of the population in the latter part of February up to a peak of 88 percent by the end of March. This rose from 49 percent up to a peak of 85 percent from late March to early April in the Philippines. This rose from 45 percent up to a peak of 86 percent in Thailand between the tail end of February and mid-April. And this rose from 56 percent in the latter stages of March up to a peak of 83 percent by late April in Vietnam.

The same basic pattern was evident in Singapore and Taiwan. In the former, self-reported public crowd avoidance increased from 44 percent of the population in the later part of February up to a peak of 86 percent by late April, whereas in the latter this rose from 49 percent up to a peak of 81 percent over the same timescale. As for Hong Kong, following mainland China's lead, crowd-avoiding behaviour was already running at 63 percent of people in the final week of February. This peaked at 83 percent during the first week of April.[70]

Staying at home and working-from-home trends for these countries during the first wave mirror those for public crowd avoidance, though at lesser scales, according to self-reports. In Malaysia, home-staying and working-from-home rates increased from eight percent of people in late February up to a high point of 70 percent by early April. In the Philippines, they increased from nine percent up to a peak of 66 percent over roughly the same duration. In Thailand, on the same timescale, they increased from 14 percent to 54 percent. And in Singapore, they rose from 11 percent also to 54 percent, again over the same period.

On a later timescale, home-staying and home-working in Vietnam rose sharply within a week from 38 percent (towards the end of March) up to a peak of 53 percent in the first week of April. Home-staying and home-working increased much less radically in Hong Kong over this period compared to the others, but only because this was already at a high level by mid-February, peaking at 51 percent by mid-April. Of the Southeast Asian countries, only Taiwan was something of an anomaly. Here home-staying and home-working rates peaked at just 28 percent during the first pandemic wave. This was in the first week of April. However, this later reached 44 percent by mid-point 2021, in response to a later upsurge of the virus.[71]

Turning now to the data for trends in personal hygiene and object avoidance in public places for these same countries. What does this reveal? This fits the general pattern for higher-than-average international compliance rates. In Malaysia, the number of people who said that they were improving their personal hygiene in response to the pandemic (by regular hand-washing and the use of sanitizers) increased from 76 percent to 88 percent from the start of March up to early April. The number of Malaysians who self-reported avoiding touching objects in public places increased from 40 percent to 75 percent over the same period.

In the Philippines, the number of people who self-reported higher levels of hand-washing and sanitizer use increased from 76 percent to 87 percent from early to late March, whereas the number of those who said they were public object-avoiders increased from 48 percent to 70 percent on the same timescale. (The number of people practising object avoidance in public places in the Philippines did not peak until mid-September at 87 percent). As for Hong Kong, rates of public compliance with pandemic-linked personal hygiene measures were in the mid-eighties percentage-wise before the start of March, where they stayed across successive pandemic waves. Object avoidance behaviour peaked at 72 percent of the population in mid-April. This too was up from higher levels than was typical even in the region (in the mid-sixties percentage-wise) since February.[72]

In Thailand, 88 percent of people self-reported enhanced attention to personal hygiene in response to the pandemic by mid-April, up from 73 percent at the tail end of February, whereas 75 percent self-reported object avoidance in public places in mid-April, up from 45 percent at the start of March. In Vietnam, 84 percent self-reported increased personal hygiene to minimize catching or passing on the virus by April's end, up from 54 percent in the second half of March. This was as 71 percent were self-reporting object avoidance outside the home by the start of May, up from 40 percent towards the end of March.

Self-report data for Taiwan over this period was very similar to that for Hong Kong since this indicates high levels of public engagement with hand-washing and sanitizing practices, even by regional standards, right from the start of the pandemic. These were already in the mid-eighties percentage bracket before February's end. The number of Taiwanese self-reporting object avoidance rose from 49 percent to 65 percent between the final week of February and the first week of April.[73] As for Singapore, the number of people self-reporting compliance with hand-washing and hand-sanitizing recommendations was already running at 81 percent of the population by the tail end of February, and this peaked at 87 percent at the start of April.

The number of Singaporeans who were self-reporting public object avoidance also increased from 40 percent at the close of February to 62 percent by the second week of April.

****

YouGov self-report data therefore indicates that public compliance with a range of NPIs during the pandemic's first wave increased rapidly and assumed high scales. This was especially in the period from March to April 2020 in the North Atlantic region and from February to April in the Asia-Pacific region. Yet the data also shows that there was considerable variance right from the start of the crisis in the public response across the world. This also shows that, in certain parts of the world, including and especially in North America, the UK, and mainland Europe, public compliance with the NPIs, that is, *self*-reported compliance, was much less impressive than it was initially represented.

In Europe and the US, most people did not switch to home-staying and home-working, even over the course of the pandemic's first wave. Here as well substantial minorities of people did not self-report conformity to other NPIs, even at the peak periods of conformity. The rate of non-conformity with avoiding crowded public spaces, at peak periods of conformity, ranged from 25 percent (in Sweden) to 10 percent (in Italy), with an average rate of non-compliance across the seven North Atlantic countries under review of around 18.7 percent. The rate of non-conformity with avoidance of touching physical objects in public places, during the peak periods of conformity, ranged from 41 percent (in the UK) to 33 percent (in Spain), with an average non-compliance rate across the seven of 38.7 percent. The rate of non-conformity with personal hygiene improvement measures ranged from 28 percent (in Germany, Sweden, and the US) to 14 percent (in Spain), at the peak periods of conformity, with an average rate of non-compliance overall of 23.3 percent across the sample.[74]

Later compliance with NPIs

But what of the fate of public responses to the NPIs beyond the rise of the pandemic's first wave? Worldwide, NPIs remained in place in the context of phased unlockings of lockdowns, albeit scaled down, and were scaled up again in the context of later lockdowns, whether local or national. This was the case in the UK from March 2020 up until mid-July 2021, though time scales varied in other countries. Throughout this period of greater or lesser restrictions, significant levels of non-compliance with NPIs were constant, with a tendency to grow. New pandemic waves would motivate temporary upward spikes in public adherence to NPIs, but at lower scales than at previous peaks, albeit to greater or lesser degrees in different places,[75] so that there was a downward trajectory overall.[76]

Similar patterns of variable compliance and non-compliance with NPIs (with a tendency for the latter to increase) have been found to be the case in previous epidemiological crises.[77] These include the H7N9 influenza outbreak (of 2013) in China, and the SARS outbreak (of 2002 and 2003) that impacted especially on

China and Hong Kong but which touched 30 countries.[78] This has also been characteristic of other recent outbreaks of dangerous viruses, such as swine flu and Ebola.[79] Norton *et al.* summarize the evidence:

> In previous pandemics, the uptake of these NPIs has been an uphill battle for the public health. In general, people routinely fail to follow handwashing recommendations. During the 2009 swine flu pandemic, people who believed that they were in the "low risk" category for infection were less likely to engage in handwashing. Another study conducted at the same time found that less than 10% of people with acute respiratory infections stayed home when symptomatic, and as many as 45% of people reported attending social events because they did not believe they were contagious. Even during highly lethal outbreaks, such as the African Ebola virus epidemic, some families sheltered sick relatives at home instead of sending them to quarantine facilities.[80]

Petherick *et al.*'s review of trajectories of compliance and non-compliance with NPIs in 124 countries, in the period from April to September 2020,[81] found that declines "in adherence were empirically meaningful and geographically widespread". This was apart from mask-wearing, which increased over the period of the study's coverage, as compliance with other NPIs dipped.

> While a low-cost and habituating behaviour (mask wearing) exhibited a linear rise in adherence, high-cost and sensitizing behaviours (physical distancing) declined, but this decline decelerated over time, with small rebounds seen in later months. Reductions in adherence to physical distancing showed little difference across societal groups, but were less intense in countries with high interpersonal trust ... In the portion of these curves showing gradual, non-linear declining adherence, we observe reductions of noteworthy magnitudes. On average, adherence in the case of self-report physical distancing (using the aggregated measure) fell by 15% ... between the baseline period (the 30-day period starting when required policies were first adopted) and the period with minimum adherence (150–180 days after first required measure) ... Considering the portion of the U-shaped curves after the inflection points, the rebounding adherence that we identify is substantively smaller than the prior declines.[82]

Among those countries that witnessed the biggest drops in NPI compliance over the course of the pandemic's first year was the US. This witnessed a substantial decrease in the national NPI index from April to June 2020. This was from 70.0 to 50.8.[83]

> All US Census regions experienced decreases ... from early April to late November, from 70.0 to 60.5 in the South, 71.5 to 62.2 in the West, 70.8 to 62.4 in the Northeast, and 70.3 to 54.4 in the Midwest. The NPI adherence

index in the final survey week was significantly lower in the Midwest than in the South, West, and Northeast.[84]

A November rally in public NPI compliance levels in the US, as the pandemic resurged, could restore the index only to 60.1. Despite the resurgence, the number of people who reported staying at home except for essential activities or exercise had fallen from 79.6 percent in April to 41.1 percent by November's end. Over the same period: the number of people who reported maintaining physical distancing from people outside their own households had fallen from 63.5 percent to 37.8 percent; the number reporting not having visitors in their homes had fallen from 80.3 percent to 57.6 percent; and the number who reported avoiding dining out in restaurants had fallen from 87.3 percent to 65.8 percent.[85]

A similar pattern existed in Germany. By October 2020, according to panel survey data, non-compliance with the major NPIs was running as follows: with stay-at-home rules, 22 percent; with physical distancing in public places, 24 percent; with public mask-wearing, 21 percent.[86] Consistent with the international direction of travel, a study carried out in Israel, also in October, reported that a substantial number of people (around 40 percent) were hostile to the idea of ramping-up NPIs to deal with new pandemic waves. This data was gathered during a time in which a fourth COVID upsurge was engulfing the country, driving up hospitalizations. Yet only 60.1 percent of people surveyed said that they would comply with another round of lockdown restrictions to bring the crisis under control.[87]

As for the UK, a large-scale study, conducted by Wright, Steptoe, and Fancourt, spanning the period from 1 April 2020 to 22 February 2021, and based on longitudinal data on self-reported compliance obtained from a sample of almost 51,000 adults,[88] found that around

15% of participants had decreasing levels of compliance across the pandemic, reporting noticeably lower levels of compliance in the second wave. Individuals with declining compliance levels were younger on average, in better physical health, had lower empathy and conscientiousness and greater general willingness to take risks.[89]

By September 2020, according to Ipsos MORI poll data, people's self-reported compliance with NPIs had dropped from the initially high rates that some surveys found in March (in the eighties or even nineties in percentage terms) to just 62 percent. An October rebound, as the second wave gathered steam in the autumn, restored the number of people who were claiming adherence to NPI norms, but only partially, to 73 percent, well below the early-pandemic thresholds.[90] "The most commonly broken rules were not abiding by social distancing rules (42%) and visiting friends or family who they aren't allowed to (19%)".[91]

At the same time, large numbers of respondents, according to Ipsos MORI's results, were now expressing scepticism about pandemic restrictions and endorsing reasons for non-compliance. When participants were asked in the poll how convincing they found a range of arguments for non-compliance with government mandates or recommendations, the following ones were well supported:[92]

People in government have not been following the rules, so why should we – 47 percent

We don't know enough about the coronavirus to know if these rules are the right thing to do – 42 percent

It's OK not to follow the rules if you need to work or look after someone – 41 percent

We need to learn to live with the coronavirus so we need to stop following these restrictions – 38 percent

The rules have gone too far and are causing more harm than good – 38 percent

People should be able to decide for themselves how much of a risk they want to take – 32 percent

The impact of coronavirus is greatly exaggerated – 29 percent

Remarkably, these responses were gathered following a period (since May of 2020) in which the UK government had taken the country out of lockdown, and in which owing to phased de-escalation of restrictions, there were actually few NPIs remaining.[93]

NPIs in the vaccination era

Even so, at no time in the pre-vaccination era of COVID-19 when NPIs were often legally mandated could self-reported public rule-following be said to be poor, notwithstanding the limitations of self-report data. Consequently, in this period, the public health protections afforded by the NPIs retained some efficacy, albeit significantly diminished. The vaccination period, however, has seen public compliance with NPIs drop away steadily in the high-income countries (as the judicial sanctioning of these has been removed), just as less radical declines have been witnessed elsewhere. This is even though the pandemic (and the harms that COVID-19 is capable of inflicting on the vulnerable) was not ended by mass inoculation. As Borchering *et al.*'s epidemiological modelling of the US pandemic (which mapped out the period ahead from April to September 2021) showed: "Even moderate reductions in NPI adherence were shown to undermine vaccination-related gains during the subsequent 2–3 months; decreased NPI adherence, in combination with increased transmissibility of some new variants, was projected to lead to surges in hospitalizations and deaths".[94]

YouGov data confirms that the vaccination era decline in public compliance with NPIs is a worldwide phenomenon, albeit at different rates and scales. In the pre-vaccination era, the US and Europe have, by and large, experienced amongst the lowest levels of public compliance with the NPIs, whereas Southeast Asia has experienced the highest. Since then, in the vaccination era, Europe and the US have also experienced some of the biggest average declines in rates of public compliance across the range of NPIs, whereas Southeast Asia has experienced the smallest. This is during the period from the start of 2021 (when vaccination programmes really got started in earnest in the high- and upper-middle-income countries) up until mid-July 2022.[95]

I will illustrate these trends by considering five case examples: the US, the UK, Spain, Malaysia, and Indonesia. Spain and the UK are selected because they represent each end of the European spectrum (higher and lower) for public compliance with NPIs. Malaysia and Indonesia are selected because these represent the higher and lower scales of public compliance with the NPIs in countries of the Asia-Pacific region. However, since the higher scales of compliance are more typical of Southeast Asia than the lesser ones are, plenty of other countries could have taken Malaysia's place.

In the US, from the start of January to the end of 2021, the number of people who self-reported avoiding crowded public places fell from 67 percent to 49 percent. The rate stabilized at these lower scales (in the higher forties and lower fifties) in January and February 2022, but thereafter slipped to 39 percent by the start of July 2022. The number of Americans who self-reported work avoidance in favour of home-working had already dipped from its mid-April (2020) peak of 32 percent to 18 percent by the end of the year. By the end of 2021, this had dropped to 12 percent, and by mid-July 2022 to nine percent. Those who self-reported improved personal hygiene (hand-washing, sanitizer use) declined from 61 percent at the start of February 2021 to 45 percent by mid-June. From there it slipped to 39 percent by mid-October of that year, and finally to a new low of 36 percent by mid-April 2022. Those who self-reported avoiding direct touching of objects and surfaces in public places fell from 48 percent at the end of January 2021 to 32 percent by the year's end, then to 25 percent by early July 2022.[95]

In the UK, the number of people who self-reported avoiding crowded public places declined from 69 percent to 53 percent in the period from mid-January to mid-July 2021. By the end of November of that year, this had dipped to 39 percent. A winter COVID-19 surge helped drive this back up to 50 percent for a month or so, but since then the decline has been uninterrupted, hitting a new low of 26 percent by mid-June 2022.[96] The number of people who self-reported they were avoiding going out to work in favour of home-working peaked at 39 percent in early April 2020. By mid-January 2021, at the height of the third pandemic wave, this stood at 27 percent. By mid-January 2022, this had fallen to 12 percent, and by the end of June of that year to just four percent.[97] Those who self-reported improved personal hygiene declined from 57 percent at the start of January 2021 to 44 percent by mid-June and then to 39 percent by the year's end. By mid-July 2022 this had reached a new pandemic-era low of 28 percent.[98] Those who self-reported avoiding directly touching objects and surfaces in public places stood at 47 percent in early January 2021. By mid-July this was reduced to 31 percent and by the year's end to 26 percent. Presently (July 2022), this stands at 17 percent.[99]

In Spain, the number of people who self-reported avoiding crowded public places peaked at 86 percent at the end of January 2021. From there it declined to 60 percent by the end of October of that year and, since then, following a winter revival in response to another pandemic wave, to 46 percent by mid-June 2022. The number who self-reported they were avoiding going out to work in favour of home-working peaked at 51 percent at the start of April 2020. This tumbled to just 10 percent by mid-September 2020. New COVID-19 waves then incentivized a partial and fitful return to home-working, with 20 percent reporting that they were doing so by the tail end of January 2021. Since then, however, the decline has been steady, dipping to five percent by April 2022. Those who self-reported improved personal hygiene peaked at 86 percent in mid-March 2020. By mid-September of that year, however, this had fallen to 65 percent, and by early July 2022, this was languishing at 49 percent. Those who self-reported avoiding direct touching of objects and surfaces in public places stood at around 54 percent at the start of 2021, down from the pre-vaccination peak of 67 percent in the last week of May the year before. By mid-September 2021, this was reduced to 37 percent, and by late July 2022 to 23 percent.[100]

Turning now to countries of the Asia-Pacific region. In Malaysia, the number of people who self-reported avoiding crowded public places peaked at 90 percent in the first week of April 2020. From there until mid-August the following year, the number of people reporting this behaviour remained mostly in the eighties percentage-wise. Thereafter, a steady decline set in, so that by mid-July 2022, this stood at 67 percent.[101] The number who self-reported they were avoiding going out to work in favour of home-working peaked at 70 percent in the first week of April 2020, thereafter, dropping to 20 percent by the end of September of that year. Through several zig-zags, those reporting avoiding working outside the home was back up at 55 percent by mid-July 2021 before a steady decline set in, so that the rate stood at 19 percent by mid-July 2022.[102] Those who self-reported improved personal hygiene peaked at 88 percent at the start of April 2020. However, thereafter, a steady though slow decline was established, so that by mid-July 2022, this was down to 70 percent.[103] Those who self-reported avoiding direct touching of objects and surfaces in public places stood at around 66 percent in mid-August 2021, down from the early-April (2020) peak of 75 percent. Thereafter, this showed an overall decline, across the usual ups and downs, so that this stood at 50 percent by mid-July 2022.[104]

In Indonesia, the number of people who self-reported avoiding crowded public places peaked at 84 percent in the last week of March 2020. This had, across various ebbs and flows, fallen to 72 percent by the first week of July, and thereafter to 49 percent by mid-July 2022. The number who self-reported they were avoiding going out to work in favour of home-working peaked at 63 percent by the end of March 2020, before a downward trend reduced this to 28 percent by the first week of June 2021. A partial revival restored this to 39 percent by mid-July, before a second long period of gradual decline reduced this to 15 percent by mid-year 2022. Those who self-reported improved personal hygiene peaked at 84 percent, also at the end of March 2020, and has since then declined, albeit slowly, through peaks and dips, to 72 percent by mid-July 2022. Those who self-reported avoiding direct touching of objects and surfaces in public places stood at around 54 percent by the end of 2020. This had fallen to around 43 percent by mid-October 2021, and from there to 33 percent by mid-July 2022.[105]

Comparing, then, the North Atlantic and Asia-Pacific regions – with regard to levels of public compliance with the NPIs in the vaccination era – what conclusions may be drawn? Both regions have witnessed significant falls in the level of self-reported public compliance with the NPIs. However, the falls have been slower and shallower in the countries of Southeast Asia than in those of the North Atlantic. Indeed, in Southeast Asia, certain of the NPIs retain the support of large minorities if not majorities of the public, whereas major public support for the NPIs has not been retained in the high-income countries of North America and Europe.

The average rate of public compliance with avoiding crowded public spaces across nine European countries (UK, Denmark, Germany, Spain, Finland, Italy, Sweden, France, and Norway) at mid-year 2022 was around 34 percent, whereas in the US this was around 39 percent. In eight countries or territories of Southeast Asia (Malaysia, Indonesia, the Philippines, Thailand, Hong Kong, Vietnam, Singapore, and Thailand), by contrast, the average rate of public compliance with this NPI was still around 62 percent by mid-year 2022. The average rate of public compliance with working from home rather than going out to work across the European nine was 5.4 percent at mid-year 2022, whereas in the US this was nine percent. By contrast, this was, by that time, 23 percent across the Southeast Asia eight. The average rate of public compliance with improved personal hygiene practices across the European nine was 35 percent by mid-July 2022, whereas in the US this was 36 percent. This compared to 73 percent across the Southeast Asia eight on that date. Finally, the average rate of public compliance with avoidance of direct hand contact with objects or surfaces in public places across the European nine and in the US was 23 percent and 25 percent respectively, whereas for the Southeast Asia eight this was 49 percent, at mid-year 2022.[106]

****

The range of studies documenting compliance and non-compliance with the NPIs cited so far in this chapter raises the legitimate concern that even though the lockdowns and persisting NPI restrictions beyond these did succeed in depressing caseloads their efficacy was probably significantly less than would have been the case if compliance was higher. This is obscured by the mere fact that lockdowns yielded positive results. For – and this is an obvious point – with stronger and higher compliance, the virus would have been reduced faster and further than it was within the limited timeframes for the lockdowns that governments brought in. This in turn would have lessened the impact of subsequent waves. Public non-compliance (or rather the non-compliance of large numbers of people) increased the number of hospitalizations and deaths. In the UK, and beyond, the pandemic is not merely a story of government failure but of community failure. This is especially a failure of the publics or peoples of the West and of the Global North – for reasons that I will discuss.

Community failure was certainly not tackled by the government. In the UK, for example, non-compliance with stay-at-home regulations during the lockdowns was hardly supported by the coercive powers of the state. There was little criminal justice backing for the normative line of defence against the pandemic in favour of reliance on the public's voluntary acquiescence. There was little attempt to police the lockdowns, which might be explained by the enormity of the task of keeping millions under home curfew. However, since in the early days of the pandemic, it was a small minority who were persistent violators of lockdown rules, this explanation would not be satisfactory. A better job could have been done of enforcing the rules or at least rendering them more visible in public spaces.

But this was not supported by a lockdown-averse (ostensibly libertarian) government, nor perhaps by police chiefs, who would see this as placing huge demands on local forces without the central funding to support it.[107] A system that later was dubbed by police chiefs as "the four Es" became the default control strategy in the UK. According to this, before fines were entertained, police would: (1) engage rule-breakers (asking why they are breaking them); (2) explain to them why they should not break the rules on public health grounds; (3) encourage them to do the right thing; and (4) impose a penalty notice only as "last resort".

Only 9,000 penalty notices were imposed nationwide for physical distancing breaches in the first month of the first lockdown. This meant that just 0.02 percent of the population in this crucial period when the lockdown needed to be bedded down were sanctioned for endangering lives in what was presented as a "proportionate" approach.[108] By mid-January 2021, two weeks into the third UK lockdown, the total number of fixed-penalty notices issued since the start of legal restrictions stood at only 65,000.[109] Only those violators who were undeterred by repeat fixed-penalty notices would risk court proceedings under this approach. It is quite feasible that the British government eschewed mobilization and buttressing of the coercive powers of the state to defend the lockdown restrictions in order to undermine them. This could then be attributed to "freedom-loving Britons" (as PM Boris Johnson described them)[110] refusing to tolerate unreasonable restrictions, thereby compelling a fast-tracked return to normality, and hence reliance on the "herd immunity" strategy that was briefly flirted with in March 2020 before being ditched when it was realized that it would sink the NHS.[111]

This might explain why the penalties for infringement of stay-at-home rules during the first UK lockdown were remarkably small – on-the-spot fines of £60 reduced to £30 if paid within two weeks.[112] These stood no chance whatsoever of discouraging the committed rule-breaker. The lack of efficacy of these sanctions was arguably revealed by the fact that, on the police's own admission, they did nothing to deter repeat offending by the same individuals. Later these penalty notices were increased in England and Northern Ireland to £200 and were deployed more readily.[113] This was as the country was faced with rising levels of non-compliance in the runup to the second circuit-breaker lockdown.[114] Part of the British government's purpose was to deflect blame for the resurgence of the pandemic from its mixed messaging and over-hasty unlocking of restrictions on the public's "fraying discipline" (as Johnson put it).[115] Another intention was to head off the danger of a more protracted shutdown later on. Either way, this belated boosting of the normative aspect of social control was too little and too late to repair the damage perpetrated on the cause of public health by the steady erosion of NPI compliance.

Predictors of compliance with NPIs

Contrary to the claims of some commentators, such as Žižek, who found themselves impressed with the initially high levels of compliance with the lockdown restrictions, public conformity to physical distancing norms or recommendations may be more or as much motivated by self-interest than by communal solidarity or support for public health services and workers. This would be fear of possible harm to oneself and to one's immediate intimates (or of harm to one's own interests) rather than of being expressive of a new collective spirit of care for unknown community others. The possibility is certainly supported by a volume of pre-COVID research exploring public responses to health and other social crises, including epidemiological ones. As studies by Markowitz and Shariff and Young and Choy have found, when faced with such crises, "collective harm minimization tends to be a weak motivator for behavior change".[116] Rather, instrumental and egoistic motivations tend to crowd out others – fear of harm to self and to intimate others.[117]

What the rational choice economists call "risk perception" is reckoned to be a more powerful behavioural motivator for complying or not complying with NPIs under emergency conditions that limit civic freedoms than would be a sense of community obligations or of moral responsibilities for others. Such was found to be the case during the H7N9 influenza epidemic in China, for example.[118] If the risks to oneself or to one's intimates of non-compliance are seen as of a certain magnitude, the rules and restrictions will be complied with. If these risks are seen as of a lesser magnitude so that the burden of compliance on self-interest is higher than that of non-compliance, however, the rules and restrictions are much more likely to be disregarded. In the latter case, egoistic risk perception may be accompanied by "responsibility shifting" rationalizations of non-compliant behaviours.[119]

> Responsibility shift refers to the belief that infected persons are particularly responsible for (not) spreading the illness, thus protecting others, whereas healthy persons are responsible for protecting themselves from becoming infected, leading to a shift in personal priorities in protective behaviors depending on one's infection status.[120]

At the start of the pandemic, as the first wave built towards its peak, the sense of risk or danger to oneself and loved ones that the disease threatened across the social spectrum was at its extreme. This, according to researchers, has incentivized risk-avoidance behaviours as well as a willingness to submit to political authority during previous epidemiological and other crises.[121] This perspective is supported by current international pandemic research investigating motivational factors of compliance with NPIs during the first-wave lockdowns and beyond.[122] Such has found compliance to be weakly and inconsistently associated with trust in government, just as this was much more strongly and consistently associated with fear stemming from risk perceptions – whether of the virus or of sanctions for flouting legally mandated NPIs.

Evidence in support of this relevant to the UK is to be derived from a study by Wright *et al.*, for example.[123] Results here were based on data drawn from a sample of 17,000 people selected from a large panel survey of 70,000 adults aged 18 and above collected for a period of 22 weeks starting from 21 March 2020. The study found that a desire to reduce harm to people in general and ease pressures on NHS staff was not absent from the self-reported motivations sustaining compliance to NPIs. However, by far the "main factors facilitating compliance were desires to reduce risk to oneself and one's family and friends".[124]

Several studies (not only of the present pandemic but of earlier epidemics) have found that some degree of increase in self-reported compliance with NPIs coincides with increased trust or confidence in government, though this is often a weak association.[125] But many have not,[126] whereas others have found the opposite to be true.[127] Indeed, for some people, *distrust* in government could motivate *increased* compliance with government-mandated NPIs, as well as additional precautions beyond these. This may be because people regard the measures as necessary, but at the same time view their political leaders' commitment to them as insincere and equivocal. Seyd and Bu summarize the results of Kooistra's and van Rooij's systematic international review of public compliance with COVID-19-motivated NPIs.[128] This "found that, among the 19 studies exploring the role of trust in government, just five identified a positive impact on compliance, while three identified a negative impact and 11 no statistically significant impact".[129]

These sorts of results challenge well-established perspectives in the motivation theory literature. These hold that, as a general rule of thumb, high trust or confidence in political authority generates high levels of compliance with legal norms, whereas low trust or confidence in political authority generates the opposite, low compliance with legal norms.[130] This is the case, it is argued, in "normal" times as well as under emergency conditions, such as pandemics.[131] However, as the COVID-19 studies have shown, what is regarded as axiomatic in the moral leadership school of thought is not terribly well supported, or not so in the context of the present crisis. This may be explained by making a distinction between abstract "trust" (of people for authority) and actual "trustworthiness" (of governing authorities). For sure, if political authority was regarded as trustworthy by the general public, people would be incentivized to follow the COVID-related rules brought in by that authority. Conversely, they would be less incentivized to do that if they regarded political authority as untrustworthy. In short, they would, under these circumstances, conform because they have trust or confidence in political leaders.

But what if untrustworthy government is common in liberal democratic states (just as it is in illiberal autocratic ones) so that public distrust in political leaders is normalized? This would be owing to their dominance by and subservience to propertied elites and money power – which has accelerated in the neoliberal age. Such would be a factor of decivilization. In that case, although people may disregard legal norms such as those which mandated the COVID NPIs, they would equally have rational reasons (instrumental and otherwise) not to. Untrustworthy governments that prioritize profits over people are not precluded from "doing the right thing" in the service of public health, however reluctantly, equivocally, or tardily they take the necessary policy steps. This is because they are placed under pressure from adverse circumstances and the demands of a concerned citizenry. Indeed, the foot-dragging of neoliberal governments (such as the UK's) in mandating the NPIs, as they were faced with the pandemic, and their enthusiasm in scaling these down hastily, actually provides people with good reasons to trust the necessity of the NPIs, just as they distrust the authority which has so grudgingly mandated them.

My book, *The Pandemic in Britain*, conveys exactly this process in one pandemic-blighted corner of the world, that is, in "Blighty".[132] In the UK, in advance of the first lockdown on 24 March 2020, the public began practising NPIs, and businesses were already by then closing their doors. This was out of step with government policy recommendations – which were trailing pandemic events. Later on, a major part of popular opinion considered, rightly, that the UK government's first unlocking of restrictions was started prematurely. Parents and teachers, for example, refused to cooperate with plans of government to fast-track school reopenings in the late spring of 2020. Resistance in the form of refusal was so great that the plans were abandoned. Parents simply did not return their children to the classrooms. Teachers simply stayed at home. This was during a period in which the peak of the first wave was just a few weeks gone by and in which hospitalization rates remained relatively high. Here people were sticking to NPIs that were to be legalized or which had been mandated by ministers and their scientific advisers because they did not trust their political leaders or government scientists to make responsible decisions on matters of public health safety.[133]

Seyd and Bu's own longitudinal study (from April 2020 until February 2021) of public compliance with COVID-19 restrictions in Austria, Germany and Britain found that this was "maintained … *in spite* [my emphasis] of declining aggregate levels of trust" in government over the course of the pandemic up to that point. This was indicative, they surmised, that "fear may indeed be doing much of the 'heavy lifting' in sustaining pro-social forms of behaviour among the population".[134] Similarly, basing their findings upon analysis of a large international community sample, Harper *et al.* conclude: "Consistently, the only predictor of positive behavior change (e.g., social distancing, improved hand hygiene) was fear of COVID-19, with no effect of politically relevant variables".[135] Specifically, this study found that

> those participants who were more concerned about COVID-19 … were those who engaged more with public health-compliant behaviors (e.g., regular hand washing, and social distancing). It is of interest that the measures of fear and anxiety symptoms were stronger predictors than moral and political orientation, all of which explained small to no variance, potentially suggesting more emotional (rather than sociopolitical) influences on compliant behavior.[136]

Yet alternatively, if not additionally, conforming behaviour may be normatively motivated.[137] Normative motives for conformity may be undergirded by trust in political or juridical authority,[138] but not necessarily so. Rather, such may be sustained simply by recognition that political and judicial authority is legitimate, and/or by social pressures that arise from that.[139] Thus, the law and the law-making authority should be obeyed, from this perspective, because it would be morally wrong (because *unlawful*) not to obey them. This is just as hedonic incentives for rule-breaking may be held in check by fear or guilt over the moral disapproval this would elicit in known others.

Normatively motivated conformity has been evidenced by studies of public attitudes in relation to other epidemiological crises that posed potential community health risks.[140] Such has also been confirmed by current pandemic research into factors accounting for public compliance with physical distancing and other public health protection rules.[141] This is inasmuch as such studies have shown that many people have complied with NPIs not for reasons of pro-sociality (empathy for or altruism towards the community Other or wider citizenry) but rather because they believe that it is right and proper to obey the law (since the law is sacrosanct) or because they are wary of legal sanction or of disapproval of peers or of significant others if they were to disregard the rules. This is the case even if the normatively motivated disagree with those aspects of law pertaining to the pandemic. For, even though particular laws may be questionable, the rule of law is not. In the latter case, instrumental motivation (fear owing to high risk perception, self-interest) merges with normative motivation, however.

This does not mean, of course, that pro-social motives for public compliance with COVID-19 restrictions were negligible, even if these were not the primary ones for those who held them, and not for most people. Pro-sociality may be defined as "a person's proneness to take the interests of others and the collective into account, even if it presents a disadvantage for themselves".[142] People may choose to behave pro-socially rather than instrumentally or egoistically or be convinced to do so.[143] That empathic concern for or altruism towards community members can be a motive for complying with physical distancing, quarantining, and personal hygiene rules has some degree of research backing.[144] For some people at least these pro-social affectual incentives are important.

Which people? Studies prior to and during the present pandemic have shown that stronger and longer compliance with NPIs is associated with people with certain "personality traits ... [and] ... pro-social motivations", that is, such behaviour is more common among those who were high in "conscientiousness" and "empathic concern". Conversely, weaker and declining compliance with COVID-19 restrictions has been "more pronounced among young people, individuals low in conscientiousness and empathic concern, and individuals with risk-seeking attitudes".[145] A study by Oosterhoff and Palmer, for example, found that American youths tended to self-report higher egoistic values than other demographic groups, just as those who did were much less inclined than others to comply with pandemic restrictions.[146]

But, in the eye of the storm of the pandemic's first wave, public compliance with NPIs was for most people in most places driven by hedonic motives (fear of the threat posed by the virus to self and known intimates) and by normative goals (acquiescence to politico-judicial authority and peer pressure), with the hedonic bolstering or solidarizing the normative. Six *et al.*'s study of the first three stages of the pandemic (March through to June 2020) in Belgium certainly supports this conclusion.[147] I will briefly summarize the chief findings.

This study found that during the first pandemic phase (March and early April 2020), "pro-socialness, trust in government, and effectiveness of rules ... [did] ... not impact compliance significantly".

> Apparently, citizens' fear of the virus and observed respect for rules have such a strong impact on the normative goal that pro-socialness becomes irrelevant. In this phase, it also makes sense for self-centered people to comply ... [I]t seems not to matter whether people trust the government or not: when fear is that high (high compatibility of hedonic goal), observed respect for rules and appropriate rules are enough to turn the rules into social norms (high salience of the normative goal).[148]

Thereafter, during the second phase of the crisis (from late April 2020), compliance to NPIs became "positively predicted by observed respect of the rules, fear of COVID-19 (both risk severity and risk proximity ... [and] ... rules that make sense (both appropriateness and effectiveness of measures)". Pro-social motives and trust in government remained in this period insignificant predictors of compliance. The former became a significant predictor of compliance with NPIs (alongside fear of the virus and perceptions of rule appropriateness and effectiveness) only during the third phase of the pandemic from the tail end of June 2020. This was during a period of de-escalation of restrictions in which general compliance levels with NPIs were dropping significantly and the fear factor that powered the compliance of many was abating owing to the success of the lockdowns in radically depressing caseloads and hospitalizations.

During the same period, trust in government was found to have "a significantly negative" relationship to compliance with NPIs, in that there were "low-trustors that comply with the rules". This was suggestive that there were rule followers who thought that "government relaxed the measures too soon, which ultimately lowered their trust in government". This was as the decline of the motivational power of fear from high risk perception that allowed non-compliance to increase sharply in the general population from late spring rendered the compliance that remained "more reliant on stable personal characteristics", including endorsement of pro-social values. In the third stage of the Belgian pandemic, therefore,

> more differentiation in groups that are more or less likely to comply starts to manifest itself ... Thus, more young people are failing to comply compared to older people; more women are complying compared to men; and more self-interested people are failing to comply compared to pro-social people ... Among those that are still complying, there are different constellations of factors influencing that compliant behavior: those that comply because of

their pro-socialness; those who believe that government is not strict enough anymore and hence do not trust government, but still comply; those that comply because of fear; and those that comply because they see others complying (in their social circles).[149]

Evidence in support of "functional fear" as the primary motivator of compliance with NPIs during the present pandemic could also be read into widespread incidents of "panic"-buying (in reality egoistic strategic-instrumental buying) that emptied supermarket shelves on the cusp of the British pandemic.[150] This behaviour coincided with initially the highest levels of public compliance with lockdown measures and it left over-pressed key workers in frontline services and those disinclined or unable to compete with the store raiders short of necessaries. By the summer of 2021, the media-orchestrated doorstep handclap in solidarity with NHS workers in the UK was a distant memory. But healthcare practitioners were by then, according to media reports, being subject to abusive behaviours and threats of violence from members of the public for knocking back their demands to jump ahead in the vaccine queue so that they could avail themselves of "Freedom Day" consumer opportunities to holiday overseas.[151]

There are, in fact, economic and cultural elements of contemporary modernity that would explain why community altruism or empathy is not generally a powerful behavioural motivator, as I have set out. Others will be elaborated over the next few pages. These are the factors of decivilization.

Normative versus moral order

Emile Durkheim's famous analysis of the relationship between the normative and moral orders of modern society whereby (on his reckoning) the former is subordinate to the latter may be pertinent to contextualizing my analysis – though not in the way that Durkheim would have seen it.[152] As we have seen, some research, albeit not much, supports the notion that compliance was rooted in empathy for and altruism towards the generalized Other. Such would evidence moral solidarity with others as part of a community "in it together" that made lockdowns work. However, as reported in the preceding, a substantial body of research suggests that concern for community welfare is not a generally strong predictor of behaviour when faced with public health crises. This is alongside research suggestive that self-interest has been a stronger motivational factor of compliance with NPIs during the current pandemic.

Durkheim's sociology of modernity would predict the former public response to pandemic restrictions rather than the latter. Social integration, for him, is secured by the "conscience collective" (the shared values and mutual moral obligations of community members) backed by the power of constraint exercised by legally sanctioned rules. Durkheim considered the moral axis (or social solidarity) to be by far the more potent source of social conformity and cohesion under modern conditions. This was much more so than in traditional society. Indeed, there is a case for affirming that Durkheim fused the moral and the normative basis of social order while also rendering the latter as epiphenomenal of the former. This is because he accounted for the authority of norms to command behaviour in terms of moral precepts that were bound to them. People obey the rules, Durkheim argued, because they identify with the moral values that the rules represent. This renders submission to politico-juridical authority a matter of moral obligation (that is, a sense of duty) and of moral desire (that is, to do the "right" thing). Under modernity, moral order (the conscience collective of shared moral values and beliefs) was the basis of normative order and of the power of judicial sanction.[153]

The reasons why Durkheim maintained this perspective on the nature of modern social order have been discussed earlier. To reiterate, this was because, he thought, the specialized division of labour in industrial society generated in potential at least a solidarity not of sameness or identity (as was the case in premodernity) but of the interdependence of roles that imbued in people an awareness of their mutual dependencies as well as of their differences. This made possible, Durkheim affirmed, a higher "organic" form of moral solidarizing as the cultural basis of social integration in modern times that was quite unlike the repressive "mechanical" solidarity (of homogeneous values and identities) that integrated pre-industrial society.

However, there is a good case for thinking, *contra* Durkheim, that the matter is much less clear-cut. It seems plausible that the moral and the normative are distinctive axes of social order. Moreover, it is also plausible that neither the moral nor the normative are the dominant or primary modes of modern authorization. Or, if not, that the normative is the stronger force of the two, owing simply to the fact that it is backed by an authority (the state) that is viewed as legitimate and which exercises powers of coercion and sanction. But, if either position were true, social cohesion would be rather less a question of social solidarity on the basis of shared moral commitments and rather more a case of acquiescence to normative regulation based on the expressive and disciplinary authority of the state. As such, conformity to physical distancing regulations would be not so much a story of a shared sense of duty of care to others but rather more an unreflective acquiescence to the force of politico-legal authority and judicial rules. This difference in motivations for compliance is not, however, straightforwardly a distinction between those based on morals and those based on rules. This is because the latter may also be expressive of a sense of moral obligation – that is, the belief that it is the duty of citizens to submit to the authority of the state and judicial rules.

Durkheim himself drew attention to the clarificatory function of normative regulation.[154] This is where people obey rules because these simply express what is expected of them and what is not. From this perspective, mandatory physical distancing rules may generate compliance less because of the deterrence effect on rule-breakers of facing legal sanctions, or because people identify morally with the rules, or on the basis of mere self-interest, but because these simply specify how people should behave. From Durkheim's point of view, this compliance would be owing to acceptance of the legitimate *moral* authority of the state, but of course, this is not necessarily so. Compliance may, as we have seen, rest on mere submission to the power of legal norms or it may be motivated by a desire to avoid social disapproval.

Either way, this would show that compliance to COVID-19 restrictions is not a matter of people exercising independent moral or practical judgement (of what is right or wrong or what works and what does not), but rather is evidence of their lack of capacity for making such judgements or lack of willingness to do so. This would be compliance to the "how's" of behaviour as expressly set out by authority, without consideration of the "why's". This in turn may be a testament to the way that, owing to the sovereignty of the normative and self-disciplinary over the moral or valuational in modern societies, contemporary citizenries (or rather large numbers of those who make them up) have been rendered passive.

If so, this would lend support to the accounts of modernity set out, in their different ways, by Norbert Elias and Michel Foucault, both of which emphasize how disciplinary norms have been internalized (as aspects of the personality system) by the modern subject or "self".[155] Moreover, as Bauman's famous analysis of the relationship between modernity and the Nazi genocide has demonstrated, this passive submission of citizenries to the normative authorizations of the state may, under certain circumstances, allow or even contribute to the perpetuation of the most horrific crimes imaginable against humanity.[156] This is because centralized normative authority (as commanded by the state) allows people to set aside independent moral judgement.

Such is not of course uniformly the case. It is not that independent moral or practical judgement disappears. Rather, the capacity or confidence of many to wield it is significantly diminished, owing to the monopolization of authorization by the state. Nor is this to deny that there was and is in the physical distancing behaviours of some if not many people a significant degree of altruism, of a sense of civic responsibility, and of moral and affectual concern for the welfare of others. Independent moral judgement was evidenced by the fact that a majority of people in the UK stated that they would continue to don their face masks after 19 July 2021's "Freedom Day", for example, when the practice was due to no longer be legally required.[157] This is significant because the scientific consensus of recent times is that wearing the mask offers protection not so much for the wearer but much more so for those whom the wearer comes into contact with.

But, on the other hand, a large minority of the population (one-third) reported in advance of "Freedom Day" that, as soon as political authority abolished this short-lived mandatory requirement, they would ditch their face coverings.[158] Given that this was already a large popular constituency, even in advance of the lifting of the mask-wearing mandate, there was at the time good reason to think that, post-"Freedom", the numbers of non-maskers and anti-maskers would grow as the habit became normalized, especially if they were to experience or perceive no immediate negative consequence from exercising this freedom. This was my own prediction at the time. And this indeed came to pass. According to YouGov data, within a couple of days of the 19 July (2021) lifting of COVID restrictions, mask-wearing among 18–24-year-olds (the least vaccinated demographic) had dipped from 58 percent to 46 percent.[159] A month after "Freedom Day", as the *New York Times* reported:

According to official survey data, about nine in 10 Britons said they had used face coverings within the past seven days when outside their homes. But anecdotal evidence suggests that compliance is much spottier, even on buses and subways in London, where wearing a mask is still compulsory ... After most restrictions were lifted, the transport police lost legal responsibility for enforcement of that rule. That left the task to transportation workers, who have been advised by one union to avoid confrontations with the public ... One government minister, Greg Hands, tweeted a picture of himself on the subway wearing a mask, but complained that only about half of the passengers around him were doing likewise.[160]

Self-reported public mask-wearing in the UK, according to YouGov data, peaked at 77 percent of the adult population in February 2021. This was still running at 71 percent by mid-July that year – on the cusp of "Freedom Day's" dismantling of legally mandated NPIs. By the end of the month, however, this had fallen to 63 percent and by the start of October to just 57 percent.

This was during a period where significant if not major gaps in vaccine coverage in the UK population still existed. A winter (2021) COVID-19 upsurge motivated an upward spike in levels of self-reported mask-wearing (up to 69 percent by mid-December), but since then the decline has been continual and dramatic. By the end of July 2022, only 21 percent of UK adults were claiming that they were wearing face masks in public spaces.[161]

The price of "freedom" (including from mask-wearing) in the UK was predictable since this coincided with a new wave of infections. On 15 July, on the cusp of "Freedom Day", more than 56,000 new cases were recorded. Somewhat surprisingly, and perhaps owing to a "freedom" motivated sharp rise in COVID underreporting (as citizens were incentivized to not take tests or report results), official daily caseloads fell back to 20,000 by the end of the month. However, that is where they stayed, before they climbed back up to 28,000 by the start of August.[162] By 24 August, there were 30,000 confirmed new cases. On that day 970 people were admitted to hospitals, and there were 133 new deaths.[163] Two months later, on October 21, the daily death had reached a vaccination-era high of 223 mortalities, alongside a new caseload on that day of in excess of 50,000. It was estimated that 1 in 55 Britons (that is, a million people plus) were infected in the week from 9 to 16 October alone. This was a higher number than was "reported in Germany, France, Italy, Spain and Portugal combined" in that period.[164]

From the perspective of personal experience (that is, of my daily to-work and from-work rail commute), even before 19 July, the typical rate of conformity to mask-wearing on the local service I use dropped from around 75 percent to 50 percent. This was from the start of June up until mid-July 2021. People were at the time, of course, being incentivized to abandon their face coverings (not merely being permitted to do so) by the UK government's mixed messaging on the cusp of "Freedom Day". Indeed, this was also legitimized by mass mask-ditching by ministers and Conservative MPs in the House of Commons post "Freedom" on their return to parliament in August after the summer recess.[165] Afterwards, mask-wearing on my local commute route dipped precipitously. So much so that, on my count, less than a quarter of observed passengers were donning face coverings on the cusp of autumn of that year. By the start of 2022, this was less than one in ten. Not untypically, and certainly not surprisingly, data to be derived from personal observations of people flows in public spaces indicates much lower real rates of mask-wearing than self-reported ones over the period – and this was a period in which COVID-19 was still inflicting major harm on public health.

Nonetheless, the British public was also receiving guidance in the runup to 19 July 2021 from Chris Whitty, the UK government's chief medical officer, which was strongly supportive of masking. Whitty presented public mask-wearing as a sensible measure that self-responsible citizens should entertain on a voluntary basis out of respect for others for the foreseeable future.[166] There were also plenty of mask-wearers who took to social media to promulgate the same message. Moreover, for all the ambivalence of government messaging in the UK context, this did for the most part convey that mask-wearing would be a case of responsible citizenship and would reduce the chances of restrictions being re-introduced. For tens of millions, this was to no avail, however. This arguably verifies the primacy of the normative over the moral for a substantial number of contemporary citizens in shaping their social conduct. As such, this demonstrates that tough and clear normative controls (reinforced by the power of sanction) would command public acquiescence when faced with pandemic situations and that these would also be more efficacious than appeals to voluntary moral solidarity in defending public health and safety from pandemic situations under modern conditions.

Of course, the negative in this is exactly that substantial numbers of modern citizens are seemingly unable or unwilling to exercise independent moral or practical judgement when faced with situations that render this imperative. The pandemic in the UK has caused enormous human suffering in damaged and lost lives – and this has been experienced disproportionately by the most vulnerable and by the most economically disadvantaged and socially excluded. These are people who clearly have not been protected as they should have been. Simultaneously, the pandemic in the UK has been "managed" by a government that has time and again taken unnecessary risks with public health in order to minimize the harm to money and business, albeit self-defeatedly.[167] Under these circumstances, a citizenry with the capacity and inclination to exercise moral and practical judgement apart from the political authority of the day, rather than one that for the most part has simply followed the twists and turns of the often bizarre rule changes, could have played an active part in its own self-protection from the pandemic. Alas, this kind of citizenry is not one that is particularly facilitated by contemporary politics and culture in countries where neoliberalism is ascendant.

All of this said, the dilution of a morally and socially self-responsible citizenry under contemporary political and cultural conditions is not a universal phenomenon – or at least this is not experienced to the same degree internationally. The problem may be a general one, but it is especially acute in the West, in the Global North, and in the high-income countries of the "developed" world, that is, in those countries in which individualized consumerist rights cultures and neoliberalized polities are most consolidated. International comparisons of public mask-wearing (and other NPIs) arguably provide some support for this perspective.

Mask-wearing and pro-sociality

Mask-wearing is a good gauge of the strength of pro-social motivations in a society because this confers health protections not so much on the wearer but more on those whom the wearer comes into proximity with. Mask-wearing, then, may be viewed as indicative of empathic concern for community others rather than as behaviour motivated by self-interest. Unlike home quarantine, mask-wearing does not (in lesser-developed countries without or with lesser furlough protections for stay-at-homers) impact adversely on the livelihoods of the wearer. Especially in the West, furloughs have minimized the economic deficits of home isolation for the quarantined, unlike in other parts of the world where people often cannot feed themselves or their families if they self-quarantine. This also makes mask-wearing a particularly good candidate for gauging pro-social behaviours. Put simply, quarantining imposes lesser economic costs on people in the Global North than in the Global South. By contrast, mask-wearing does not impose economic burdens on anyone. The personal costs of mask-wearing for everyone are those of mere inconvenience.

Now, throughout the global pandemic to date (by mid-year 2022), public rates of mask-wearing have been generally much higher outside the West, beyond the North. They have been highest – and consistently so – in the countries of Southeast Asia. This is even though NPIs are legalized in them to different degrees and these countries have highly variable rates of vaccine coverage. Here are several examples.

Rates of self-reported mask-wearing in Hong Kong stood at 90 percent towards the end of February 2020, and these thresholds have been maintained ever since. By mid-July 2022, 86 percent of adults were still self-reporting mask-wearing in public places. Public mask-wearing in Thailand was also very robust right from the start of the pandemic. This stood at 73 percent in early March 2020, rising to 90 percent from the start of April. From that point onwards, right up to October 2021, self-reported public mask-wearing fluctuated, at high scales, between a low of 76 percent (in September 2020) and a high of 88 percent (in July 2021). With the de-escalation of restrictions, as COVID-19 rates were radically suppressed, public mask-wearing dipped substantially, albeit for short periods. This was in early November and towards the end of December (2021). However, faced with the threat of new pandemic waves, mask-wearing has been rapidly restored to the earlier high rates (between 77 and 83 percent of adults) since the start of 2022.[168]

In Indonesia, at the start of the pandemic, initial mask-wearing was much lower than in Hong Kong and Thailand. In early March, 47 percent of adult citizens self-reported wearing a face covering. Towards the end of April 2020, however, this had risen to 81 percent. Since then, between May 2020 and July 2022, the level of public mask-wearing has, through various ebbs and flows, declined only marginally. Presently (mid-year 2022), this stands at 79 percent. Similarly, in Malaysia, initial pandemic mask-wearing was self-reported by 55 percent of adults. Subsequently, this increased to 86 percent by April (2020's) end. Subsequently, public mask-wearing has never dipped beneath 75 percent, and typically has been in the eighties percentage bracket.[169]

The same basic pattern exists as well for the Philippines, Vietnam and Singapore. In the Philippines, by mid-March 2020, 59 percent of adults were self-reporting mask-wearing. In Vietnam, this was also 59 percent, towards the end of March that year. By early April, in the Philippines, compliance had increased to 84 percent, where it has remained, on average, ever since. Similarly, in Vietnam, levels of mask-wearing fluctuated between 72 percent and 87 percent in the period from April 2020 to December 2021. Thereafter, with the relaxation of other pandemic controls, rates were reduced until these plateaued at 60 percent by mid-June 2022, before climbing back up to 72 percent by mid-July of that year. Singapore is unusual, in that initial mask-wearing was reported by just 20 percent of the adult population, at the start of March 2020, much lower than elsewhere in Southeast Asia. However, the discrepancy disappeared within a month, as mask-wearing rose rapidly to 90 percent by April (2020's) end. Since then, from May 2020 through to December (2021's) end, rates of mask compliance fluctuated between the upper eighties and lower nineties in percentage terms. This dropped to a low point of 67 percent by the start of May 2022 but has since climbed back up to the mid-eighties.[170]

****

Comparing the Southeast Asian experience with the history of public mask-wearing in North America and Europe over the course of the pandemic to date is instructive. I will address first of all the US experience. At the start of March 2020, as the US pandemic accelerated, the number of American adults who self-reported public mask-wearing was just seven percent. By the start of April, this was still less than 30 percent as the pandemic reached its first wave peak. Eventually, by mid-November 2020, the number of American adults who self-reported public mask-wearing peaked at 83 percent – a level significantly lower than in Southeast Asian countries. Thereafter, there was a long-drawn process of decline, however, so that by mid-July 2021 only 48 percent of people were still donning their face masks in public spaces. In response to new COVID-19 upsurges, rates of mask-wearing twice recovered, but only up to the lower sixties in percentage terms. This was in late September 2020 and mid-January 2021. Since then, however, public mask-wearing has steadily tailed off, reaching a new low self-reported level of 40 percent by the start of July 2022.[171]

As for Europe, here the UK has delivered the lowest rates of public mask-wearing over the course of the pandemic in comparison with the leading EU countries – Germany, France, Italy, and Spain. As we have seen, the rate of self-reported compliance peaked at 77 percent in February 2021 but at mid-year 2022 is languishing at just 21 percent. But none of the European countries have come close to matching the levels of public compliance with this particular NPI of the Southeast Asian countries, or indeed of most elsewhere in the Global South.

Of these, Italy and Spain have managed by far the better results. By mid-March (2020), only five percent of adults self-reported as public mask-wearers in Spain. In Italy, at this same stage, 26 percent of people did so. Mask-wearing peaked at 91 percent in Spain at mid-point of April 2021, having touched 90 percent at the end of July the year before. In Italy, this peaked at 89 percent in mid-April 2020. In Spain, high levels of public masking were maintained for the better part of 16 months (these never dropping below 80 percent) – an impressive performance by European standards. But these have tailed off since the start of 2022, dipping to 52 percent by July's end. In Italy, the higher rates were maintained for a shorter period than in Spain before the decline set in. By mid-February 2021, self-reported mask compliance was reduced to 72 percent, and by the start of July 2022, to 53 percent.[172]

In comparison, Germany and France have fared significantly worse than their EU neighbours. In Germany, by mid-April 2020, only 17 percent of adults self-reported donning face coverings in public spaces, whereas towards the end of the month, this was still less than 40 percent. Public face-masking did not peak (at 75 percent) until mid-February 2021, 11 months into the European pandemic, and since then has been on a downward curve, dipping to 40 percent by the end of July 2022. In France, pretty much the same pattern is evident, though the results are a little better than for Germany. At the start of March 2020's, only five percent of adults self-reported masking-up in public places. By mid-April, this had climbed to 43 percent, and by July's end (2020) this peaked at 85 percent. Mask-wearing was stable at these higher scales for several months, before a gradual decline set in over the course of 12 months. This has accelerated since mid-February 2022, so that by mid-July of that same year only 38 percent of people self-reported as public maskers.[173]

The marked difference in rates or levels of public compliance with public mask-wearing in the North Atlantic region compared to the Asia-Pacific region during the pandemic has been found to be replicated in the case of other NPIs. Remarkably, this is true even of home quarantining, despite the harms to livelihoods this causes, which are bound to be more acute in middle-income countries compared to high-income ones. From the start of the pandemic right up to July 2022's end, people in the Asia-Pacific region have consistently self-reported much higher rates of compliance to stay-at-home restrictions than people in North America and in Europe. Indeed, Europe and the US have been the least compliant regions to stay-at-home restrictions internationally, according to self-report data, despite furlough protections.[174] The same pattern over the same period holds in the case of personal hygiene behaviours (washing hands regularly, using hand sanitizer), refraining from touching objects when in public spaces, avoiding where possible crowded places, avoiding contact with tourists, and so on. In each case, people in the Asia-Pacific countries have self-reported the highest compliance rate internationally to these precautionary behaviours, whereas people in the North Atlantic countries have self-reported the lowest.[175]

This evidences not simply more effective, proactive pandemic management policies (at the centre of which are the various NPIs) in the Asia-Pacific region compared to those in the North Atlantic region but also a higher degree of public acceptance of and support for such policies in the former than in the latter. The point is well made by Jeffrey D. Sachs, Director of the Center for Sustainable Development at Columbia University:

> The publics of the Asia-Pacific have … endorsed tough public policy measures by the government. According to … YouGov survey data, the publics in the Asia-Pacific has consistently supported two core pillars of NPIs: quarantining all inbound airline passengers and quarantining (or locking down) locations in regions hit by infection. Such strong measures are key to suppressing transmission, and public support is vital for implementation, but these measures do not garner majority backing in many countries in the North Atlantic region.[176]

The fact that the citizenries of the Asia-Pacific countries have been more receptive to and accepting of the range of NPIs than have those in the North Atlantic countries may also be gleaned, as Sachs suggests, from the fact that, over the course of the pandemic's first year, these countries experienced only one mass protest against the COVID-19 restrictions. This was in New Zealand – one of the two most Westernized countries of the region (Australia, of course, being the other). By contrast, there were several mass protests in the North Atlantic region. These were, as Sachs says, "against even the most basic public health measures, such as wearing face masks, with agitators rejecting mask mandates in the name of 'liberty'."[177] Up until January 2021, this pattern held up, during which time there were 11 large-scale protests against pandemic restrictions involving clashes with the police and arrests in the North Atlantic region (mostly in Europe).[178]

Further evidence (albeit inconclusive) of higher degrees of public buy-in to pandemic NPIs in the Asia-Pacific countries, especially those of Southeast Asia, compared to those of the North Atlantic, may be based on making comparisons between *other*-report data on compliance with NPIs across the two regions. Again, Sachs, basing his analysis on YouGov survey data,[179] draws our attention to the fact that, even though rates of reported *self*-compliance were not radically dissimilar in all countries of the two regions over the period of study (ranging from 77 percent to 94 percent), people nonetheless reported that the compliance of *others* was much lower than their own. However, the variation between *self*-reported compliance and *other*-reported compliance was markedly different in the two regions:

> Interestingly, the five locations in the Asia-Pacific region (Australia, China, Hong Kong, Indonesia, and Singapore) score an average of 67.4% for "most people" following COVID-19 rules, while the nine locations in the North Atlantic region (Denmark, France, Germany, Italy, Poland, Spain, Sweden, United Kingdom and United States) score an average of 55.4%.[180]

A good explanation, therefore, for the greater public acceptance of and compliance with pandemic NPIs in the Asia-Pacific region than in the North Atlantic region is simply that pro-sociality is more prevalent and deeply embedded there in public attitudes than it is in the West and the North. As Sachs puts it: "COVID-19 … has exposed the shortcomings and outright failures of pro-sociality in many countries, including many of the richest countries, for which lack of material resources is not an issue".[181] Why is this the case? My argument, which is shared by Sachs, is that this is because the cultures of the Asia-Pacific countries – especially those of Southeast Asia – are rather less individualized than those of the West and of the Global North more generally. This is likely a major reason why these countries have out-performed those of the North Atlantic in terms of minimizing both public health and economic harms, as Serena Nanda and Michael Ryan surmise.[182] As Ryan elaborates:

> On a more global level, the data shows that more collectivist cultures and countries have typically fared better – economically, yes, but also in terms of loss of lives and livelihoods – than more individualistic cultures and countries. China, for example, is often criticized for being overly collectivist, and yet they have fared extraordinarily well during the pandemic. Their economy actually grew in both 2020 and 2021 (by 2.3% and 8.1% respectively) and their relative infection and death rates were (almost suspiciously) low until recent outbreaks at the beginning of 2022 (which are also relatively minor on a per capita scale). On the other hand, the USA, widely recognized as a highly individualistic culture, has fared terribly. With only roughly 4% of the global population, that country accounts for roughly 16% of both confirmed infections and confirmed deaths as a result of the virus.[183]

My argument that variations in compliance rates with NPIs between countries in the two regions are accountable in terms of their respective degrees of collectivism and individualism has been verified in quite an empirical way drawing on statistical tools. Iveta Silova, Hikaru Komatsu, and Jeremy Rappleye have attributed the resistance by publics and governments in the West to legally mandated NPIs as resulting from what they define as "excessive individualism".[184] Their study draws upon a cross-country scale of degrees of individualism in different parts of the world inspired by Hofstede *et al.*'s ideal types.[185] These degrees or levels of individualism are enumerated, with a score of 100 attributed to countries that could in theory manifest "complete individualism" and a score of 0 attributed to those that could in theory manifest "complete collectivism".

Based on this comparative-statistical analysis, Silova *et al.* attributed a mean score of 38.3 to the Asia-Pacific countries on the individualism-collectivism scale. This compared with a mean score of 64.9 that was attributed to the North Atlantic countries.[186] As Sachs points out:

> The difference is statistically significant at the 0.01 level. All of the Asia-Pacific countries score below 50 (that is, are more collectivist) except for Australia (90) and New Zealand (79). In contrast, all of the North Atlantic

countries score above 50 (that is, are more individualist) except for Greece (35) and Portugal (27).[187]

Silova *et al.*'s analysis correlated the excess individualism of the North Atlantic cultures with lower public support for physical distancing and other pandemic restrictions, including mask-wearing in public places. Conversely, more public support for the NPIs in Asia-Pacific countries was correlated with the higher degree of collectivism *vis-à-vis* individualism of their cultures.[188]

Yet perhaps the issue is not so much that there is "too much" individualism, especially in the West and in the North, in its corrosive impact on pro-sociality. Rather, perhaps the issue is more that of the particular modes of individualism that are excessive. As I have argued (Chapter 3), some forms of individualism would not necessarily be corrosive of the community bond upon which robust collective responses to pandemic events must depend. However, certain modes of modern individualism (economic, consumerist, wholly rights-based, etc.), which are culturally ascendant in Westernized cultures, undoubtedly are. This is because these are egocentric to the core.

Notably, as Michael Ryan has observed, whereas at the start of the pandemic "there was an unprecedented amount of discussing 'us' and expressing feelings of collectivity" since then "there has been a growing debate around individual rights, with almost no mention of collective responsibilities".[189] Certainly, there was much talk of mutual obligations at the start, of being "all for one and one for all", on the cusp of the lockdowns and beyond, even though the heavy lifting work on behalf of compliance was carried out elsewhere. Over the longer *duree*, however, even the semantics of solidarity have slipped, as the Western cultural norm reasserts its grip. The reason for this could be that once the fear factor that secured high initial compliance to NPIs was majorly reduced, there was just not enough pro-sociality "in the tank", in the North Atlantic societies, to bind people to the restrictions.

Silova *et al.* would appear to endorse my emphasis on the corrosive forms of modern individualism on NPI compliance, rather than on individualism *per se* since they also define this "excess" individualism quite explicitly as *neoliberal* individualism. They offer a stark warning of its dire planetary consequences:

In fact, both the coronavirus pandemic and the climate catastrophe clearly signal that the most immediate crisis we face is the crisis of (neo)liberal individualism, which not only prioritizes personal freedoms and individual gains above all else, but also undermines support for collective action and coordinated policy intervention. Our survival may well depend on our capacity to make a cultural shift by rearticulating Western modernity's dominant concept of self (that is, independent self). This necessarily entails reconfiguring our way of being towards more interdependent, relational approaches. Ultimately, these interdependent relationships extend beyond humans and include the Earth's broader ecological community. Even if this cultural shift does not reverse or even mitigate the effects of the climate crisis, it will increase the chances of survival for those who remain.[190]

The role of decivilizing modes of individualism in accounting for people's *non-compliance* with the pandemic restrictions will be explored in the analysis that follows.

Explaining non-compliance with NPIs

How might non-compliance with NPIs be interpreted? I touched on the latter at the start of the chapter and of course at various parts thereafter (because compliance and non-compliance are two sides of the same coin). But now I will go into some detail.

Research informed by psychology into rule conformity and rule breaking, including under circumstances where this would be supportive or injurious to the cause of public health, links such behaviour to personality traits, or even to personality types. By such means, rule conformity and rule-breaking are individualized, since this is detached from the prevailing ensemble of cultural and social relations in which this is situated. From this perspective, greater rule conformity to pandemic restrictions is correlated with personality traits such as introversion, neuroticism, and conscientiousness, whereas lesser rule conformity is correlated with other personality traits, such as extraversion, impulsiveness, and risk-taking.[191] Now, COVID-19-focused studies into compliance and non-compliance with NPIs informed by psychology have tended to discover evidence that these associations hold. These are indeed among the predictors of compliance and therefore of non-compliance with pandemic restrictions – along with those of age, gender, income level, employment status, and so on.

However, reliance on static personality traits or types to explain greater or lesser conformity to pandemic restrictions has obvious limitations. One of these is that public responses to pandemic regulations are dynamic rather than fixed.[192] Personality traits borne by individuals cannot explain the shifting social patterns of conforming and non-conforming behaviour over the course of the pandemic. The other limitation of significance is that personality traits and their assemblage into supposedly determinate personality types are not fixed or given in any historical or cultural sense. Such "mentalities" or "spiritualities" are shaped by elements of social structure (the constraints, enablements, and inducements placed on people by the kinds of social relations they inhabit and their positioning in these social relations) and by the forces of cultural sensibility that historically specific modes of material sociality have facilitated.

For sure, then, the behaviour of people in any particular time and place is linked to personality factors. For sure, too, certain of these personality factors, under certain circumstances (such as those facing us today during the present pandemic) may be less compatible with conformity to specific rules (such as those setting out pandemic restrictions). But what rather drops off the radar in this "empirical" and rather contextless account is simply the lesson to be learned from cultural history. This is that our subjectivities, which shape our agency, are powerfully conditioned by the kinds of social and cultural worlds in which we are adapted or acclimatized to living.

So, if the "egoistic self" or the "risk-averse personality" (by definition a variant of the egoistic type) is to function as part of the explanation for the disregard shown by many for COVID restrictions intended to save lives and defend public health, as psychologists contend, how are we to explain the prevalence of these elements of personality in contemporary individuals under modern conditions that have generated this unhappy result? The answer, I have argued, is simply that our society and culture are rather better adapted to supporting and nurturing egoistic selves (or controlling elements of egoism in human personality and motivation) than these are to supporting and nurturing empathic community-affirming selves (or an altruism of self that extends beyond kin as controlling elements of personality or motivation). A society that is organized for economic competition, for the individualized pursuit of money success, for the subordination of public life to markets and private interests, cannot easily maintain a robust sense of itself as community. Such a society will always struggle to function as a collective whose members are bound together by ties of mutual moral obligation in support of each other's well-being.

Part of the explanation for community failure faced with the challenges of the pandemic, then, would be that public life itself has been undermined in the neoliberal era, albeit to varying degrees depending on the degree of neoliberalization in different countries. Such has resulted from the retrenchment of the welfare state,[193] the legal emasculation of the trade unions,[194] the privatization or marketization of public services (such as health, housing, education and social care),[195] and (in the UK) more than a decade of austerity politics.[196] This attack on public or collective life has reinforced the tendencies of the capitalist mode to atomize or individualize the citizenry on the terrain of economistic and consumerist self-interest. This is by basically dismantling social-welfare support structures for people's lives, thereby forcing these into greater reliance on strategies of self-reliance and self-care.[197]

Neoliberal reforms have thus weakened the institutional and cultural redoubts against instrumental individualism that were constructed in the developed countries in the postwar era. Those people who have been most adversely impacted by the assault on public life (especially on social and welfare support services) are especially vulnerable to decivilizing pressures. This is in the sense that the community-bonding rhetoric of national togetherness spun by governments when faced with the pandemic does not chime with their experiences of marginalization and exclusion from civil society and disregard by the state. As we shall see, there is evidence that non-compliance with pandemic controls has been more common among the poor or economically deprived and oppressed ethnic minorities than among others.

The undermining of community life or collective solidarity by the neoliberal culture of libidinal consumerist and "rights-based" individualism, by radical marketization, and by the hollowing out of public welfare and social support services, also perhaps explains the apparent prevalence of citizens who have "low involvement" in the pandemic. They are, in effect, disinterested in and disengaged from the pandemic and matters arising from it, such as policy responses. The phenomenon was noted in Kaine *et al.*'s research into compliance and non-compliance with the pandemic NPIs in New Zealand.

These people are likely to have little knowledge, or even awareness, of the policy outcome and are likely to have limited knowledge of the policy measure, and to have weak attitudes towards it, if any at all. [They] … may appear to be either detached (i.e. they have other interests and concerns) or "know-nothings" (people who do not particularly care about or have no interest in the outcome).[198]

Such a citizen was regarded by the researchers as posing special problems for the cause of public health in the context of the pandemic. This was not by actively resisting or thwarting NPIs, but by drifting into inadvertent non-compliance with them "simply because they are not paying attention".[199] Where their involvement is low (in policy goals and means), people simply *fail to notice*.

Messages are not necessarily deliberately ignored; they simply fail to catch the attention of those with low involvement (they are not noticed). In the context of Covid-19 measures, this means that people with low-to-mild involvement with eliminating Covid-19 and with the measures for preventing the spread of Covid-19 may fail to notice or properly process promotional messages about Covid-19 and the measures. They may, for example, be entirely unaware of lockdown rules (or even what level of lockdown is in play). This increases the risk that people with low involvement may inadvertently be non-compliant, especially if changes are made to lockdown rules, or new lockdown levels are introduced.

The researchers mull over how those with low involvement in the pandemic can be made attentive to the cause of the NPIs. Promotional campaigns, after all, would struggle "to meet with success among people who have low-to-mild involvement with Covid-19 … as they are unlikely to pay proper attention to such promotional messages unless they are designed in such a way as to capture their attention".[200] How might their attention be grabbed? The researchers suggest that the best strategy would be to try and make the pandemic "relatable" to them personally somehow.

If so, what does this tell us about those who are uninvolved in the pandemic? Arguably, it tells us that this is a peculiar *type of citizen*, the "disinterested" or "uninvolved" citizen, who is simply disengaged from matters beyond his or her own circles, concerns or interests, and who "tunes in" to the wider public world only where matters there appear as relatable to his or her personal world. This is the citizen who is otherwise detached from matters of "politics" at the societal level. Now, although (in the context of a global public health emergency that has killed millions), lack of involvement in the pandemic seems a remarkable feat, just as the figure of the "uninvolved citizen" appears as unlikely as it is preposterous, these alas have their conditions of possibility in modern individualism and in decivilization.

Despite decivilizing processes, however, for many (if not most) people, physical distancing and other community-protection behaviours were more or less respected, in the pre-vaccination era, especially during the pandemic's first and second waves. Nonetheless, for many others, they have not been, in part or in whole. This is arguably because a culture of especially egoistic-instrumental individualism makes it easier for people to see it as their right and liberty to determine whether or not they should obey lockdown and physical distancing rules, based on consideration only of their own best interest. Such a "rational" calculus would be made on the basis of judgement on the likelihood or odds that they themselves (or those dear to them) could become ill-balanced against the personal inconvenience of compliance.

This is why when people's "risk perceptions" of viral hazards are reduced, as tends to happen over time, as they evade serious illness, or as they perceive known others evading serious illness, they are incentivized to reduce or abandon their compliance with NPIs, in effect leaving the "vulnerable others" to their fate. Consequently, the belief that COVID-19 is low risk is one of those factors most commonly associated with non-compliance, and this is why people who believe it is low risk have the "lowest self-reported compliance overall", according to research.[201] This is also one important reason why non-compliance in the present pandemic is much more associated with young adults than with senior and elderly people: young people are simply those least likely to be made seriously ill by contracting COVID-19. Pandemic management policies, in the context of decivilization, are therefore placed under pressure to compromise the stringency of NPIs (which is shown to be necessary to curb outbreaks, ease pressures on healthcare systems, and save lives) in order to maintain higher levels of public compliance with lesser measures that are experienced as less burdensome.[202]

A culture of narrow rights-based individualism also licenses people to adopt techniques of neutralization by which they may rationalize their disregard of personal restrictions. This may be on the grounds of special-case pleading (predicated on the prioritization of personal needs over social needs) for exemption from certain NPIs, for example. "I am lonelier than others, so I need to meet with people". "I have mental health issues, so I cannot be expected to self-isolate". "I have young children, who should not be cooped up, and who cannot understand why they are, whereas others do not, so I must facilitate their need to be with other children", etc. This also renders the free-rider problem of *homo economicus* especially acute. This is because non-compliance may be justified by people on the grounds that, since most others (or enough others) will comply with the restrictions, the risk of transmitting the virus by virtue of their own non-compliance with NPIs would be negligible.

Ölcer *et al.*'s research examined the attitudes to the pandemic of those people who self-identified as non-compliant with physical distancing as these were expressed on three social-media platforms. Responses included: scepticism about media reports of the seriousness of the crisis owing to the untrustworthiness of the corporate media; scepticism over the motives of government (which were seen as exploiting the crisis for their own ends); incredulity over the notion that the virus was inter-generational in its negative impacts – and so was harmful to people other than old folk; and lack of confidence over the efficacy of the existing restrictions (if these will not succeed why follow them?). Certain of these attitudes were consistent with the phenomenon of declining popular trust in and growing public disengagement from political institutions and politicians (as well as other key elements of established authority) characteristic of the neoliberal era, which has been reported, for example, by Social Attitudes surveys in the UK.[203]

Commonly posted reasoning for flaunting restrictions, however, was the need to uphold individual freedoms – especially freedom of association (e.g. "this is an attack on our rights; specifically, the right to peacefully assemble is being infringed") and freedom of consumer and leisure opportunities (e.g. "this is America ... I'll do what I want").[204] As I have noted beforehand, even the "liberty" of disregarding mask-wearing mandates was upheld by some as integral to citizenship. This close identification of personal liberty with unbridled freedom to pursue the libidinal pleasures or to avoid minor personal inconveniences, in the tooth and claw of the pandemic, was aptly expressed by an American poster who declared that "at the end of the day, I'm not gonna let it stop me from partying".[205]

Such libertarians, or rather some of their number, would be those who would engage in a series of anti-lockdown protests, in several Western countries. As well as giving voice to pandemic denialism and conspiracy theories of different kinds and to varying degrees, these protestors found common cause in their view "that governments had no authority to restrict movement or enforce mask usage and that doing so was a direct violation of their civil rights and liberties".[206] Others, in different contexts, would resort to extreme acts of violence when confronted or restricted over their non-compliant behaviour. For example, as reported by Griffiths, Albinsson, and Perera, "disgruntled customers fatally shot a security guard in Flint, Michigan, shot and injured McDonald's employees in Oklahoma City, and attacked store managers in Pennsylvania and Michigan for restricting their access ... when they refused to wear a mask".[207]

This arguably evidences the corrosive impact of the individuated rights culture as mediated by consumerism on public receptiveness to those social restrictions that were intended to protect those community members at the highest risk from serious illness or death from catching COVID-19. As Sachs wryly observes:

Nobody explained to these would-be libertarians that the first dictum of classic libertarianism is that the right to liberty does not include the right to harm others. John Stuart Mill famously put it this way: "The only purpose for which power can be rightfully exercised over any member of a civilized community, against his will, is to prevent harm to others."[208]

This evidence accords well with my personal experience of life under lockdown. Everyone has tales of lockdown incivilities to tell. Speaking of my own, I will relay just two. Firstly, on each and every one of my outdoor exercise excursions during the first British lockdown, I beheld groups of people socializing without physical distancing (varying in size from six to a dozen or more), which owing to their size and composition could not have been from a single household. These were in parks and on the beach and in the town centre of my homeplace. These were by no means solely gatherings of young people. Often they were multigenerational. Alcohol consumption was frequent.

Secondly, quite early on during the first lockdown, I ventured forth for the first time to the main supermarket for the weekly shop. Upon entry, I beheld several shoppers (a dozen in all) disregarding the one-way system that was set up to prevent congestion and making no effort to maintain physical distance from other customers. I perceived incidents of such behaviours in each and every aisle. When I raised the matter with two staff members who witnessed one such incident, asking why they did not intervene to encourage compliance, they responded (apologetically) that they had abandoned such attempts because these were responded to with abuse. They were, they said, instructed to "f*** off", "chill out", or "mind their own business".

There can surely be no more telling illustration of the cultural grip of solipsistic individualism (which recognizes no legitimate interest or concern other than that which is owned by one's own self) than the words "mind your own business". By those words, matters of public concern or community interest are simply dissolved. These have no right to encroach on the actions or motives of the sovereign consumer monad. My conversation with the two staff members motivated me to raise with the store manager the matter of how staff experiencing this kind of hostile behaviour from customers were being supported and how abusive shoppers were being dealt with. Providing staff support, he said, was catered for by his instruction that staff refrain from challenging non-compliers (which would also put a stop to the abuse, but which would hardly serve the purpose of public health). My first lockdown visit to the supermarket was my last, in order to save myself from rising blood pressure.

Returning from anecdote to Ölcer *et al.*'s results. These verify that an important motivation for physical distancing non-compliance among many is indeed this narrow individualized or subjectivized perception of (usually consumer-focused) rights and entitlements that leaves no room for recognizing communal or social obligations. Individualized rights-consumerism is thereby established as a force of decivilization in that this subordinates the social to the personal and in doing so undermines collective well-being and community solidarity.

But, as Ölcer *et al.* also show, there was a class dimension as well to the social-media postings of physical distancing hostiles in that some commentators cited fear of redundancy or loss of vital income ("money to survive" in opposition to protecting health) as reasons for disregarding stay-at-home guidance or restrictions. As one commented: "Life and death are tied to the economy. Not just viruses." And as another posted: "I know of too many people being threatened with unemployment if they do not attend work when they are not a key worker."[209]

This chimes with research evidence that "labor market status" has had "a sizeable influence on non-compliance" with NPIs during the pandemic. As Ganslmeier *et al.* found in their analysis of compliance and non-compliance in the UK, for example:

> The unemployed had a 5.6% predicted probability of non-compliance compared to 3.6% for individuals with a full-time contract. Similarly, respondents

with more precarious contracts (part-time and others) tended to have higher predicted probabilities of non-compliance than workers in more standard employment.[210]

Non-compliance in the US would also be motivated by the failings of the pandemic furlough and assistance schemes to support workers who were forced home or laid off owing to the lockdowns. These were of course "minimalist", to say the least, offering only partial compensation for loss of income, in sharp contrast with the astronomical sums of public money that were allocated to big business in subsidies and bailouts to cushion them through the pandemic.[211] The lockdowns radicalized the impoverishment of America's poor and its deeply entrenched inequalities of "race" and class. Migrants without rights of citizenship or residency were particularly hard hit (since they were not entitled to economic assistance), as were Native Americans, who are amongst the most disadvantaged of America's poor.[212]

In the lower-income countries, where there was even less state assistance for workers released from employment owing to lockdowns, the levels of precarity were more precipitous, and those migrants without rights of residency or citizenship were again especially vulnerable to impoverishment.[213] These adverse circumstances would certainly incentivize non-compliance with certain of the NPIs, such as stay-at-home orders in favour of illegal cash-in-hand working, just as this would render sticking to distancing more difficult. Furlough protection for stay-at-home workers and assistance for laid-off workers in the EU and UK during the lockdowns was much better than in the US. But, even so, all furloughed workers would have seen a drop in income, possibly of 10–20 percent, owing to the fact that governments would not bankroll the wages bills of employers in their entirety, whereas the newly unemployed everywhere (12 million in Europe, 40 million in the US) who were forced to draw on welfare benefits experienced substantial losses of household income. Millions of others (especially in lower-income and lower-status jobs) were switched by employers from permanent to impermanent contracts, and from full-time working to part-time working, with associated loss of earnings.[214]

Precarity, low pay, and low work status (in a word, economic marginalization of denizens of the G-economy, which is connected to the substantial increases in wealth and income inequality of neoliberal times) are also likely predictors of personal life dissatisfaction – which according to some research is a predictor of non-compliance with NPIs.[215] People who are dissatisfied with their lot in life, especially if they view this as resulting from the injustice of blocked opportunities for economic advance or security, are likely to experience weaker ties than others with the normative order of society, according to a particular school of thought in the sociology of deviance founded by Robert K. Merton.[216] Economic marginalization and the social exclusion that may stem from this would then be supportive of deviance "in general" – and if so why not also of deviation from NPIs that are experienced as disadvantageous? Decivilizing processes are those which weaken or undermine people's identification with normative order.

The personally dissatisfied may also, for these reasons, experience a lesser sense of being members of a unitary citizenry that would allow them to build social bonds with institutions and with other people beyond their immediate circles. Again, persons who have not formed social bonds, or who have become detached from social bonds, are those most likely to engage in deviant behaviours generally, according to one influential criminological theory that has a substantial empirical base in research.[217] Again, if this is so, one may reasonably surmise that deviation from NPIs is, for those with weaker or lesser connections to the controls on conduct provided by social bonds, likely to be included among the non-conforming behaviours.

Scepticism over the efficacy and sufficiency of support for stay-at-home workers was also expressed by the subjects of Ölcer *et al.*'s study. Government aid was thought to be skewed towards big business and the wealthy rather than towards the ordinary folk and the genuinely needy. Hence, comments included:

they will throw money like water at the rich to make sure they do not suffer

Everything that should be invested in the emergency program in the social area is blocking!

If you really want to protect ... freeze rent now! And if you really want people to stay home, protect those without housing.[218]

Such postings not only expressed class realities and their attendant grievances. They also embodied a lively anti-corporate and anti-neoliberal sensibility. This was hardly arbitrary but was evidence-based and experiential.[219] Such is indicative of how the divisions, inequalities, and exclusions of class (addressed elsewhere in this book) that have been widened in the neoliberal era fracture the societal bond and undermine the force of appealing to a unitary community ("we're all in it together"), which has been the narrative spun by governments (such as the UK's) to solidarize the public response to the pandemic. The pandemic exposed that there was no unitary community in the sense of a people united by a common experience of privation and restriction. Decivilizing processes are those that weaken or undermine the sense of a collective bond that would bolster community-level obligations or commitments.

The subsequent spectacle played out over the course of the British pandemic of ministers and MPs repeatedly managing to contract COVID-19 and being caught flouting physical distancing rules and other aspects of the official guidance in the midst of lockdown (as such events were paraded in the media) will have done nothing to ease the grievances or suspicions or scepticisms that motivate certain of the NPI rebels.[220] The hypocrisy of those in authoritative roles in the state for failing to practice what they preach (manifestly undermining the "stand together" or "all for one and one for all" public health messaging) was likely to have been a force corrosive of physical distancing generally, but this could only bolster the rebels and refusers.[221]

As I have summarized, according to research, factors that would account for behaviour that is either compliant or non-compliant to physical distancing and other

NPIs include: (1) the degree of trust that people have in government or authority, local and national (with low trust sometimes, but not always, associated with low compliance and high trust sometimes more often associated with high compliance); (2) people's perception of personal risk and of risk to nearest and dearest of becoming ill or worse from the virus (with low risk perceptions associated with non-compliance and high risk perceptions associated with compliance); (3) people's income and education level (with higher income and education associated with compliance and low income and education associated with the opposite); and (4) whether or not and to what degree people experience a sense of being part of a community as opposed to feeling detached from one (that is, whether or not they can draw on "civic capital" and by how much) – with those low in civic capital associated with non-compliance, whereas those high in it associated with compliance.[222]

These findings are consistent with my hypothesis associating non-compliance with those who have most absorbed or been most absorbed by the individualized rights culture. This is obviously true of (2) since decisions on whether or not to acquiesce to NPIs are made dependent on judgements of personal rather than social or public risk. But much of this is also compatible with a social-class frame of analysis. Low socioeconomic status radicalized and exacerbated by racial disadvantage and oppression has been shown by research to be strongly associated with the highest risks and rates of COVID-19 infection, hospitalization, and mortality. This also exposes the limits of social solidarity as a redoubt of community defence against the virus. By far the worst-hit communities and groups have been the poor, including and especially the ethnically oppressed poor (who tend to be the poorest) – and they can hardly be unaware of the fact.[223]

This particular vulnerability of the have-nots (especially of certain oppressed minorities) to the disease is owing to a complex array of social and cultural factors associated with inequality and injustice.

> While no medical explanation for the difference in infection has been established, it may be in part explained by differentials in socioeconomic status, living conditions and educational attainment or greater occupational exposure to the virus (since ethnic minorities are disproportionately represented in the health and care services workforce in the UK). In addition, the difference between ethnic minorities and White ... people specifically in rates of infection, rather than severity of the illness once infected, may be associated with variations in preventive behavior (that may be themselves linked to life circumstances).[224]

Relevant causal factors accounting for both greater vulnerability to infection and higher ill-effects from infection may be briefly summarized as follows. Firstly, lower levels of general health, fitness, and well-being – and hence of disease resistance – compared to members of higher-status groups. This is due to income constraints and associated ill-effects. These include substandard housing conditions – including poorly insulated and heated homes; poorer diet; higher exposure to occupational- and lifestyle-related diseases (including those that especially compound the risk of becoming seriously ill or dying from COVID); less access to leisure and well-being opportunities; and so on. Secondly, higher infection risks – including of vulnerable persons – than those faced by members of other social classes. These include higher exposure than others to densely populated workplaces and crowded homeplaces (which are more likely to be multigenerational homes); lesser access than others to private transport (and so greater reliance on busy public transport to get people to and from work); fewer opportunities for home-working compared to others – especially professionals; and greater economic pressures than others to go to work in spite of stay-at-home guidance.[225]

But another important factor explaining vulnerability may be that people with low socioeconomic status and from marginalized groups tend to be less *voluntarily* compliant than the members of higher-status groups with NPIs.[226] The reason for this would be that those people who are most likely to have lower trust or confidence in government or authority or "expertise" (since this is placed in the service of the state from which they are estranged) and who are most vulnerable to feelings of detachment from the community – factors associated with voluntary non-compliance – are exactly those who are least included in and who are most marginalized, economically, politically and culturally, from the life of society.

So, certain "predictors" of non-compliance with NPIs established by studies cited earlier (distrust of medical experts, not obtaining regular updates from health authorities)[227] may be grounded or contextualized in a theory of decivilization. Those at the wrong end of the widening class divide are also those people who would be most lacking in civic or "associational" capital – another factor of non-compliance,[228] which may be attributed to decivilization mechanisms. This fits the profile of the "precariat" – the casualized or semi-casualized ranks of the lower working class, the denizens of the G-economy, whose members are drawn especially from the most ethnically oppressed among the BAME populations.

As I noted beforehand, research also indicates that in societies with stronger collectivist values (e.g. South Korea), compliance with NPIs generally was higher than in those with individualistic values (e.g. the US). Earlier I cited a study of compliance and non-compliance with COVID-19 restrictions in Greece, the results of which were indicative of higher levels of compliance than was typical across the North Atlantic zone.[229] Interestingly, if not instructively, Greece is also unusual in that (as Sachs points out) it scores much more highly for collectivism on the individualism-collectivism scale than other countries in the Global North do.[230] Higher levels of compliance in more collectivist societies are sometimes attributed to the fact that people in those are more likely to trust the government's guidance, though as we have seen compliance and trust or confidence in government do not always align. Yet people in the US who were represented by researchers as being "horizontally collectivist" in their values were sometimes found to be those most likely to be non-compliant with NPIs.[231]

This probably had something to do with the fact that Donald Trump led the government in question.[232] Basically, non-compliance for some was mandated by a normative authority that expressed pandemic scepticism and was therefore accepted by those who supported that authority. Trump successfully represented himself for many poorer Americans as anti-establishment, anti-corporate, and anti-globalist. Non-compliance then fitted with the confirmation bias (that mask-wearing was of little utility) of those who would rather avoid the personal inconvenience and discomfort of donning the mask. Trump, of course, spent much of the pandemic's first six months minimizing its impact. This included comparing it to the flu and claiming that 99 percent of people would not get sick from it and that children were immune. He also repeatedly asserted that the virus was "fading away" or "getting under control" and would not need the help of a vaccine to see it off.[233]

Moreover, Trump acted to undermine scientific guidance on pandemic management. For example, for much of 2020, he refused to be seen wearing a face covering, and he did not relent until mid-July. Trump did "advise" mask-wearing in April of that year, but then promptly undermined the guidance by declaring he would not wear one and that doing so was "*only* [my emphasis] a recommendation".[234] At the same time, mask-avoidance was tolerated at the White House. This may partly explain why science scepticism is a factor that has been associated with non-compliance in the US but not so much elsewhere.[235] At one point Team Trump was even saying that the pandemic was a conspiracy of spin or "fake news" by Democrats and left-wing media to undermine his "America first" policies and re-election prospects.[236] Those Republican states in which Trump supporters were most populous had the lowest level of compliance with physical distancing and other NPI measures – and the highest rates of infection.[237]

US research also revealed clear divisions in cultural attitudes towards wearing a face covering. These were between supporters (reputedly motivated by altruism, empathy or solidarity) and opponents (supposedly motivated by self-interest and self-reliance).[238] These tended to cluster in particular places or regions. Political orientation was the major predictor of attitudes towards or beliefs about mask-wearing. A large number of people (the "conservatives") viewed mask-wearing in classic liberal terms as symbolic of "government overreach … and … an infringement on personal freedom".[239] These people embraced the values of individualism interpreted as the right to pursue self-interest with as few normative restrictions as possible. They "often considered the pandemic less severe and the response disproportional, with experts being considered less than competent, and public health measures, such as wearing a mask being misguided or ineffective".[240] Ryan and Nanda cite other studies that, similarly and unsurprisingly, have linked these differences in attitude towards mask-wearing (and indeed to a range of other NPIs) to party-political affiliations in America, with Republican sympathizers being less likely than Democrat sympathizers to comply with hand-washing and crowd avoidance as well as with mask-wearing.[241]

A large number of these people also viewed mask-wearing as lacking in honour because it denoted individual weakness, a loss of status, and as ruinous of their self-image as someone "to be reckoned with". Such honour "cultures tend to arise in economically challenging environments in which the influence of government and law enforcement is relatively weak, forcing individuals to fend for themselves".[242] This contrasted with the beliefs or attitudes of "liberals". Liberals tended to endorse the values of "relational interdependence" or "collective inter-dependence". In doing so they tended to regard mask-wearing as civic duty and as normative.

> Not only were respondents from collectivistic states more likely to report having worn masks, but respondents from such states also perceived greater utility in mask wearing, they considered it more normative, were more likely to derive social recognition from wearing masks, and were more likely to agree that masks may make other people feel protected.[243]

However, this was not necessarily because these liberals were weighing things up and exercising personal judgement on the efficacy of mask-wearing. Rather, this was because the practice was mandated by collective authority or was seen as a communal expectation:

> Unexpectedly, conservatism was also related to the perception of higher lev-els of voluntariness. Whereas conservatives had a much less favorable view of masks and mask wearing than was the case for liberals, they were also less likely to wear masks regularly. The greater perceived voluntariness of mask wearing may be because conservatives reject ... the social expectation that otherwise seems to have produced very high levels of mask wearing; instead, they might assert their own agency in deciding when (and when not) they are willing to wear masks. By contrast, liberals might be wearing masks habitu-ally; hence, for liberals mask wearing may simply not be the subject to any reasoned voluntary decision-making process.[244]

Again – such findings are hardly incompatible with the decivilization thesis. These evidenced that "rights" individualism was a force that obstructed mask-wear-ing behaviour that would have significantly reduced the negative impacts of the pandemic. The brand of individualism embraced by those absorbed by "honour culture" was an especially negative force since this encouraged people to view mask-wearing as exhibiting a lack of agency and status.

This was especially associated with people from economically marginalized communities and regions because these are people whose experience of political governance under the neoliberal state has been essentially negative. For them, the "authority" of the state is not protective or facilitative. Rather, this has been expe-rienced as a remote irrelevance, since it provides little collective support for their individual or community lives. Consequently, the influence on the behaviour of the "honour individualist" of political public safety messaging contrary to his or her preconceptions during much of the pandemic was always likely to be weak. To repeat, factors of decivilization are not only those that undermine community solidarity by untrammelled "rights" individualism (economic and cultural) but are also those that loosen the grip of liberal state normative authority on those who have good reason to mistrust it.

The pandemic and NPIs in low-income countries: the case of Africa

So far my analysis has focused on the public or people's response to the pandemic NPIs in the North Atlantic region, with some attention paid to those in the Asia-Pacific region. Especially in the case of the former, though not exclusively so, this analysis upholds the decivilization thesis, in that the concept (as I have theorized it) provides an account that integrates the various factors of compliance and non-compliance within a critical explanatory framework that situates these in contemporary-modern sociostructural and sociocultural environs. But what about the pandemic and the people's response to the efforts of governments to combat it in the low-income or least economically developed countries? What has been the success and public reception of the NPIs in these parts of the world that are less touched by capitalist modernization? Does the concept of decivilization here retain efficacy in explaining whatever non-compliance with the NPIs there has been? To address this matter, I will focus briefly on the COVID-19 crisis in Africa.

Such a strategy immediately encounters a constraint, however. This is simply that, as Hiwote Solomon and his colleagues observe,[245] the data to base it on is somewhat limited:

How successful NPIs were in limiting disease spread in Africa, especially in the first year of the COVID-19 pandemic has been underexplored in the literature. The degree of implementation and the impact of these NPIs during the COVID-19 pandemic has largely been studied in high-income countries, and there has been limited data in the literature focused on low- and middle-income countries, especially in Africa.[246]

However, Solomon *et al.*'s own case study of government and people's responses to the pandemic in three African countries – Nigeria, Rwanda, and Zambia – provides insights that illuminate the issues. Before addressing these, I will offer a few words on policy context.

The responses of governments of the AU to the pandemic mirrored those in most other parts of the world and on more or less the same timescales. As Solomon *et al.*, basing themselves on other studies,[247] relay:

By early March 2020, several countries in Africa (affected and unaffected by COVID-19) began mobilizing in response to the pandemic. This included prompt case identification, information campaigns to sensitize citizens, and building laboratory capacity. Some countries relied on innovative strategies such as using locally produced cloth masks, soaps, and hand sanitizers, developing inexpensive diagnostic tests, testing pooled COVID-19 samples, and using drones to transport test kits and samples to and from hard-to-reach areas.[248]

Most of these countries introduced border controls, suspending flights from destinations that were experiencing escalating caseloads. This was accomplished before the end of March 2020.[249] Thereafter, in April and May, most had closed their borders to all international travellers, except for purposes of essential cargo or freight trade and to allow the return of overseas citizens or the departure of foreign nationals. Many countries sealed their borders proactively, that is, in advance of any local COVID-19 cases being officially ratified.[250] At the same time, right across the continent, within-border legally sanctioned NPIs were brought in, as they were everywhere else.[251] These included the closure of schools and workplaces, radical curtailments of public gatherings and freedom of movement, virtual-working where feasible, household quarantine, stay-at-home orders, nighttime curfews, and so on.

The adverse economic and social impacts of these NPIs in the African context have been extreme. This is for reasons connected to much of the continent's generally rudimentary level of economic development and low per capita income, which stems from the region's subordinate and marginal status in the capitalist world economy. The harms inflicted on livelihoods and life chances and on GDP performance by the more radical of the NPIs (that is, by lockdown policies) have been considerably greater in Africa than those experienced even in middle-income countries. And they are separated by a chasm from those experienced in the high-income countries.[252]

This is because the governments of low-income countries (as most of those of the African Union are) simply could not afford the protections and compensations of furlough schemes and the like for home-quarantined and curfewed and travel-restricted workers or indeed the financial compensation schemes for businesses that were rolled-out elsewhere. At the same time, millions of workers in Africa depend on day-to-day wages and cash-in-hand simply in order to avoid destitution, which simply dried up when the pandemic and lockdowns arrived.[253] Consequently, unemployment skyrocketed, just as businesses were bankrupted. The price of staple foods rose as supplies dwindled, forcing families to drastically scrimp on household consumption.[254] As Solomon *et al.* describe:

> Almost three-quarters (71%) of Africans work in the informal sector and thus encountered severe economic hardship with the enforcements of lockdowns and border closures. With the implementation of certain measures, some countries had food shortages, social unrest, and economic instability. Economic instability was felt across the African continent; however, Zambia became the first African country to default on its Eurobond national debt during the pandemic. The pandemic caused the Zambian economy to enter its deepest recession in history with the economy shrinking by 4.2% in 2020 … Resource-poor settings [were placed at] … especially increased risk, with some data showing income reduction as great as 70% and reduction in consumption expenditure by 30%.[255]

These purely economic deficits of lockdown and border closure policies were so severe that these have, arguably, to date, outweighed the harms to public health caused by the pandemic itself. To be clear, this does not support the idea that African countries would have done better by eschewing the more "expensive" or burdensome NPIs, in favour of the lower-cost ones economically, such as reliance on mask-wearing and maintaining physical distance in public places. This is because lockdown policies have surely succeeded in majorly reducing caseloads (and therefore hospitalizations and deaths), which would not have happened if governments had relied on less strict and fewer NPIs. Cost-benefit analysis of COVID-19 harms versus lockdown harms is scarcely feasible because the scale of the harms that would have been generated if there was reliance on fewer and less strict NPIs can only be guessed at.

The tragedy of Africa, then, is not that it sought to implement NPIs that were common currency elsewhere in order to curb a pandemic that potentially threatened the lives of millions. Rather, the tragedy is that these exerted such a high price on livelihoods (and therefore on public health) because of the chronically reproduced inequalities of the capitalist world economy that preserve international relations of domination and subordination to the advantage of the high-income countries and to the detriment of the low-income countries. There was, of course, no coordinated economic assistance programme courtesy of the G7 to ameliorate pandemic and lockdown harms across Africa, as the continent was buffeted by repeated COVID waves, any more than there will be any kind of a "Marshall Plan" to restore the continent's economic fortunes when the pandemic is done.

Solomon *et al.*'s own case study of NPIs in Nigeria, Rwanda and Zambia revealed significant variation in the strictness and stringency of enforcement of the restrictions brought in by the respective governments:

> Rwanda had far more consistent and stringent measures compared to Nigeria and Zambia … There were … major differences between countries when examining the degree of implementation of the CHI [containment and health index] which measured … containment and closure NPIs and … health system NPIs. In Rwanda, the overall average score for the CHI was 58.5 (SD = 25.3, median = 71.4) … In contrast, the average scores in Nigeria and Zambia were 38.3 (SD = 32.2, median = 16.7) and 31.1 (SD = 20.8, median = 40.5), indicating lower stringency and levels of implementation compared to Rwanda … .Rwanda's success in implementing COVID-related measures was partly due to strong enforcement and having a population that generally follow the recommendations of their government.[256]

The better public health outcomes with regard to COVID-19 were accordingly found in Rwanda, with lesser ones in Nigeria and Zambia.

The researchers also mobilized a wealth of qualitative data, courtesy of in-depth "key informant interviews" (KIIs) with "decision-makers and experts involved in the COVID-19 response". These were "officials of Ministries of Health, Africa CDC Regional Collaborating Centers, and WHO African Regional Office (AFRO)".[257] The qualitative data illuminated the immense practical difficulties in implementing and enforcing NPIs in the three countries. These include those resulting from lived environments that problematize physical distancing, that is, public transportation systems [that] are often overcrowded, dense shanty towns and informal settlements [that] are part of the physical infrastructure, and [of] many people [who] do not have the luxury to self-isolate even if they are positive, as many homes face overcrowding.

These also include limited access to clean running water that often rendered the protocol of frequent hand-washing unrealistic. "In rural areas, many households share sanitation facilities and have only access to water from a communal tap".[258] Involuntary pressurized non-compliance with NPIs for these reasons has been and will continue to be a significant if not major phenomenon in low-income countries. This is far less the case in high-income countries.

There was of course also the problem of voluntary as well as involuntary public non-compliance with the NPIs. The qualitative data gathered from the KIIs is suggestive that this has been far from negligible. Indeed, there are good reasons to think that there may have been higher levels of voluntary non-compliance than was the international norm, and higher levels of non-compliance than even in the worse-performing of the North Atlantic countries, especially in Nigeria and Zambia (and quite likely many others). Solomon *et al.*'s interviewees sometimes report "mass defiance" of government mandates (on public gatherings, stay-at-home restrictions, curfews, travel restrictions, even mask-wearing) in certain places and among certain citizen groups – especially among the urban poor in the densely populated shanty towns.[259]

This was owing to much less strict enforcement of the NPIs by the coercive arm of the state in Rwanda than in the other countries, and greater decentralization and devolving of political authority in Nigeria and Zambia, in contrast to tighter central control of the provinces in Rwanda.[260] In Rwanda, lockdowns and curfews were actively policed and violators were much more likely to face legal sanctions than in Nigeria and Zambia. Voluntary non-compliance here may be motivated by distrust of ruling parties and of state machines that are perceived to be self-serving, beholden to foreign powers or local tribalisms, and riddled with cronyism and corruption (since cronyism and corruption are often acute in economically hard-pressed or marginalized countries in our hyper-competitive interstate system dominated by imperial powers). One of Solomon *et al.*'s interviewees reported the problem of pandemic denialism motivated by suspicion that political authorities had "hidden agendas" rooted in self-interest in imposing lockdowns.[261] Involuntary non-compliance may also be incentivized by the radicalization of subsistence poverty that NPIs generate in such economically hard-pressed places. People break the rules simply because they need to meet basic subsistence needs.

The structures and processes of the global political economy that generate these outcomes for certain places and for some peoples may quite reasonably be construed as decivilizing mechanisms. For sure, decivilization here is much less for most people a story of the negativities of an individualism of rights (without obligations) – especially of consumerist rights – as it is in the West and in the North and perhaps among elites and urban middle classes generally. But this is decivilization, nonetheless.

Compliance and non-compliance with test-and-trace

Non-engagement of many people with physical distancing and other public safety guidelines over the course of the pandemic extends beyond those NPIs already discussed. In the UK, there were also high rates of public non-engagement with the NHS test-and-trace system (NHSTT). I have discussed elsewhere the dysfunctions of NHSTT as an aspect of British exceptionalism. These of course substantially undermined it.[262] But the system was also undermined by the huge variations in public response to it. Substantial numbers of people who were contact-traced neither took a test nor self-isolated. As was reported by the parliamentary accounts committee on 18 January 2021:

> National and local government have tried to increase public engagement with tracing, but surveys suggest that the proportion of contacts fully complying with requests to self-isolate might range from 10% to 59%. NHST&T acknowledges that non-compliance poses a key risk to its success and has taken steps to increase levels of self-isolation, for example by making follow-up calls to people while they are self-isolating. For as long as compliance is low, the cost-effectiveness of NHST&T's activities will inevitably be in doubt.[263]

Since its inauspicious beginnings, engagement of the British public with NHSTT showed a gradual tendency to improve, up to the point at which the UK government lost interest in the system in the runup to and aftermath of 19 July (2021) "Freedom Day". By May 2021, 82 percent of those who were contact-traced were disclosing those with whom they had been in close contact.[264] But this still left a sizeable minority of people who were not cooperating with the system. "Freedom Day", however, for all practical purposes, fatally compromised the system, since this basically declared the end of the British pandemic. Even before then, as the Health Foundation put it, "the ongoing changes to policy on testing – including testing for people without symptoms, the use of PCR tests, and the role of testing for people who are fully vaccinated – makes it ever more challenging to interpret trends in test use and case numbers".[265]

NHSTT was formally terminated by the UK government on 24 February 2022.[266] But, before then, for much of its short-lived history, in the three key areas – self-isolating if experiencing symptoms, requesting a test if symptomatic, and sharing details of close contacts – responses were insufficient to enable the system to deliver on its own stated public protection goals. For starters, rarely was it the case that more than half of those who were symptomatic self-isolated:

> Combining data from 14 April 2020 to 27 January 2021, ... of those who reported having experienced symptoms of covid-19 in the past seven days (excluding those who reported receiving a negative covid-19 test result since having developed symptoms), only 20.2% ... said they had not left home since developing symptoms. The percentage of people who reported full self-isolation was largely stable until October 2020 and then increased ... In the

latest wave of data collection ... the percentage of people who reported not leaving home after symptoms developed was 31.3% ... From 26 October 2020 to 27 January 2021 ... duration adjusted adherence to full self-isolation was 42.5% ... In the latest wave of data collection (... 25–27 January 2021), duration adjusted adherence was 51.8%.[267]

As was later reported by the Health Foundation (June 2021), a number of surveys estimated that non-compliance with homestay orders for the full 10 days could be running at anywhere from 10 to 60 percent of those people who had tested positive for COVID-19.[268]

As for requesting a test if symptomatic, in the period spanning the first and second UK pandemic waves, less than a quarter of people complied:

When data from 26 May 2020 to 27 January 2021 ... were combined, of those who reported experiencing covid-19 symptoms in the past seven days, only 18.0% ... reported requesting a test. In the latest wave of data collection ... , the percentage of people requesting a test after symptoms developed was 22.2%.

Finally, although a huge majority of people expressed intent that they would share details of close contacts if they were to come down with the virus, those who delivered on the intention were significantly fewer than that. This was the case in the pre-vaccination age, in the teeth and claw of the pandemic.

When data from 1 June 2020 to 27 January 2021 ... were combined, of those who had not experienced covid-19 symptoms in the past seven days, 79.1% ... reported that they probably or definitely would share details of close contacts with the NHS contact tracing service if they tested positive for covid-19 and were prompted by the NHS contact tracing service. Intention to share details of close contacts increased slightly over time. In the latest wave of data collection ... 81.9% ... intended to share details of close contacts. [But] ... According to NHS Test and Trace, 25% of people who test positive for covid-19 do not provide details of any close contacts, suggesting a slight degree of underreporting.[269]

Part of the reason for low public engagement with NHSTT is likely to have been public scepticism over its efficacy. A failing system, after all, may be considered as hardly worth the bother – especially when there are economic and other costs to bear when doing the bother (that is, quarantining oneself and family members and potentially close contacts). However, for the first few months of 2021, in the context of lower caseloads, there is evidence that NHSTT began to improve its contact performance so that up to 91 percent of cases were reached.[270] Despite this, as a House of Commons committee review (of 27 October 2021) reported:

Around 16% of people who have tested positive for COVID-19, and around 20% of their contacts, do not fully meet self-isolation requirements ... Only a minority of people experiencing COVID-19 symptoms get a test. Between

18% and 33% of people who experience COVID-19 symptoms report getting a test. Some groups, such as older people, men, and certain ethnic minorities, are much less likely to request tests. While it recognises that some groups of people are underrepresented in the testing programme NHST&T's test and trace data is not sufficiently robust to establish a baseline against which progress can be measured.[271]

Consequently, the more important motives for public non-engagement with the test-and-trace system are likely to be exactly those which are elaborated earlier as reasons for non-compliance with NPIs generally. These are factors of decivilization. The culture of egoistic rights-based individualism, which would prioritize private interests over public ones, and which would elevate the desire to avoid personal inconvenience to the status of "citizenship right", would be one such factor, of course. But another would be the economic hardship that would be incurred on those positive-tested who just happen to be on the wrong side of the social-class divide from having to self-isolate for 10 days.

The financial burden of home quarantine on members of the "precariat", on the denizens of the G-economy, would be especially acute. This is especially so in the UK, owing to austerity politics, which have followed hot on the heels of decades of welfare retrenchment under successive neoliberal governments. As the Health Foundation reported, in the summer of 2021, the "UK has the lowest sick pay in the OECD, and the government's current self-isolation support payments are insufficient, offering only £500, and rejecting two-thirds of applicants".[272] A failing of NHSTT was that it actually exacerbated class and racial-class inequalities in healthcare. This was due to the fact that the system was less successful in contact tracing people who were poor and who lived in the most rundown areas than those who were better off and lived in more affluent areas.[273] But this failure dovetailed with the lack of a sufficient welfare safety net that would minimize the financial penalties on the economically hard-pressed and insecure by complying with stay-at-home rules. The poor and oppressed minorities were doubly disadvantaged.

Now, the UK's suboptimal test-and-trace performance was not simply a case of British exceptionalism, though here public engagement with this NPI was particularly poor by international standards. Lesser rates of public buy-in to test-and-trace policies and systems also characterized other high-income countries of the Global North. As Sachs explains:

> Many individuals in Europe and the United States were simply unwilling to disclose personal information, even their contacts, to public health officials … A survey of attitudes to contact-tracing across 19 countries in August [2020] found that nearly three-quarters of respondents would be willing to provide contact information. But rates varied. In Vietnam, only 4% of participants said that they wouldn't provide this information. In the United States and Germany, the proportion was 21%, and in France, it was 25% … Similarly, the public in North Atlantic countries rejected phone applications

to signal proximity to COVID-positive individuals, with such apps widely criticized as invasions of privacy.

As Sachs aptly concludes: "Though considerations of privacy are important, the failure of testing, tracing, and isolating in the North Atlantic countries has had devastating consequences on mortality rates, suggesting that claims of liberty have been carried too far".[274]

Vaccine hesitancy

In more recent times, of course, non-compliance of many people on COVID matters has extended beyond NPIs and embraced the key pharmacological intervention – the vaccines. The issue of vaccine hesitancy has been foregrounded in the present pandemic as tens of millions of people who have had the opportunity to be COVID-vaccinated have not taken it. The WHO succinctly defines vaccine hesitancy as "delay in acceptance or refusal of vaccination despite availability of vaccination services".[275]

Vaccine scepticism in the UK

A significant proportion of the UK population has been vaccine-hesitant, based on this definition, since even before the vaccination programme got started. Freeman *et al.*'s OCEAN I survey (based on self-report data gathered between 24 September and 17 October 2020) illuminated the extent of the problem, the reasons for it, and who was most associated with it.[276] This found that "71.7% ... were willing to be vaccinated, 16.6% ... were very unsure, and 11.7% ... were strongly hesitant".[277] Vaccine hesitancy, according to the survey, was associated with negative "beliefs about the collective importance, efficacy, side-effects, and speed of development of a COVID-19 vaccine". Such was also associated with what the researchers call "excessive mistrust", that is, with "conspiracy beliefs, negative views of doctors, and need for chaos".[278] Who were the vaccination doubters, according to the survey? "Vaccine hesitancy was associated with lower age, female gender, low education, lower income", and with "black and mixed ethnicities", with "age explaining the highest amount".[279]

Denford *et al.*'s small-scale qualitative study of the attitudes of vaccine-hesitant adults towards getting jabbed reported similar findings to Freeman *et al.*[280] This was with regard to people's reasons for not taking up vaccination opportunities. The researchers interviewed 70 people, 35 aged 18–29, who were unvaccinated, and 35 people aged 30–49, who had not yet taken up their second vaccine opportunity. This was between 10 September and 22 October 2021. Yet, unlike Freeman *et al.*'s (much larger and much earlier) study, this one did not reveal respondents who were "strongly hesitant", that is, actually opposed to getting vaccinated. Denford *et al.*'s vaccine sceptics were not anti-vaxxers. They were usually cognisant of the general benefits of vaccination and indeed of the COVID-19 vaccines. Rather, these people were simply uncertain, with this motivated mainly by concern about negative side-effects, scepticism over efficacy, and mistrust of the motives especially of government. As Sarah Denford summarized the study's chief conclusions:

> What we found is that, overall, participants were not opposed to taking the COVID-19 vaccine but that they had a number of concerns, which can be viewed as barriers to uptake. Most people we spoke to were actively engaged in weighing up the relative risks and benefits. It was concerns around safety, efficacy and trust in government and science that acted as barriers and contributed to their hesitancy.[281]

The concern of participants with negative health impacts, primarily on themselves, was based on their perception that there was insufficient research on potential side-effects, both immediate and longer-term, due to the speed at which the vaccines were developed. As one participant explained:

> I had concerns that there was not enough time to allow for any side-effects to actually happen. I thought that the vaccine was a bit rushed into, you know, being widely available …[282]

Participants expressed concern that the vaccines would impact adversely on matters of importance, such as fertility or mobility, and relayed social-media stories or anecdotes of known others suggestive of dramatic ill-effects – including of people being disabled or killed by it.[283]

The scepticism over efficacy was conveyed by beliefs that the vaccines did not prevent infection and transmission. As one participant in the study put it, "even if I had the vaccine I still might pass it [the virus] on. I still might catch it. You just never know and that's the thing". As another opined:

> Obviously, different strains are immune to the vaccine, or at least the vaccine's not as strong against them, so I suppose I'm quite sceptical as to how the vaccines are working and whether or not it's actually causing that much of an impact or whether it's going to be a bit of an issue further down the line as [variants] become more and more immune.

Remarkably, one participant considered vaccination as superfluous due to lack of efficacy because a relative had died from COVID-19 despite being double-jabbed. This was despite the fact that the vaccination programme had clearly caused hospitalizations and mortalities to tumble and that 100 percent protection had never been claimed by scientists for the vaccinations.[284]

Younger participants in particular were sceptical of efficacy. This was also because they considered vaccination (whether first vaccination or second vaccination) as superfluous to their own needs, since they were unlikely to become ill from COVID-19, just as the vaccines would not prevent them from catching the virus.[285] For example, responses included:

I just feel like I don't need [the vaccine] ... I suppose I've just heard that people have said it's not necessary, you don't really need it, that's what I've heard from other people ... so I just feel like it's not necessary for me ...

Yes. I don't really understand what the vaccine is going to do. Okay. It says it's not going to hospitalise me, but then, it didn't do that to me in the first place, and neither did it do anything to all the other of my friends who got it at the same time as me ...

When they talk about the survival rate once you've contracted it, why are we vaccinating so much for something that survival rate's something like 99% or 98% or something like this? That, to me, doesn't add up ...

Vaccine hesitancy for many was also motivated, as the researchers reported, by "a lack of trust in government, and misunderstanding of science".[286] Arguably, for reasons I have discussed, the mistrust of government is easier to make sense of (that is, in the sense of being credible) than are the apparent scientific misunderstandings. As one participant put it:

I don't believe half what they [the government] say anyway so it goes in one ear and out the other. Look how often we get lied to by the government about stuff, so I just think I can't trust a word they say.

However, other justifications for distrust of government were the stuff of wild conspiratorial conjecture. These included speculations that ministers were hard-selling vaccination in order to make money for pharmaceutical companies or to place the public under state surveillance, or that they were tardy in implementing NPIs in order to legitimize mass inoculation.[287] For example:

Is this all just a ploy to get us all home and under government control?

Why did [the government] take so long to lock down the country? Why did they take so long? Did they want more people to be infected? ... Is that a promotion for more people to get ill and get vaccinated?

They're just trying to get more money. They get money per vaccination ... .

As for the "misunderstandings" of science, these are clear from certain of the above-cited rationalizations offered by participants for their vaccine hesitancy. The main purpose of mass vaccination, of course, is to protect the vulnerable (the elderly and those with health-related vulnerabilities), not people in general, or the young person without health complications who receive the jab. Why then was it confusing for these participants to behold that hospitalization from COVID-19 for people like them was unlikely even before vaccination and that this remained the case afterwards?

Vaccination is not simply a matter of what lies in the interests of the "I" or the "me", or of a specific "us", but also of the wider community or public interest, as ought to have been apparent to Denford *et al.*'s respondents. A 99 percent "survival rate" from COVID-19, after all, is equivalent to 600,000 plus people in the UK dying from the disease. And what of the "survival rate" for the elderly and those with underlying health conditions that would make, for them, catching the disease potentially life-threatening? Such considerations were not much in evidence amongst these vaccine sceptics. But why do people manifest this peculiar insularity of outlook? Such may be accounted for as a consequence of decivilization as individualization. I will revisit this argument shortly.

Freeman *et al.*'s survey, conducted at the start of the vaccination rollout in the UK, demonstrated that vaccine hesitancy of various degrees was an attitude of almost a third of UK adults. If translated into vaccine refusal, this would undermine the efficacy of the vaccination programme. A later study by Chaudhuri *et al.* reported survey data that was even indicative of an increase and hardening of vaccine hesitancy. This was as the vaccination programme got started.

> Within the UK by the 18 February 2021, 34% of 18,855 participants of OCEANS II/III study confirmed that they were either doubtful or strongly unwilling to opt for the vaccine. Similar mistrust was also noted amongst a higher risk category namely the 'keyworkers' with 23.9% of the 579 keyworkers surveyed responding that they are uncertain or will refuse to take the vaccine. These rates of COVID-19 vaccine hesitancy have remained relatively stable since earlier studies conducted by January 2021 suggesting around 50–60% of individuals would be willing to receive a vaccine.[288]

A more positive outlook has been revealed by other surveys, however. According to ONS data, 91 percent of adults surveyed between 13 January and 7 February (2021) said they were positive about the vaccines. Even so, nine percent said they were not – a significant cohort of sceptics numbering more than five million.[289] In the later period from 23 June to 18 July 2021, according to ONS data, the proportion of adults who said they were positive about the vaccines increased to 96 percent, so that the proportion of self-declared vaccine sceptics was more than halved.[290] Nonetheless vaccine sceptics then still numbered more than two million adults, according to this data. Again, if translated into vaccine refusal, this would be tantamount to a significant breach of the vaccine wall, potentially injurious to the cause of public health.

The ONS report on vaccine hesitancy rates in the UK covering the period from 23 June to 18 July 2021 was, as far as I can tell, the last one in the series. Others were seemingly mooted but did not come to pass. However, data on vaccination take-up rates in the UK since then may be obtained from other ONS reports, from the UK Health Security Agency, and also from GOV.UK's Coronavirus Dashboard. These can cast light on the issue of vaccine hesitancy up to the time of writing (or rather updating) this chapter.

The UK Health Agency estimated that 89 percent of eligible persons (that is, persons of 12 years of age and above) had been once-jabbed and 80 percent had been double-jabbed by early December 2021. Based on ONS population estimates, this would mean that up to six million eligible people were unvaccinated at that time. The majority of those who had not taken their second vaccination were under 40 years of age. Only 60 percent of those aged 40 or under were by then double-jabbed. Of these, the least twice-vaccinated were 16–17-year-olds (26 percent) and the next least twice-vaccinated were 18–24-year-olds (67 percent).[291] According to a later ONS report on vaccination rates among people aged 18 years and above by sociodemographic characteristics and occupation, "66.6% had received three coronavirus … vaccinations as of 31 December 2021; of those who had received two vaccinations by 30 September 2021, 79.6% had continued on to receive a third vaccination".[292] This report was, unfortunately, the last one to date in that particular ONS series.

According to the UK Coronavirus Dashboard, though, by mid-year 2022 (19 July), 53,682,329 people had received their first COVID-19 vaccination, 93.3 percent of the population aged 12 and above. By then, 50,395,333 people (87.6 percent of the plus 12 population) had received their second jab and 40,141,657 (69.8 percent of the plus 12 population) their booster.[293] Such data obviously suggests significant persisting vaccine hesitancy among adults, though its exact magnitude amongst them cannot be gleaned from this data. This was especially with regard to first-jab take-up (since probably between three and five percent of adults were still without any vaccine protection), but also with regard to second-jab take-up, since by then, all members of adult cohorts had long been offered both opportunities. The Public Accounts Committee estimated that, by the end of May 2022,

> 2.98 million adults in England remained unvaccinated with a further 1.5 million only having had one dose of a covid-19 vaccine. Although 90% of the adult population has received two doses of vaccine, the uptake for the first booster, for which all adults are eligible, is only 73%.[294]

At the same time, vaccination of children, especially of the 5–11 age group (which had been started in March 2022) but also of the 12–15 age group (which had been started in September 2021), was languishing at low thresholds, as parents were vaccine-hesitant on their behalf.[295] By then, only seven percent of the former had received a jab and only 24 percent of the latter. The Public Accounts Committee also reported that "by the end of May 2022 only 55% of young people aged 16 and 17 had received two doses and only 38% of 12 to 15 year olds".[296]

The vaccination of children and teenagers has limited public health benefits for them themselves. But the benefits for them are potentially significant, nonetheless. It is unknown to what extent young people (including children) could be impacted later on by "Long Covid", for example. But the greater importance in vaccinating the young is the pro-social one of protecting older people (especially vulnerable older people) who would contract the disease from the youngsters, not least because unvaccinated cohorts can be the incubators of new variants – some of which may be more virulent or better adapted to evade vaccination protections. For this reason, parental vaccine hesitancy on behalf of their offspring will pose significant public health risks for as long as the pandemic lasts.

Vaccine scepticism worldwide

Vaccine reluctance is by no means, of course, a case of British exceptionalism. This is also prevalent in the US, for example, where it has a political colouration, dividing up on party-political lines, with much lower take-up among Republican supporters than among Democrat supporters. Thus,

> as of August 2021, 86% of Democrats reported having received at least one dose of a vaccine compared to only 60% of Republicans. Further, the 20 states with the highest vaccination rates were all won by Biden in the 2020 election, while 15 of the 16 states with the lowest vaccination rates were all won by Trump. An additional poll showed that, as of April 2021, 43% of Republicans had indicated that would never be willing to get a vaccine, compared to 5% of Democrats and 22% of independents.[297]

This may have a lot to do with the fact that Republicanism under Trump sought to build popular support by masquerading as a representative of an anti-corporate, anti-establishment politics, and because Trump himself, as we have seen, expressed a vociferous pandemic denialism, which could only encourage vaccine scepticism of various degrees among his supporters.[298] This may also be due to the fact that more Republican supporters than Democrat supporters (and certainly more Trump supporters) fit the definition of "honour individualism" that I addressed earlier.

But, of course, vaccine hesitancy extends beyond the US and UK. This is, in fact, a global phenomenon, as has been reported by major international reviews of vaccine scepticism research. One of these was Cascini *et al.*'s.[299] This review, as Chaudhuri *et al.* describe it, drew together "information on all validated cross-sectional surveys examining vaccine hesitancy". In doing so it "identified 53 studies from Europe alone, identifying similar rates of vaccine hesitancy to the UK in countries such as Italy, Poland, France, Germany and Greece".[300] Another international review of vaccine hesitancy conducted by Jeffrey Lazarus and his colleagues (published in the summer of 2022) found that 24.8 percent of 23,000 respondents reported themselves as vaccine refusers.[301] Vaccine resistance is even prevalent amongst certain frontline healthcare workers. An international review of 51 studies investigating vaccine take-up by nurses in 36 countries, for example, found that almost 20.7 percent of nurses surveyed were vaccine refusers.[302] Such is obviously deeply concerning for reasons that hardly require stating.

Vaccine hesitancy has declined over time in the high-income countries, as the vaccine rollouts have proceeded relatively smoothly since the start of 2021 with few reports of adverse side-effects surfacing in the media. This is according to Lazarus *et al.*'s follow-up study to their earlier survey drawing on data gathered from 160,000 participants in 23 countries. This study, published at the start of 2023, compared public acceptance levels in 2022 and 2021. The researchers reported an overall or aggregate increase in favourable or accepting views on the vaccines of 5.2 percent over the period of coverage. However, a decline in vaccine scepticism was not experienced across all of the countries under review. This was the case for 15, but others (eight), including the UK, witnessed an increase in hesitancy in

2022 compared to 2021. Amongst the study's findings was that a large number of people who had been vaccinated were also vaccine sceptics. Of these, 12 percent reported that they were undecided about if they would get a second or third dose, with a large number of these reporting that they were unlikely to do so.[303]

Whether or not hesitancy is reducing, the problem appears deeply embedded and resistant to reform. The number of people who self-report as unvaccinated, according to another study, presently stands at around 13 percent of the adult populations of the UK, Canada, Germany, France, Italy, Japan, and the US, taken as an aggregate. In the UK, US, and Japan, 16 percent are unvaccinated, according to self-report data. In France, Italy, Germany, and Canada, it is 11 percent.[304] These were among the findings of a survey of vaccine take-up among a sample of 23,000 participants in the G7 countries conducted under the auspices of the British Academy in the spring of 2022.[305] Notably, this estimated a much higher percentage of unvaccinated persons in the UK than the other studies I have cited. A reason for the discrepancy could be that ONS population estimates are significant undercounts.

The survey also found that alongside self-reported vaccine refusal was, unsurprisingly, high levels of distrust of the vaccines. This was right across the G7 but was more pronounced in some countries than others.

> Nearly a fifth of people in the G7 said they do not trust the vaccines. France was the least trusting, where only 67% said they trusted the vaccine, followed by the USA at 71%, with Italy and the UK the most trusting, both at 85%.[306]

Finally, the survey found evidence of a hardening of anti-vaccination sentiments among the unvaccinated minority (since most of them claimed to be unvaccinated by choice), so that vaccine sceptics are now outright refusers. As the study concludes:

> In our survey, which is representative of the populations in G7 countries, we find that 13% of people remain unvaccinated. The vast majority of the unvaccinated say they did not want to receive the vaccine (87%). People who have still not received any COVID-19 vaccination are becoming harder to reach and to persuade.[307]

This suggests that further progress in the immunization programmes may have reached its limits.

"Race", class, and vaccine hesitancy

Vaccine hesitancy (which includes outright resistance or refusal) also maps on to the class and ethnic divides of contemporary society, that is, from those divides generated by class exploitation and racial oppression. Research in the UK indicates that "those of Black and ethnic minority background and lower socioeconomic households or those currently unemployed ... have ... even greater rates of hesitancy".[308] This was inasmuch as actual vaccine take-up, as well as self-declared intention to be vaccinated, has been much lower among certain BAME groups (especially among Black people of African and Caribbean descent followed by Asian people of Pakistani and Bangladeshi descent) and among those people (of all ethnicities) who are economically disadvantaged.[309] Hussain *et al.*'s recent review of 24 British studies of vaccine take-up and hesitancy reported that all but one of these found lower rates of vaccine take-up and higher levels of self-reported vaccine hesitancy amongst these minority ethnic populations than amongst majority White populations.[310]

The UK government was up until mid-year 2021 a world leader in the race to vaccinate its population. By mid-May 2021, 92.6 percent of White Britons under 40 years of age had been vaccinated. But this at that stage compared to 78.6 percent of Bangladeshi Britons, 70.3 percent of Pakistani Britons, 67.8 percent of Black-African Britons, and 63.6 percent of Black-Caribbean Britons who had been vaccinated. In the period from 13 January to 7 February (2021), 44 percent of Black adults reported that they were vaccine-hesitant compared to eight percent of White adults. In the period from 23 June to 18 July 2021, 21 percent of Black adults reported that they were vaccine-hesitant compared to four percent of White adults. Over the same period, vaccine hesitancy "was higher for adults identifying Muslim (14%) … as their religion, compared with adults who identify as Christian (4%)".[311]

As for class differentials in rates of vaccination and in expressions of vaccine hesitancy, though these were less radical than those by ethnicity, they were nonetheless radical. Adults from the poorest groups and communities by mid-May 2021 were 1.75 times less likely to have been vaccinated than those from the wealthiest groups and communities. By then, 93.6 percent of adults of 40 years plus in the top quintile of earners were vaccinated compared to 84.1 percent of those in the bottom quintile.[312] One in six adults (16 percent) from the most economically deprived areas of the UK expressed vaccine scepticism in the survey period from 16 January to 7 February 2021 compared to just one in more than 14 (7 percent) of those from the least deprived areas.[313] Later on, in the survey period from 23 June to 18 July 2021, the basic pattern was unbroken. Now adults resident in the most economically deprived areas were four times more likely (eight percent overall) to express vaccine scepticism than those resident in the most economically well-off areas (two percent overall).[314]

More recent ONS data shows that inequalities in vaccine take-ups by "race" and class remain stubbornly entrenched, albeit at higher vaccination thresholds. These are now most apparent in the statistics for booster vaccinations.[315] By the start of 2022, of people aged 18 years and above, almost 67 percent had received three jabs (two vaccines plus one booster). However, on the same timescale, 39.9 percent of Black-Caribbean people, 37.8 percent of Pakistani people, and 37.9 percent of Black-African people, aged 18 plus, had received their three doses, which they had been invited to take. Presently (mid-July 2022), the overall picture of vaccine inequity by ethnicity shows no sign of being undermined. As the Public Accounts Committee reported in May 2022: "Compared with people of white British origin, people of black, black British, and Pakistani origins were less than half as likely to have had their boosters".[316] Indeed, these data were actually indicative of a widening of vaccine inequality by "race" and ethnicity since the start of the year.

Similarly, as for social-class differentials, by the start of 2022, the

> proportion of people who had received three vaccinations was lower among those in less advantaged socio-economic groups; people living in more deprived areas, those who have never worked or are long-term unemployed, those with no qualifications and those who do not own their own home all had lower coverage for third vaccinations than people in more advantaged socio-economic positions.

Only 54 percent of people in Quintile 1 of the ONS study (that is, among people who make up the most economically deprived group) had by then taken all three vaccinations. This is compared to 73 percent of people in Quintile 5 (that is, among those who were the most well-off economically) who had by then done so.[317]

These data obviously evidence the salience of the "intersectionality" of class and racial inequality (and oppression) in accounting for the variability of vaccine take-up in the UK. On the face of it, they also appear to demonstrate the greater salience of inequality by "race" than by class in the interaction of the two in accounting for the asymmetries. Despite appearances to the contrary, however, vaccine hesitancy can be seen legitimately as more of a class issue than an ethnic one. This is even though it manifestly has a "racial" aspect that is causally efficacious in deterring vaccine take-up among minorities.

This is not simply because vaccine hesitancy is a phenomenon of all groups and communities of low socioeconomic status. Rather, this is also because those ethnic groups and communities in which vaccine hesitancy is most prevalent are exactly those that have disproportionately lower proportions of people of higher socioeconomic status along with the highest rates and concentrations of people living under conditions of precarity, deprivation, and marginalization.[318] Vaccine hesitancy has been especially concentrated in Black-African, Black-Caribbean, Bangladeshi, and Pakistani groups and communities because here all of the injuries of class (inequality and injustice) that foster alienation from state authority are concentrated and condensed. Indeed, these injuries of class are actually radicalized, just as they are compounded by others, owing to the discriminatory and oppressive impacts of the various domains of racism (institutional, structural, communal, etc.) as these are undergirded by systemic racism.[319]

Such may encourage profound suspicion of the machinations of all "White" authorities and institutions. Trust may also be damaged by the fact that members of BAME groups have been "under-represented within health research, including vaccines trials, which can influence trust in a particular vaccine being perceived as appropriate and safe".[320] Vaccine resistance especially in Black communities perhaps is motivated as well by distrust of healthcare organizations (owing to a perception of them as "culturally insensitive")[321] and healthcare-related scientific practices ("due to historical issues of unethical ... research")[322] to which Black people in particular have been subjected. Moreover, as Razai *et al.* point out, disregard for non-Christian religious festivals may further undermine trust, just as "residential segregation ... affects health and access to resources to enhance health in multiple ways, creating conditions that amplify mistrust".[323]

Razai *et al.* affirm that vaccine hesitancy in minority communities – which is, as they say, "characterised by uncertainty and ambivalence about vaccination" – is a "legitimate viewpoint". This was also encouraged by "the failure or lack of effective public health messaging" in the UK. They point out that mischievous "anti-vaxxers" "have capitalised on ... concerns to spread misinformation, adding to the historical mistrust of government and public health bodies that runs deep in some ethnic minority groups". The chief motives for vaccine scepticism that they would distil from social research findings are "concerns about side effects and the long term effects on health, and lack of trust in vaccines, particularly among Black respondents".[324]

These are the same sorts of motives for vaccine scepticism amongst certain BAME groups that have been uncovered by other (and more recent) studies, such as Naqvi *et al.*'s, for example.[325] This research, a small-scale qualitative study of the reasons for vaccine hesitancy among persons from minority ethnicity cohorts in the UK, focused exclusively on those who had self-identified as vaccine sceptics. Vaccine-hesitant BAME persons were the only participants in the study, who were all interviewed in depth. By these means, Naqvi *et al.* confirmed Razai *et al.*'s findings:

> General and long term side effects and speed of development of the COVID-19 vaccinations were the most common reasons, followed by the "belief in your own immune system" and concerns regarding the ingredients in the COVID-19 vaccine. Five of the twelve participants cited both side effects and long term side effects as concerns, while two of the twelve participants cited side effects generally, and a further two participants cited long term side effects specifically as concerns. Concerns regarding period irregularities, infertility and breastfeeding were recurring themes in three interviews.[326]

In keeping with other research findings as well, participants cited mistrust of "official sources" of information on the pandemic and on the vaccines as contributing to their hesitancy or scepticism, in favour of greater reliance on social-media sources. This of course exposed them to the views of anti-vaxxers who have a significant online presence:

> The participants discussed receiving anti-vaccination content concerning topics of extreme side effects such as blood clots, inflammation and negative effects on the immune systems. Participants also cited "conspiracy theories", including the idea that COVID-19 is not real and microchips were used in vaccines for tracking purposes. While some participants found these theories to be exaggerated, scaremongering or false, others thought there was some truth in them.

Hesitancy was also motivated by doubt over the benefits of vaccination for one's own protection. This was the "trust one's own immune system" judgement call.[327] As one participant expressed it:

> In the long term, I am thinking what is the point of putting a dormant version of the virus in me that could cause more complications down the line, because my body seems to be fighting COVID-19 fine at the moment.

Razai *et al.* might have added that the prevalence of vaccine hesitancy especially in minorities would also likely be a consequence of the younger demographic of these groups compared to the majority White population. In the UK, for example, vaccine sceptics are disproportionally found among younger adults. Around 17 percent of people aged from 16 to 29 years reported vaccine hesitancy during the period from 13 January to 7 February 2021.[328] Later on, this showed signs of reducing, though this remained much higher than for other age groups. Thus, during the period from 23 June to 16 July 2021, "vaccine hesitancy was 11% among those aged 16 to 17 years (14% in the previous period), 5% among those aged 18 to 21 years (9% in the previous period) and 9% among those aged 22 to 25 years (10% in the previous period)".[329] The average (median) age of the White population is 41 compared to 30 for Black people and 29 for Asian people. More than 43 percent of British Asians and 35 percent of Black Britons are aged from 18–39. This compares to almost 29 percent of White Britons.[330]

Most of Razai *et al.*'s and Naqvi *et al.*'s conclusions about reasons or motives for vaccine hesitancy also dovetail with those of an earlier qualitative ONS survey.[331] This explored the reasons of refusers from *all* those groups where vaccine resistance was especially widespread, not simply minority ethnicity groups. As well as eliciting the views of minority ethnicities, those of young people, people on low incomes, those with lower educational attainment, and those who were clinically vulnerable, were also sought.[332] The respondents gave two main reasons for vaccine refusal.

The first reason was concerns over the vaccines' immediate side-effects and longer-term health consequences. This was especially given the speed at which the vaccines were developed and rolled out. The second reason was their belief that COVID-19 did not pose a significant threat to them because they were confident they would not catch it (owing to their own personal precautions) or would not become ill from it if they did catch it.[333] Secondary concerns were diverse. These included worries over the unknown ingredients the vaccines contained (which were rumoured to be animal remains or foetal elements) and distrust of the agendas of the pharmaceutical companies and of the government. Some respondents thought that the scale and harm of the pandemic was exaggerated by ministers (to control, manipulate, or experiment on the public),[334] which undermined the necessity of mass vaccination.[335]

Now, again, these British results are not anomalous, since similar findings have been derived from studies worldwide. As Chaudhuri *et al.* point out, these have been corroborated by those from the US and France, for example.[336] In the US, also in keeping with the British findings, vaccine hesitancy has been especially linked to people from ethnic minority backgrounds, "especially younger Blacks, who resist being vaccinated more than older people do". But here, according to Ryan and Nanda, these sceptics are motivated by "distrust [of] the government, based on the history of previous medical experiments using Black subjects, related to sexually transmitted diseases".[337] Jaspal and Breakwell cite other US studies indicating that "unemployed and African American respondents were least likely to be accepting of vaccination", whereas "older adults and college and graduate degree holders" were most likely.[338] As for France, which has probably the highest proportion of the vaccine-hesitant internationally, the resistance of minorities, especially of Black minorities, to getting jabbed is doubtless an especially concentrated version of the anti-establishment and anti-pharma libertarian sensibility that is common there in many population groups.[339]

Vaccine hesitancy has also been revealed as a significant issue in the nations of sub-Saharan Africa, though here this problem of hesitancy is dwarfed by that of scarcity of supply. This is owing to the colonial legacy issues which, as Ryan and Nanda observe, make many Africans distrustful of the motives of Western governments and corporations, and fearful that they will treated as vaccine "guinea pigs".[340] Of greater efficacy, perhaps, there is also, for Africa's poor, the prohibitive practical difficulties (arduous travel) and financial costs (taking time off work) incurred by actually attending vaccination centres.

However, Abba-Aji *et al.*'s systematic international review of ethnic minority groups' and migrants' access to and acceptance of COVID-19 vaccines uncovered a more nuanced pattern.[341] This review screened a total of 248 relevant studies, of which 33 were selected for analysis because these were turned into peer-reviewed journal articles. Most of these were conducted in the US (17) and UK (10). Others were conducted in France, Israel, China, and Qatar, whereas another study spanned several countries. The majority of studies (more than two-thirds) were quantitative, whereas others were qualitative or based on mixed methods. The review found that elevated vaccine hesitancy was indeed strongly associated in most studies with Black ethnic minority groups, replicating the US and UK results. This too was accounted for by "low confidence in COVID-19 vaccines … driven by mistrust and safety concerns", which were higher in these groups than in others, thus constituting "a major barrier to COVID-19 vaccine uptake".[342]

But higher levels of vaccine hesitancy and lower rates of vaccine take-up were not found to be universally the case for Asian minorities in the UK. For some groups, it was higher, for others lower, for others the same (as for Whites). Where this was lowest, this was among the poorest or most economically hard-pressed minority ethnicity groups. Similarly, in the US, the same pattern was true of Hispanic minorities. Abba-Aji *et al.*'s review also found that

Asians in the US had the highest COVID-19 vaccine acceptance compared to other ethnic groups. There was higher vaccine acceptance among migrant groups in Qatar and China than in the general population. However, migrants to the UK experienced barriers to vaccine access, mainly attributed to language and communication issues.[343]

Yet these misgivings over the COVID-19 vaccinations, which are expressed also by the poor as well as by members of BAME communities, are not exclusive to these groups. Rather, they are, for reasons already discussed, simply especially common here. This is no exceptionalism of the poor and racially oppressed minorities. International surveys and studies investigating the motives or reasons for vaccine hesitancy have tended to find, as Lazarus *et al.* point out, that across all countries and all population groups "vaccine hesitancy is associated with a lack of trust in COVID-19 vaccine safety and science, and skepticism about its efficacy".[344] Such is also true of the worldwide vaccine scepticism of healthcare frontliners. The major motives for COVID-19 vaccine refusal among nurses, according to Khubchandani *et al.*'s international survey, for example, are their "concerns about vaccine safety, side effects, and efficacy; misinformation and lack of knowledge; and mistrust in experts, authorities, or pharmaceutical companies".[345]

****

On the face of it, based on sources such as the qualitative survey data mobilized by the *COVID-19 vaccines refusal study UK*, vaccine hesitancy does not appear strictly continuous with the refusal of NPIs discussed earlier in this chapter. At the level of appearances, this also does not fit as closely with the thesis of decivilization. Indeed, some anti-vaccine respondents claimed in the IFF/ONS study that they practised physical distancing and other safety measures as an alternative to vaccination. This, however, should be treated with scepticism, not least because such ought to have committed them (at the time they expressed these views) to *indefinite* distancing, whereas most of them expressed a desire to see a speedy return to normal life.[346] On a deeper level, or on closer inspection, however, such responses are indicative of attitudes that arguably are at least compatible with decivilization, for reasons I will set out. The "legitimacy" of vaccine-refusal motives (on moral and rational grounds) is questionable.

The respondents articulated quasi-rational grounds for some concern over the long-term health impacts of the vaccines that motivated their vaccine resistance. This was owing to the fast-tracking of the development and approval process. Typically, vaccines may take years to develop and evaluate, but the COVID-19 vaccines were in mass production barely a year since the start of the pandemic. Some respondents regarded this as troubling. The quasi-rationality of these motives for vaccine refusal would also be stronger for younger people than for older people, because most younger people are indeed at minimal risk of becoming seriously ill from the virus, whereas the risk of harm to older people is significantly higher. Many of the vaccine-refusing respondents in this IFF/ONS survey were younger people.

Yet there was more than a hint of confirmation bias in the responses of those who considered the scale and impact of the pandemic to be exaggerated by the government in order to browbeat everyone into vaccine compliance. (This perspective of vaccine sceptics has, as we have seen, been identified by several studies). So much so that one cannot help thinking that this must have been for many of them rationalization (or technique of neutralization) rather than reason – or if it was not it really ought to have been. This perspective hardly fitted the pattern of government mismanagement of the crisis in the UK, as spelt out in my book on *The Pandemic in Britain*, for example.[347]

Sceptics of "authority" in the UK for its supposed enthusiasm for lockdowns in order to big up COVID-19 and scare people into vaccine compliance surely ought to be alive to the wretched mess that British authority has made of the pandemic. This was a mess generated by lockdown-*aversion* rather than its opposite. Nor could any rational motive other than the termination of the pandemic be attributed to government support everywhere for mass vaccination policies. Why would governments commit themselves to enormously costly vaccine procurements if these were unnecessary to defend public health? Why would they act (however reluctantly) to shut down much of economic life in the pre-vaccine period if they considered the pandemic as anything less than (potentially) disastrously injurious to public health? This was manifestly not a remotely defensible perspective owing simply to its glaring logical shortcomings.

As for the two main reasons offered by the respondents for their vaccine resistance, these arguably fitted to some degree the mould of decivilization as individualization, notwithstanding that these were also (for respondents from minority communities) shaped and skewed by scepticism generated by structural and systemic aspects of decivilization – those of class and "race". (The IFF/ONS survey, like others, found higher levels of general suspicion and scepticism towards the government, media, and pharmaceutical businesses among respondents from minority ethnicities than among other participants). This was simply because these were not expressive of any sort of concern with actually protecting the wider public or indeed protecting a specific community. These were, rather, mostly concerns *of* the self *for* the self: firstly, concern to avert all risk to oneself (however small) of theoretical vaccine side-effects and of speculative longer-term harms; and secondly, to accept a higher risk of COVID infection for others (including vulnerable others), since this was the inevitable consequence of their own vaccine refusal.[348]

This was not even a rational calculus of the ratio of self-risk to public risk, because the former was merely possibility, whereas the latter was reality. In fact, the former was not even *reasonable* concern, to be considered against incorrigible fact. This is because concern over *potential* long-term health ill-effects is a concern of mostly young people over what are *unknowable unknowns*. There are no particular reasons based on any specific knowledge for why this concern supporting COVID-19 vaccine refusal exists. This is merely an abstract (and for the most part unsupported, unevidenced) concern. But, at the same time, the respondents were well aware, unless they were among the "unconcerned" or "uninvolved" citizens that I discussed earlier, that the virus was immediately, verifiably injurious to the lives and well-being of millions of older and more vulnerable people. Yet this knowledge obviously was not yet sufficient to morally incentivize a change of mind on the issue.

For sure, in the past, Black people have been subject to inappropriate scientific studies, and minorities have not always been included in vaccine trials. But, on the other hand, there was the immediate crisis, which was a calamitous one (a pandemic that was killing millions worldwide – and disproportionately minorities at home), hence an urgent need for fast-tracked vaccines. These were fast-tracked as much for White majorities as they were for Black and Asian minorities, so that there was no question of greater risks being taken with the lives or well-being of the latter. Not only that, respondents in the IFF/ONS survey (whether White or Black) did not mostly convey that their vaccine scepticism was motivated by colonial "legacy issues" that explicitly linked to medical science, pharmacology, or vaccine trial studies.[349] Hardly anyone in the IFF/ONS survey expressed their vaccine resistance as generated by concerns that the COVID-19 drugs were developed or trialled in such a way that this would make their use by ethnic minorities riskier than for White majorities.[350]

Nor were most of these vaccine sceptics anti-vaxxers generally. They accepted the full range of other kinds of vaccines which were developed, trialled and mass produced also by the self-same pharmacology and pharmaceutics. Thus, as the IFF/ONS survey found:

> All participants had, to their knowledge, received their childhood vaccinations, such as for meningitis, hepatitis B, the BCG tuberculosis jab, polio, and MMR. Many participants had received vaccines in their adulthood such as the flu jab, as well as those required for travel to certain countries, such as vaccinations against malaria and yellow fever. Overall participants did not have any hesitation about vaccines in general and were positive about their role in protecting against disease. Many parents interviewed also ensured their children were vaccinated.[351]

As for militant anti-vaxxers, who would make up part of the refusing 13 percent in the G7 countries, based on estimates of the British Academy study, their motives would seemingly align with decivilization in a more clear-cut, less controversial, way than would the motives of the softer vaccine sceptics. This is encapsulated by those members of the anti-vaccine protest movement who in demonstrations carry aloft banners displaying slogans that declare the absolute primacy of the "I" over the "we" or "they" or "us", or of the absolute priority of the individual over the collective, as justification enough for vaccine refusal.

From this perspective, no public health interest may be permitted to veto preferences of the self whatever collective harms may result from these preferences. Consequently, for the radical libertarian anti-vaxxer, no actual reason beyond *this is what I want* is required to explain or legitimize vaccine refusal, though plenty of others may be advanced. Wants, inasmuch as these pertain to one's own body, are necessarily sacrosanct, that is, matters of right. Justificatory arguments that vaccination is ineffective, or that this serves sinister agendas of state control, or that this will deliver harmful side-effects, are then superfluous. "My body, my choice", or my "bodily sovereignty", as protestors memorably put it.[352]

Decivilization and the future of NPIs

I conclude that it is feasible, if not probable, that vaccine hesitancy along with non-compliance or inconsistent or variable compliance by large numbers of people to legally or normatively mandated NPIs, has adversely impacted the cause of public health protection during the COVID-19 pandemic to date. By how much is hard to estimate, but in terms of mere statistics, this is likely to be significant, whereas in qualitative human terms, the cost would of course be much heavier. In the UK alone, for example, this may have been at the price of several thousand lost lives and thousands of others that are permanently damaged, with these disproportionately found among minorities and the poor. By and large, success in terms of protecting lives and defending health services has been claimed for lockdown policies and for the NPIs. That these have had a considerable degree of efficacy is undeniable. However, this success has also been overstated. The protections afforded by physical distancing norms and practices have been diluted owing to the variability of public engagement with them.

Compliance variability is partly explainable in terms of weak and ambivalent public health messaging from political authorities, which reflects the reluctance of capitalism-friendly state actors to prioritize public health over profits. This is certainly true of the UK, as I have discussed in my book on *The Pandemic in Britain*.[353] But it is at least feasible that this is also accountable in terms of decivilization mechanisms that are integral to modern capitalist societies (as defined in the previous chapter and as applied in this one to make sense of limited engagement or non-engagement by substantial numbers of people with NPIs and aspects of vaccine resistance). These mechanisms have been radicalized in the neoliberal era owing to the commodification of culture as consumerism, the de-legitimization of services that serve public rather than private interests, and the steady erosion of the protections afforded to ordinary folk and the poor by welfare states that have been downsized.

This is a matter of considerable concern because, for reasons that I explore in my *Contagion Capitalism*, we are entering an era of what may be described as zoonotic accelerationism. This is an age in which pandemics are likely to become more frequent and hence in which certain of the diseases that convey them are likely to be more virulent and pathogenic than COVID-19 has been. Public health protection will thus depend again on the re-introduction of the NPIs before another vaccine fix is to hand. Yet neoliberal politicians and media opinion-formers in their race to forget the pandemic and to embrace "normality" are, as I write these words, already embracing quasi-scientific notions that the lockdowns and strict implementation of NPIs to counteract COVID-19 were excessive, draconian, surplus to (public health protection) requirements, indeed of little efficacy in preventing deaths, while incurring huge economic and other costs.[354] Indeed, such notions were doing the rounds, in a blaze of media publicity, much in advance of the vaccine fix.[355]

Epidemiologist Mark Woolhouse has made perhaps the most sophisticated anti-lockdown case on these sorts of grounds (relatively speaking). This is in his critique of the UK government's pandemic response. Typically, liberal economists rather than scientists or public health professionals have made retrospective critiques of lockdown policies, so Woolhouse's interventions are likely to carry greater authority in opinion-forming. Woolhouse "even-handedly" rejects a strategy of generalized NPIs as well as the UK government's purportedly herd immunity strategy of complete unlocking of restrictions after 19 July 2021. This is in favour of shielding policies for the elderly and vulnerable and reliance on test-and-trace policies. This is how the British government could and should have managed the pandemic, he opines. Such is based on the commonplace observation that COVID-19 is a radically discriminate rather than indiscriminate virus in that it is far more injurious to the elderly and those with specific underlying health conditions that render them vulnerable than to "ordinary" folk.[356]

Woolhouse's account is seasoned with the usual myths about the supposedly calamitous and irreparable harms perpetrated on public mental health and well-being and on children's education (as additional ill-effects to the economic ones) by the lockdowns to bolster his critique. As he explains, when promoting his book in an interview for the *Observer* newspaper:

> We did serious harm to our children and young adults who were robbed of their education, jobs and normal existence, as well as suffering damage to their future prospects, while they were left to inherit a record-breaking mountain of public debt … All this to protect the NHS from a disease that is a far, far greater threat to the elderly, frail and infirm than to the young and healthy … We were mesmerised by the once-in-a-century scale of the emergency and succeeded only in making a crisis even worse. In short, we panicked. This was an epidemic crying out for a precision public health approach and it got the opposite.[357]

But there are other problems with Woolhouse's polemic worthy of note. Firstly, he is far too dismissive of pandemic harms beyond the elderly and vulnerable. In fact, COVID-19 was capable of harming anyone, which his talk of "small risk" to most rather covers up. As Nazneen Khan illuminates, in the US, during the delta wave, which coincided with school reopenings, hundreds of children were killed by the virus, most of whom did not have underlying vulnerabilities, and many more were hospitalized.[358]

> The Centers for Disease Control and Prevention (CDC) reported a dramatic ten-fold increase in COVID-19 related hospitalizations amongst children ages 0–4 and a five-fold increase amongst all children aged 18 and under upon circulation of the delta variant. As of November 2021, approximately 6.8 million children had tested positive for COVID-19 in the USA, with over one million of those positive tests occurring during a four-week timeframe connected to the early fall 2021 peak of the delta. In conjunction with school reopenings, delta proved dangerous, even deadly, for children. As of November 2021, 712 child deaths (ages 0–18) have been reported by the National Center for Health Statistics, but cumulative child deaths nearly

doubled due to the delta surge. From July to October 2021 alone, nearly 300 child deaths were reported.[359]

Secondly, in the UK at least, there was no test-and-trace system that could function as an alternative to blanket NPIs. This was the case in advance of and throughout the calamitous first wave and beyond.[360] A third problem with Woolhouse's account, however, is that it fails to grasp that, irrespective of the discriminatory nature of COVID-19, blanket (that is, indiscriminate) physical distancing controls were needed to prevent it locating and killing exactly those people that it particularly discriminated against. Those people at least risk of becoming seriously ill from COVID are, after all, perfectly capable of passing it on to those who are at most risk.

Finally, Woolhouse's critique errs in that he simply fails to demonstrate that the UK lockdowns were unnecessary. Rather, he asserts that since many people in the UK, in the absence of government directives to physically distance in the runup to the first lockdown, were voluntarily embracing a measure of precautionary distancing, this demonstrates that lockdowns were superfluous. Yet, what this rose-tinted judgement rather misses is that many other people were not embracing such voluntary measures and that the voluntary embrace by some people of NPIs (even if a majority of people) was not stopping rapidly escalating caseloads.[361] The British lockdowns were not errors motivated by blind panic, as Woolhouse prefers to believe. Rather, these were matters of necessity to save the healthcare system from caseloads that would overwhelm it. These too were in accordance with guidance from the UK government's own Scientific Advisory Group for Emergencies (SAGE) scientific advisers.[362]

Swedish exceptionalism?

Woolhouse also draws inspiration for his perspective from the Swedish government's refusal to implement lockdown policies, which he (wrongly) claims resulted in a much better public health outcome than elsewhere. His choice of Sweden as a role model is remarkable in that the Swedish government not only eschewed lockdowns but most other NPIs (including border controls, quarantining, restrictions on the size and type of public gatherings, and – right up until December 2020 – recommendations that people wear face masks in public).[363] This approach was presented by its political artificers as placing trust in the public to take on self-responsibility for NPIs without the need for a government mandate or steer. In reality, however, it was intended to allow COVID-19 to rip unchecked through the population in pursuance of a publicly unacknowledged herd immunity strategy in order to avoid business harm.[364]

Nonetheless, in spite of this callous and reckless experiment with public health, Sweden has recorded a remarkably lower rate of excess deaths in comparison with most European and other developed countries, especially in comparison with Italy, Spain, the UK and the US. This was also much below the global average of excess deaths over the course of the pandemic up until the end of 2021.[365] This has naturally emboldened lockdown critics in British politics, who are especially well represented in the ruling Conservative party. Jeremy Hunt, former health secretary and recently appointed chancellor of the exchequer, is the highest profile of these to date, opining that "Britain has a lot to learn" from the Swedish government's decision not to opt for mandatory lockdowns in response to the crisis in favour of allowing citizens to decide if they will or will not comply with NPIs and to what degree.[366]

However, public health experts have attributed Sweden's success at least in part to demographic factors peculiar to the Nordic countries, including low population density, a much higher proportion of single-person households, and a lower proportion of multigenerational households than is typical in the more populous countries.[367] The relatively low mortality rate thus probably had nothing to do with Sweden's "laid-back" pandemic policies. On the contrary, there are very good reasons for thinking that these policies have generated a far higher mortality rate than would have been the case if ministers had implemented stringent mandatory NPIs as their neighbours did. This becomes clear if we compare like with like, which Woolhouse fails to do. The Nordic countries share not only similar demographics but are also economically, socially and culturally similar. As Irfan *et al.* rightly say: "The limited ... differences between and within these countries make them the ideal setting for comparing the effect of different strategies to tackle the COVID-19 pandemic".[368]

By the end of January 2021, Sweden's mortality rate from COVID-19 stood at almost 11,000 compared to Norway's rate of 540. As Camelia Dewan has remarked: "Even if we doubled the Norwegian number to account for population size, Sweden would still have ten times more deaths than their Scandinavian neighbour".[369] Moreover, by the end of summer 2021, Sweden had a death rate from COVID-19 that was from four to ten times higher per capita than any of its Nordic neighbours, all of which except Iceland introduced lockdowns alongside a full battery of other health protection measures.[370] (Iceland did not go into lockdown, "but instead relied on an aggressive strategy of mass-testing, contact tracing, quarantine, and isolation", also in stark contrast with government policy in Sweden). In the period from 1 January 2020 to 3 January 2021, "case fatality was 0.9% on average (0.5%-5%) for the other Nordic countries, and 2.2% for Sweden". Sweden also had much higher rates of infection, hospitalizations and ICU admissions than the others over the same period.

> The CFR of confirmed cases was highest for Sweden (2.2%) followed by Finland (1.5%) and lowest for Iceland (0.5%) among the Nordic countries ... The test positivity ratio was around 10% for Sweden, and below 2% in all other Nordic countries (in line with other reports), also indicating restricted testing in Sweden and probably the largest proportion of un-diagnosed cases in the Nordic region. These results are similar to other COVID-19 studies in Nordic countries, including a comparative analysis of epidemiological indicators that included Sweden, Norway, Denmark, and Finland.[371]

Unsurprisingly, under the circumstances, the elderly and vulnerable were especially ill-served by the Swedish government's pandemic denialism. As Diderichsen reports:

The government had an explicit priority to protect the elderly in nursing and care homes but failed to do so. The staff in elderly care are less qualified and have harder working conditions in Sweden, and they lacked adequate care for the clients. Sweden has in recent years diverged from the Scandinavian welfare model by strong commercialization of primary care and elderly care.[372]

By 2020's end, 90 percent of COVID-19 mortalities in the country were aged 70 and higher.[373] Before then, by August 2020, the vast majority of Sweden's then 5,800 COVID-19 deaths "were elderly people, including a significant number in care homes". By comparison, "Norway, with around half of the population of Sweden, did much better with less than 300 deaths in the same period".[374]

Pandemic denialism (that is, of the necessity of lockdown) is therefore rooted in ideology rather than in facts. But, despite the big holes in the case for it, such is likely to become increasingly popular retrospectively among corporate power-holders and neoliberal politicians (as Jeremy Hunt's headline-grabbing comments have shown). This of course supports the idea that every effort should be made not to repeat such policies if faced with new pandemics. Such is part of the political work of massaging public opinion in favour of a more business-friendly or profits-before-people herd immunity policy approach in advance of the next epidemiological crisis. The variability of popular engagement with NPIs this time may even be convenient for this cause since this is likely to be weaponized by political leaders and the corporate media to argue for a less "draconian" policy response next time. After all, Boris Johnson's "freedom-loving Brits" (he could equally have said "freedom-loving consumers" or "freedom-loving hedonists") are unlikely, they would say, to stomach another round of stringent pandemic restrictions. Decivilization, alas, makes this scenario plausible.

12 September 2021 (updated July 2022 and May 2023)

Notes

1   Ding, H. (2014). 'Transnational quarantine rhetorics: public mobilization in SARS and in H1N1 Flu'. *Journal of Medical Humanities*, 35 (2), pp. 191–210; Durham, D.P., and Casman, E.A. (2012). 'Incorporating individual health protective decisions into disease transmission models: a mathematical framework'. *Journal of the Royal Society Interface*, 9 (68), 562–70; Glass, R.J., Glass, L.M., Beyeler, W.E., and Min, H.J. (2006). 'Targeted social distancing designs for pandemic influenza'. *Emerging Infectious Diseases*, 12 (11), pp. 1671–81; Karimi, E., Schmitt, K., and Akgunduz, A. (2015). 'Effect of individual protective behaviors on influenza transmission: an agent-based model'. *Health Care Management Science*, 18 (3), pp. 318–33; Kelso, J.K., Milne, G.J., and Kelly, H. (2009). 'Simulation suggests that rapid activation of social distancing can arrest epidemic development due to a novel strain of influenza'. *BMC Public Health*, 9 (117), pp. 1–10; Lewnard, J.A., and Lo, N.C. (2020). 'Scientific and ethical basis for social distancing interventions against COVID-19'. *Lancet Infectious Diseases*, 20 (6), pp. 631–33; Weston, D., Hauck, K., and Amlôt, R. (2018). 'Infection prevention behaviour and infectious disease modelling: a review of the literature and recommendations for the future'. *BMC Public Health*, 18 (336), pp. 1–16.

2 See for example: Askitas, N., Tatsiramos, K., and Verheyden, B. (2021). 'Estimating worldwide effects of non-pharmaceutical interventions on COVID-19 incidence and population mobility patterns using a multiple-event study'. *Scientific Reports*, 11 (1972), pp. 1–13; Banholzer, N. *et al.* (2021). 'Estimating the effects of non-pharmaceutical interventions on the number of new infections with COVID-19 during the first epidemic wave'. *PLoS ONE*, 16 (6), pp. 1–16; Brüggenjürgen, B. *et al.* (2023). 'Impact of public health interventions to curb SARS-CoV-2 spread assessed by an evidence-educated Delphi panel and tailored SEIR model'. *Journal of Public Health: From Theory to Practice*, 31 (4), pp. 539–52; Chu, D.K. *et al.* (2020). 'Physical distancing, face masks, and eye protection to prevent person-to-person transmission of SARS-CoV-2 and COVID-19: a systematic review and meta-analysis'. *Lancet*, 395 (10242), pp. 1973–87; Dandekar, R.A., Henderson, S.G., Jansen, M., Moka, S., Nazarathy, Y., Rackauckas, C., Taylor, P.G., and Vuorinen, A. (2021). 'Safe blues: a method for estimation and control in the fight against COVID-19. *Patterns*, 2 (3), pp. 1–9; Fair, K.R., Karatayev, V.A., Anand, M., and Bauch, C.T. (2022). 'Estimating COVID-19 cases and deaths prevented by non-pharmaceutical interventions, and the impact of individual actions: A retrospective model-based analysis'. *Epidemics*, 39 (100557), pp. 1–9; Flaxman, S. *et al.* (2020). 'Estimating the effects of non-pharmaceutical interventions on COVID-19 in Europe'. *Nature*, 584, pp. 257–61; Flaxman. S. *et al.* (2020). 'Report 13: estimating the number of infections and the impact of non-pharmaceutical interventions on COVID-19 in 11 European countries. *Nature*, 584, pp. 257–61; Giordano, G. *et al.* (2020). 'Modelling the COVID-19 epidemic and implementation of population-wide interventions in Italy. *Nature Medicine*, 26, pp, 855–60; He, Y. *et al.* (2022). 'The impact of multi-level interventions on the second-wave SARS-CoV-2 transmission in China'. *PLoS ONE*, 17 (9), pp. 1–12; Hsiang, S. *et al.* (2020). 'The effect of large-scale anti-contagion policies on the COVID-19 pandemic'. *Nature*, 584, pp. 262–67; Khataee, H. *et al.* (2021). 'Effects of social distancing on the spreading of COVID-19 inferred from mobile phone data'. *Scientific Reports*, 11 (1661), pp. 1–9; Kucharski, A.J. *et al.* (2020). 'Early dynamics of transmission and control of COVID-19: a mathematical modelling study'. *Lancet Infectious Diseases*, 20 (5), pp. 553–58; Kupferschmidt, K., and Cohen, J. (2020). 'Will novel virus go pandemic or be contained?' *Science*, 367 (6478, pp. 610–11; Mohammadi, Z., Cojacaru, M.G., and Thommes, E.W. (2022). 'Human behaviour, NPI and mobility reduction effects on COVID-19 transmission in different countries of the world'. *BMC Public Health*, 22 (1594), pp. 1–19; Neufeld, Z., Khataee, H., and Czirok, A. (2020). 'Targeted adaptive isolation strategy for COVID-19 pandemic'. *Infectious Disease Modelling*, 5 (5), pp. 357–61; N'Konzi, J-P.N., Chukwu, C.W., and Nyabadza, F. (2022). 'Effect of time-varying adherence to non-pharmaceutical interventions on the occurrence of multiple epidemic waves: A modeling study'. *Frontiers in Public Health*, 10 (3389), pp. 1–11; Pozo-Martin, F. *et al.* (2021). 'The impact of non-pharmaceutical interventions on COVID-19 epidemic growth in the 37 OECD member states'. *European Journal of Epidemiology*, 36 (6), pp. 629–40; Salje, H. *et al.* (2020). 'Estimating the burden of SARS-CoV-2 in France', *Science*, 369 (6500), pp. 208–11.

3 Tomczyk, S., Rahn, M., and Schmidt, S. (2020). 'Social Distancing and Stigma: Association Between Compliance With Behavioral Recommendations, Risk Perception, and Stigmatizing Attitudes During the COVID-19 Outbreak'. *Frontiers in Psychology*, 11 (1821), pp. 1–9. See p. 2.

4 N'Konzi, J-P.N., Chukwu, C.W., and Nyabadza, F. (2022). "Effect of time-varying adherence to non-pharmaceutical interventions on the occurrence of multiple epidemic waves: A modeling study'. *Frontiers in Public Health*, 10, pp. 1–11.

5 N'Konzi *et al.* (2022), p. 1.

6 Bish, A. and Michie, S. (2010). 'Demographic and attitudinal determinants of protective behaviours during a pandemic: a review'. *British Journal of Health Psychology*,

15 (4), pp. 797–824; Perra, N. (2021). 'Non-pharmaceutical interventions during the COVID-19 pandemic: a review'. *Physics Reports*, 23 (913), pp. 1–52.

7 Bishi and Michie (2010); Galasso, V. *et al.* (2021). 'Gender differences in COVID-19 attitudes and behavior: Panel evidence from eight countries'. *Proceedings of the National Academy of Sciences of the United States of America (PNAS)*, 117 (44), pp. 27285–91; Ganslmeier, M., Van Parys, J., and Vlandas, T. (2022). 'Compliance with the first UK covid-19 lockdown and the compounding effects of weather'. *Scientific Reports*, 12 (3821), pp. 1–10; Perra (2021); Tomczyk, S., Rahn, M., and Schmidt, S. (2020). 'Social Distancing and Stigma: Association Between Compliance With Behavioral Recommendations, Risk Perception, and Stigmatizing Attitudes During the COVID-19 Outbreak'. *Frontiers in Psychology*, 11 (1821), pp. 1–9.

8 Borgonovi, F. and Andrieu, E. (2020). 'Bowling together by bowling alone: social capital and COVID-19'. *Social Science & Medicine*, 265 (113501), pp. 1–39; Grossman, G., Kim, S., Rexer, J.M., and Tirumurthy, H. (2020). 'Political partisanship influences behavioral responses to governors' recommendations for COVID-19 prevention in the United States'. *Proceedings of the National Academy of Science*, 117(39), pp. 24144–53; Jørgensen, F., Bor, A., and Petersen, M.B. (2021). 'Compliance without fear: Individual-level protective behaviour during the first wave of the COVID-19 pandemic'. *British Journal of Health Psychology*, 26 (2), pp. 679–96; Olsen, A.L. and Hjorth, F. (2020). *Willingness to distance in the COVID-19 pandemic*. OSF Home (online). [Preprint]. (30 March); Seale, H. *et al.* (2020). 'COVID-19 is rapidly changing: Examining public perceptions and behaviors in response to this evolving pandemic'. *PLoS ONE*, 15 (6), pp. 1–13; Van Rooij, B. *et al.* (2020). *Compliance with COVID-19 mitigation measures in the United States*. Social Science Research Network (SSRN). [Preprint]. (1 May); Rasul, I. and Giuliano, P. (2020). *Who complies with social distancing measures in the pandemic?* Economics Observatory (online). (20 August).

9 Bonell, C. *et al.* (2020). 'Harnessing behavioural science in public health campaigns to maintain "social distancing" in response to the COVID-19 pandemic: key principles'. *Journal of Epidemiology and Community Health*, 74 (8), pp. 617–19; Heo, S., Lim, C.C., and Bell, M.L.(2020). 'Relationships between local green space and human mobility patterns during COVID-19 for Maryland and California, USA'. *Sustainability*, 12 (22), pp. 1–16; Patel, J.A. *et al.* (2020). 'Poverty, inequality and COVID-19: the forgotten vulnerable'. *Public Health*, 183 (June), pp. 110–11.

10 Bish and Michie (2010); Papageorge, N, *et al.* (2021). 'Socio-demographic factors associated with self-protecting behavior during the Covid-19 pandemic'. *Journal of Population Economics*. 34 (2), pp. 691–738; Ganslmeier *et al.* (2022); Webster, R.K. *et al.* (2020). 'How to improve adherence with quarantine: rapid review of the evidence'. *Public Health*, 182 (May), pp. 163–69.

11 Pfattheicher, S. *et al.* (2020). 'The emotional path to action: empathy promotes physical distancing and wearing of face masks during the COVID-19 pandemic'. *Psychological Science*, 31 (11), 1363–13; Young, S.D. and Goldstein, N.J. (2021). 'Applying social norms interventions to increase adherence to COVID-19 prevention and control guidelines'. *Preventive Medicine*, 145 (106424), pp. 1–6.

12 Blagov, P.S. (2020). 'Adaptive and dark personality in the COVID-19 pandemic: predicting health-behavior endorsement and the appeal of public-health messages'. *Social Psychological and Personality Science*, 12 (5), pp. 6970–77; Zajenkowski, M., Jonason, P.K., Leniarska, M. and Kozakiewicz, Z. (2020). 'Who complies with the restrictions to reduce the spread of COVID-19? Personality and perceptions of the COVID-19 situation'. *Personality and Individual Differences*, 166 (110199), pp. 1–7.

13 See London Metropolitan University (2020). *Mind the gap? Social distancing in North London*. LMU (online). (14 September).

14 Randerson, J. (2020). 'Swedish deputy PM warns of counter reaction to harsh lock-down measures'. *Politico* (26 April); Halpern, D., and Harper, H. (2020). 'Behavioural insights, the WHO and Covid-19'. *The Behavioural Insights Team* (online). (21 May); Harvey, N. (2020). 'Behavioral fatigue: real phenomenon, naïve construct, or policy contrivance?' *Frontiers in Psychology*, 11 (589892), pp. 1–6; Mahase, E. (2020). 'Covid-19: Was the decision to delay the UK's lockdown over fears of "behavioural fatigue" based on evidence?'. *British Medical Journal*, 370 (3166), pp. 1–2.

15 The problem with the concept of "pandemic fatigue" (or "NPI fatigue" – which would have been a more accurate term) was not so much that this was implausible, though when it was advanced it was not supported by research but was simply intuitive. Of course, over the long *duree*, people may become increasingly stressed from the bur-den of social restrictions, which may foster motives for non-compliance. Rather, the problem with the concept was that it was advanced to justify (in Sweden and the UK) tardy and tepid policy responses, at the outset of the crisis, long before anyone could be experiencing "fatigue" over complying with NPIs.

16 Fetzer, T.R. *et al.* (2020). *Global Behaviors and Perceptions at the Onset of the COVID-19 Pandemic*. National Bureau of Economic Research (online). NBER Working Paper No. 27082. (May), p. 3.

17 Jackson, J. (2020). *The lockdown and social norms: why the UK is complying by consent rather compulsion*. LSE (online). (27 April). The study was illuminating rather than author-itative because, although large-scale sampling was deployed, this was not representative.

18 Ganslmeier *et al.* (2022).

19 *BBC News* (2020). 'Clap for Carers: UK in "emotional" tribute to NHS and care work-ers'. (27 March); *ITV News* (2020). 'Clap for our carers: Nation to show appreciation for NHS workers and carers amid coronavirus crisis'. (9 April); *ITV News* (2020). 'UK gives mass round of applause thanking key coronavirus workers in nationwide Clap For Our Carers'. (7 May); Addley, E. (2020). 'Clap for our Carers: the very un-British ritual that united the nation'. *Guardian*. (28 May).

20 As the LSE's webpages summarized these. See LSE (2020).

21 Ipsos MORI (2020). *Coronavirus polling*. (20 October). Available at: www.ipsos.com /en-uk/britons-increasingly-abiding-covid-19-rules-social-responsibility-and-nhs-pri-mary-drivers. The conclusion was rather fast and loose, however. The poll found that "preventing the spread to those most vulnerable, stopping friends and family catching the virus, and ensuring the NHS is not overwhelmed (all 87%) are the most convinc-ing arguments for following the rules". This was based on tick-box responses to fixed motive statements. This method did not allow respondents to offer their own views nor did it allow the strength or importance of their endorsed motives to be measured.

22 Žižek, Z. (2020). *Pandemic! COVID-19 Shakes the World*. Cambridge: Polity Press, pp. 3–4, 21–22.

23 Creaven, S. (2023). *The Pandemic in Britain: COVID-19, British Exceptionalism, and Neoliberalism*. London and New York: Routledge, pp. 56–57.

24 Ganslmeier *et al.* (2022), p. 2.

25 Jean-Francois Daoust and his co-researchers have estimated a rate of "compliance infla-tion" with the pandemic NPIs of ten percent. This is based on a review of self-report data in 12 countries. See Daoust, J.F. *et al.* (2020). 'How to survey citizens' compliance with COVID-19 Public Health Measures: evidence from three survey experiments'. *Journal of Experimental Political Science* (7 July), pp. 1–8; Daoust, J.F. *et al.* (2021). 'A guilt-free strategy increases self-reported noncompliance with COVID-19 preven-tive measures: Experimental evidence from 12 countries. *PLoS ONE*, 16 (4), pp. 1–10.

26 Sachs, J.D. (2021). 'Reasons for Asia-Pacific Success in Suppressing COVID-19'. J. Helliwell *et al.* (Eds.) *World Happiness Report, 2021* (online), pp. 92–106 (p. 98).

27 Hills, S. and Eraso, Y. (2021). 'Factors associated with non-adherence to social dis-tancing rules during the COVID-19 pandemic: a logistic regression analysis'. *BMC Public Health*, 21 (352), pp. 1–25. See Hills and Eraso (2021), p. 6.

28 Hills and Eraso (2021), p. 23.
29 Quoted by: London Metropolitan University (2020).
30 Tomlinson, J. (2022). 'What did the public really think about lockdown law?'. *Prospect*. (22 September).
31 Sykes, G. and Matza, D. (1957), 'Techniques of neutralization: a theory of delinquency'. *American Sociological Review*, 22 (6), pp. 664–73.
32 ONS (2021). *Coronavirus and compliance with government guidance, UK: April 2021*. GOV.UK (online). (12 April).
33 ONS (12 April, 2021). Students on the ONS survey offered this rationalization fairly commonly. The non-complying behaviour of other students on campus undermined the purpose of their own.
34 Tomlinson (2022).
35 ONS (12 April, 2021).
36 ONS (12 April, 2021). This type of reasoning was especially associated with high-income professionals who were knowledgeable of the rules they were legally required to follow.
37 Wright, L. and Fancourt, D. (2021). 'Do predictors of adherence to pandemic guidelines change over time? A panel study of 22,000 UK adults during the COVID-19 pandemic'. *Preventive Medicine*, 153 (106877), pp. 1–9.
38 Wright and Fancourt (2021), p. 7.
39 Lennon, R.P. *et al.* (2020). 'Public intent to comply with COVID-19 public health recommendations'. *Health Literacy Research and Practice,* 4 (3), pp. 160–65; Block, R., Berg, A., Lennon, R.P., Miller, E.L., and Nunez-Smith, M. (2020). 'African American adherence to COVID-19 public health recommendations'. *Health Literary Research and Practice.* 4 (3), pp. 166–70. Lennon *et al.*'s review was based on data gathered from 9,000 surveys in over 70 countries from 9–15 April 2020.
40 Roques, L. *et al.* (2020). 'Impact of lockdown on the epidemic dynamics of COVID-19 in France'. *Frontiers in Medicine*, 7 (274), pp. 1–7.
41 Peixoto, V.R. *et al.* (2020). 'Rapid assessment of the impact of lockdown on the COVID-19 epidemic in Portugal'. *MedRxiv.* (27 May), pp. 1–14.
42 Röst, G. *et al.* (2020). 'Early phase of the COVID-19 outbreak in Hungary and post-lockdown scenarios'. *Viruses*, 12 (708), pp. 1–30.
43 Lau, H. *et al.* (2020). 'The positive impact of lockdown in Wuhan on containing the COVID-19 outbreak in China'. *Journal of Travel Medicine*, 27 (3), pp. 1–14; Sardar, T., Nadim, S.S., Rana, S., and Chattopadhyay, J. (2020). 'Assessment of lockdown effect in some states and overall India: A predictive mathematical study on COVID-19 outbreak'. *Chaos Solitons Fractals*, 139 (110078), pp. 1–11.
44 Krishan, K. and Kanchan, T. (2020). 'Lockdown is an effective "vaccine" against COVID-19: A message from India'. *Journal of Infection in Developing Countries*, 14 (6), pp. 545–46.
45 de Bruijn, A.L. *et al.* (2020). *Why did Israelis comply with COVID-19 Mitigation Measures during the initial first wave lockdown?* Amsterdam Law School. Research Paper No. 2020-52.
46 Hoeben, E.M. *et al.* (2021). 'Social distancing compliance: A video observational analysis'. *PLoS ONE*, 16 (3), pp. 1–20.
47 Hoeben *et al.* (2021).
48 Hoeben *et al.* (2021).
49 Hoeben *et al.* (2021).
50 Tomczyk, Rahn, and Schmidt (2020).
51 Kamenidou, I.E, Stavrianea, A., and Liava, C. (2020). 'Achieving a Covid-19 Free Country: Citizens Preventive Measures and Communication Pathways'. *International Journal of Environmental Research and Public Health*, 17 (13), pp. 1–18.
52 Ölcer, S., Yilmaz-Aslan, Y., and Brzoska, P. (2020). 'Lay perspectives on social distancing and other official recommendations and regulations in the time of COVID-19: a qualitative study of social media posts'. *BMC Public Health*, 20 (963), pp. 1–9.

53 Ölcer *et al.* (2020), p. 2.
54 For example: Allegretti, A. (2020). 'Coronavirus: "This isn't a normal bank holiday" – Britons warned to stay home'. *Sky News.* (10 April); *ITV News* (2020). 'Coastguard sees surge in call-outs as people flout lockdown rules'. (9 May); Martin, H. (2020). 'Even the cold weather couldn't put them off! Revellers ignore social distancing to hit pubs and bars across Britain as they celebrate a boozy Bank Holiday'. *Mail.* (30 August); Redford, C. (2020). 'Thousands ignore pleas to stay away and head to coast'. *Lincolnshire World.* (26 May); Russell, B. (2020). 'Lockdown rules: Police crack down on people flouting Covid restrictions ahead of bank holiday weekend'. *I-News.* (5 April); Stubley, P. (2020). 'VE Day conga line criticised as public "ignore UK lockdown" over bank holiday weekend despite PM's pleas'. *Independent.* (9 May); *Sky News* (2021). 'COVID-19: Hundreds fined over New Year's Eve parties as coronavirus rules ignored'. (1 January).
55 Hengartner, M.P., Waller, G., and von Wyl, A. (2022). 'Factors Related to Noncompliance With Non-pharmaceutical Interventions to Mitigate the Spread of SARS-CoV-2: Results From a Survey in the Swiss General Adult Population'. *Frontiers in Public Health*, 10 (828584), pp. 1–7.
56 Hengartner *et al.* (2022), p. 4.
57 Lang R. *et al.* (2021). 'Characterization of non-adopters of COVID-19 non-pharmaceutical interventions through a national cross-sectional survey to assess attitudes and behaviours'. *Scientific Reports,* 11 (21751), pp. 1–14; Plohl, N. and Musil, B. (2021). 'Modeling compliance with COVID-19 prevention guidelines: the critical role of trust in science'. *Psychological Health Medicine*, 26, pp. 1–12; Seale H. *et al.* (2020). 'Improving the impact of non-pharmaceutical interventions during COVID-19: examining the factors that influence engagement and the impact on individuals'. *BMC Infectious Diseases*, 20 (607), pp. 1–13; Shumway, S.G. *et al.* (2021). 'Predictors of compliance with COVID-19 related non-pharmaceutical interventions among University students in the United States'. *PLoS ONE*, 16 (6), pp. 1–24.
58 Hengartner *et al.* (2022), p. 5.
59 Kaine, G., Greenhalgh, S., and Wright, V. (2022). 'Compliance with Covid-19 measures: Evidence from New Zealand'. *PLoS ONE*, 17 (2), pp. 1–23.
60 Kaine *et al.* (2022), p. 10.
61 Kaine *et al.* (2022), pp. 10–12.
62 Kaine *et al.* (2022), p. 8.
63 Kaine *et al.* (2022), pp. 5–6.
64 YouGov (2022). *Personal measures taken to avoid COVID-19* (online). Accessed: 30 September 2022.
65 YouGov (2022).
66 YouGov (2022).
67 YouGov (2022).
68 YouGov (2022).
69 YouGov (2022).
70 YouGov (2022).
71 YouGov (2022).
72 YouGov (2022).
73 YouGov (2022).
74 YouGov (2022).
75 Such has spurred researchers to hypothesize not only the reasons for non-compliance but also those for variability in compliance (and hence non-compliance) rates in different places. See for example: Briscese, G., Lacetera, N., Macis, M., and Tonin, M. (2023). 'Expectations, Reference Points, and Compliance with COVID-19 Social Distancing Measures'. *Journal of Behavioral and Experimental Economics*, 103 (101983), pp. 1–22; Ding, X., Brazel, D.M., and Mills, M.C. (2021). 'Factors affecting

adherence to non-pharmaceutical interventions for COVID-19 infections in the first year of the pandemic in the UK'. *BMJ Open*, 11 (10), pp. 1–7; Du, Z. *et al.* (2022). 'Pandemic fatigue impedes mitigation of COVID-19 in Hong Kong'. *Proceedings of the National Academy of Science (PNAS)*, 119 (48), pp. 1–3; Ge, Y. *et al.* (2022). 'Impacts of worldwide individual non-pharmaceutical interventions on COVID-19 transmission across waves and space. *International Journal of Applied Earth Observations and Geoinformation*, 106 (102649), pp. 1–9; Lilleholt, L., Zettler, I., Betsch, C., and Böhm, R. (2023). *Shedding Light on Pandemic Fatigue*. ResearchGate (online); Michie, S., West, R., and Harvey, N. (2020). 'The concept of "fatigue" in tackling covid-19'. *British Medical Journal*, 371 (4171), pp. 1–2; Nzaji, M.K. *et al.* (2020). 'Predictors of non-adherence to public health instructions during the COVID-19 pandemic in the Democratic Republic of the Congo'. *Journal of Multidisciplinary Health Care*, 13, pp. 1215–21; Reinders Folmer, C.P. *et al.* (2021). 'Maintaining compliance when the virus returns: understanding adherence to social distancing measures in the Netherlands in July 2020'. Research Paper No. 2020-53. University of Amsterdam: School of Legal Studies. Social Science Research Network (SSRN); Reinders Folmer, C.P. *et al.* (2021). 'Social distancing in America: understanding long-term adherence to COVID-19 mitigation recommendations'. *PLoS ONE*, 16 (9), pp. 1–39; Santos, J.V. *et al.* (2023). 'Factors associated with non-pharmaceutical interventions compliance during COVID-19 pandemic: a Portuguese cross-sectional survey'. *Journal of Public Health*, 45 (1), pp. 47–56; Yan, B., Zhang, X., Wu, L., Zhu H., and Chen, B. (2020). 'Why do countries respond differently to COVID-19? A comparative study of Sweden, China, France, and Japan'. *American Review of Public Administration*, 50 (6–7), pp. 762–69.

76 Petherick, A. *et al.* (2022). 'A worldwide assessment of changes in adherence to COVID-19 protective behaviours and hypothesized pandemic fatigue'. *Nature Human Behaviour*, 5 (September), pp. 1145–60.

77 Bish, A., and Michie, S. (2010). 'Demographic and attitudinal determinants of protective behaviours during a pandemic: a review'. *British Journal of Health Psychology*, 15 (4), pp. 797–824; Brug, J. *et al.* (2004). 'SARS risk perception, knowledge, precautions, and information sources, the Netherlands'. *Emerging Infectious Diseases*, 10 (8), pp. 1486–89; Leung, G.M. *et al.* (2003). 'The impact of community psychological responses on outbreak control for severe acute respiratory syndrome in Hong Kong'. *Journal of Epidemiological Community Health*, 57 (11), pp. 857–63; Quah, S.R. and Hin-Peng, L. (2004). 'Crisis prevention and management during SARS outbreak, Singapore'. *Emerging Infectious Diseases*, 10 (2), pp. 364–68; Rubin, G.J., Amlôt, R., Page, L., and Wessely, S. (2009). 'Public perceptions, anxiety, and behaviour change in relation to the swine flu outbreak: cross sectional telephone survey'. *British Medical Journal*, 339 (2651), pp. 1–8.

78 Matthews Pillemer, F., Blendon, R.J., Zaslavsky, A.M., and Lee, B.Y. (2015). 'Predicting support for non-pharmaceutical interventions during infectious outbreaks: a four region analysis'. *Disasters*, 39 (1), pp. 125–45; Wang, F., Wei, J., and Shi, X. (2018). 'Compliance with recommended protective actions during an H7N9 emergency: a risk perception perspective'. *Disasters*, 42 (2), pp. 207–32.

79 Gilles, I. *et al.* (2011). 'Trust in medical organizations predicts pandemic (H1N1) 2009 vaccination behavior and perceived efficacy of protection measures in the Swiss public'. *European Journal of Epidemiology*. 26, pp. 203–210; Mitchell, T. *et al.* (2011). 'Non-pharmaceutical interventions during an outbreak of 2009 pandemic influenza A (H1N1) virus infection at a large public university, April-May 2009'. *Clinical Infectious Diseases*. 52 (1), pp. 138–45; Pfattheicher, S., Strauch, C., Diefenbacher, S., and Schnuerch, R. (2018). 'A field study on watching eyes and hand hygiene compliance in a public restroom'. *Journal of Applied Social Psychology*, 48 (4), pp. 188–194; Shultz, J.M., Baingana, F., and Neria, Y. (2015). 'The 2014 ebola outbreak and mental

health'. *Journal of the American Medical Association,* 313 (6), pp. 567–68; Steelfisher, G.K. *et al.* (2012). 'Public response to the 2009 influenza A H1N1 pandemic: a polling study in five countries'. *Lancet,* 12 (11), pp. 845–850.

80 Norton *et al.* (2021), p. 2.

81 Petherick *et al.* (2021).

82 Petherick *et al.* (2022), pp. 1145, 1152.

83 Crane, M.A., Shermock, K.M., Omer, S.B., and Romley, J.A. (2021). 'Change in Reported Adherence to Nonpharmaceutical Interventions During the COVID-19 Pandemic, April–November 2020'. *Journal of the American Medical Association* (*JAMA*), 325 (9), pp. 883–85.

84 Crane *et al.* (2021), p. 883.

85 Crane *et al.* (2021), p. 883.

86 Brüggenjürgen, B. *et al.* (2021). 'Impact of public health interventions to curb SARS-CoV-2 spread assessed by an evidence-educated Delphi panel and tailored SEIR model'. *Journal of Public Health: From Theory to Practice,* 31 (4), pp. 539–52.

87 Bodas, M. *et al.* (2022). 'Lockdown Efficacy in Controlling the Spread of COVID-19 May Be Waning Due to Decline in Public Compliance, Especially among Unvaccinated Individuals: A Cross-Sectional Study in Israel'. *International Journal of Environmental Research and Public Health,* 19 (4943), pp. 1–11.

88 Wright, L., Steptoe, A., and Fancourt, D. (2022). 'Trajectories of Compliance With COVID-19 Related Guidelines: Longitudinal Analyses of 50,000 UK Adults'. *Annals of Behavioral Medicine,* 56 (8), pp. 781–90.

89 Wright *et al.* (2022), p. 781.

90 Ipsos MORI (October 2020).

91 Ipsos MORI (October 2020).

92 Ipsos MORI (October 2020).

93 Creaven (2023), pp. 96–109.

94 Borchering, R.K. *et al.* (2021). 'Modeling of Future COVID-19 Cases, Hospitalizations, and Deaths, by Vaccination Rates and Nonpharmaceutical Intervention Scenarios – United States, April–September 2021'. *Morbidity and Mortality Weekly Report,* 70 (19), pp. 719–24.

95 YouGov (2022).

96 Only Sweden, Norway, and Denmark – countries with much lower population densities than in the UK – had lower rates.

97 The average rate of compliance within the more populous countries excluding the UK (Germany, France, Italy, and Spain) was 5.5 percent at mid-July 2022.

98 The average rate of compliance within the more populous countries excluding the UK (Germany, France, Italy, and Spain) was 45.5 percent.

99 YouGov (2022). By contrast, for Germany, France, Italy, and Spain, it was around 26 percent.

100 YouGov (2022).

101 The lower threshold for this NPI of mid-year 2022 was, though above the regional average, fairly typical for Southeast Asia countries at this time.

102 This was a little below the average for self-reported compliance with outside work avoidance across the region as a whole for mid-year 2022.

103 This too was marginally below the regional average for Southeast Asia at mid-year 2022.

104 YouGov (2022). This was fractionally above the regional average for Southeast Asia at mid-year 2022.

105 YouGov (2022).

106 YouGov (2022).

107 But UK police chiefs did voice concern during the first lockdown that the government was not providing them with the operational capacities nor powers of sanction to

deter rule-breakers. See Evans, M. (2020). 'Police fear they do not have the powers to enforce the lockdown'. *Telegraph.* (10 May).

108 Brunt, M. (2020). 'Coronavirus: 9,000 fines issued to people flouting lockdown – with 400 repeat offenders'. *Sky News.* (30 April).

109 Casciani, D. (2021). 'Coronavirus: What powers do police have if people break Covid rules?' *BBC News* (12 January).

110 Murray, J. and Sparrow, A. (2020). 'UK coronavirus: Boris Johnson says, "there have been too many breaches" and warns restrictions could go further'. *Guardian.* (22 September).

111 Creaven (2023), pp. 39–43.

112 Brunt (30 April, 2020). Later these penalty notices were increased in England and Northern Ireland to £200 faced with rising levels of non-compliance at the start of the second circuit-breaker lockdown amid press reports of illegal house parties. See Casciani, D. (2021). 'Coronavirus: What powers do police have if people break Covid rules?' *BBC News.* (12 January).

113 Casciani (12 January, 2021).

114 *BBC News* (2021). 'Covid-19: Rule-breakers "increasingly likely" to be fined – Cressida Dick'. (12 January).

115 Murray and Sparrow (2020).

116 As summarized by Norton *et al.* (2021). Self-interest is a stronger predictor. See Norton, J.O. *et al.* (2021). 'Why Do People (Not) Engage in Social Distancing? Proximate and Ultimate Analyses of Norm-Following During the COVID-19 Pandemic'. *Frontiers in Psychology*, 12 (648206), pp. 1–12. For the cited studies see Markowitz, E.M. and Shariff, A.F. (2012). 'Climate change and moral judgement'. *Nature Climate Change*, 2 (28 March), pp. 243–247; Yong, J.C., and Choy, B.K.C. (2021). 'Noncompliance with safety guidelines as a free-riding strategy: an evolutionary game-theoretic approach to cooperation during the COVID-19 pandemic'. *Frontiers in Psychology,* 12 (646892). (16 March), pp. 1–8.

117 Cheng, C. and Ng, A.-K. (2006). 'Psychosocial factors predicting SARS-preventive behaviors in four major SARS-affected regions'. *Journal of Applied Social Psychology*, 36 (1), pp. 222–47; Leppin, A. and Aro, A.R. (2009). 'Risk perceptions related to SARS and Avian influenza: theoretical foundations of current empirical research'. *International Journal of Behavioral Medicine*, 16 (1), pp. 7–29; Kwok, K.O. *et al.* (2020). 'Community responses during the early phase of the COVID-19 epidemic in Hong Kong: risk perception, information exposure and preventive measures'. *Emerging Infectious Diseases*, 26 (7), pp. 1575–79; Tang, C.S.-K. and Wong, C.-Y. (2003). 'An outbreak of the severe acute respiratory syndrome: predictors of health behaviors and effect of community prevention measures in Hong Kong, China'. *American Journal of Public Health*, 93 (11), pp. 1887–88; Tang, C.S.-K. and Wong, C.-Y. (2005). 'Psychosocial factors influencing the practice of preventive behaviors against the severe acute respiratory syndrome among older Chinese in Hong Kong'. *Journal of Aging and Health*, 17 (4), pp. 490–506.

118 Wang *et al.* (2018).

119 Morrison, L.G. and Yardley, L. (2009). 'What infection control measures will people carry out to reduce transmission of pandemic influenza? A focus group study'. *BMC Public Health*, 9 (258), pp. 1–11

120 Tomczyk *et al.* (2020), p. 2.

121 Bish, A. and Michie, S. (2010), 'Demographic and attitudinal determinants of protective behaviours during a pandemic: a review'. *Health Psychology*, 15 (4), pp. 797–824; Brewer, N.T. *et al.* (2007), 'Meta-analysis of the relationship between risk perception and health behavior: the example of vaccination'. *Health Psychology*, 26 (2), pp. 136–45; Chang, H-J. *et al.* (2004). 'The Impact of the SARS Epidemic on the Utilization of Medical Services: SARS and the Fear of SARS'. *American Journal of Public Health*, 94

(4), pp. 562–64; Lerner, J.S. and Keltner, D. (2001). 'Fear, Anger, and Risk'. *Journal of Personality and Social Psychology*, 81 (1), pp. 146–59; Marcus, G.E., Neuman, W.R., and MacKuen, M. (2000). *Affective Intelligence and Political Judgment*. Chicago: University of Chicago Press; Robertson, E., Hershenfield, K., Grace, S.L., and Stewart, D.E. (2004). 'The Psychosocial Effects of Being Quarantined Following Exposure to SARS: A Qualitative Study of Toronto Health Care Workers'. *Canadian Journal of Psychiatry*, 49 (6), pp. 403–7; Rosenstock, I.M. (1974). 'Historical origins of the Health Belief Model'. *Health Education Monographs*, 2 (4), pp. 328–35; Vasilopoulos, P., Marcus, G.E., Valentino, N.A., and Foucault, M. (2019). 'Fear, Anger, and Voting for the Far Right: Evidence from the November 13, 2015 Paris Terror Attacks'. *Political Psychology*, 40 (4), pp. 679–704.

122 Barrios, J.M. *et al.* (2020). *Civic capital and social distancing during the Covid-19 pandemic*. Working Paper 27320. National Bureau of Economic Research, Cambridge, MA; Brouard, S., Vasilopoulos, P., and Becher, M. (2020). 'Sociodemographic and psychological correlates of compliance with the COVID-19 public health measures in France', *Canadian Journal of Political Science*, 53 (2), pp. 1-6; Chua, H.C. and Sim, K. (2020). 'Narrative Synthesis of Psychological and Coping Responses Towards Emerging Infectious Disease Outbreaks in the General Population: Practical Considerations for the COVID-19 Pandemic'. *Tropical Journal of Pharmaceutical Research*, 61 (7), pp. 350–56; Cruwys, T. (2020). 'Risk Perception'. J. Jetten *et al.* (Eds.) *Together Apart: The Psychology of Covid-19*. London: Sage Harper; Dryhurst, S. *et al.* (2020), 'Risk perceptions of COVID-19 around the world'. *Journal of Risk Research*, 23 (7–8), pp. 994–1006; Guglielmi, S. *et al.* (2020), 'Public acceptability of containment measures during the COVID-19 pandemic in Italy: how institutional confidence and specific political support matter'. *International Journal of Sociology and Social Policy*, 40 (9–10), pp. 1069–85; Harper, C.A., Satchell, L.P., Fido D., and Latzman, R.D. (2021). 'Functional fear predicts public health compliance in the COVID-19 pandemic'. *International Journal of Mental Health and Addiction*, 19 (5), pp. 1875–88; Raude, J. *et al.* (2020). 'Are People Excessively Pessimistic about the Risk of Coronavirus Infection?' *PsyArXiv Reprints* (online); Weinberg, J. (2022). 'Can political trust help to explain elite policy support and public behaviour in times of crisis? Evidence from the United Kingdom at the height of the 2020 coronavirus pandemic'. *Political Studies*, 70 (3), pp. 543–65; Woelfert, F.S. and J.R. Kunst (2020), 'How political and social trust can impact social distancing practices during COVID-19 in unexpected ways'. *Frontiers in Psychology*, 11 (572966), pp. 1–16; Zettler *et al.* (2022). 'The Role of Personality in COVID-19 Related Perceptions, Evaluations, and Behaviors: Findings across Five Samples, Nine Traits, and 17 Criteria'. *Social Psychological and Personality Science*, 13 (1), pp. 299–310.

123 Wright, L., Elise, P., Steptoe, A., and Fancourt, D. (2021). 'Facilitators and barriers to compliance with COVID-19 guidelines: a structural topic modelling analysis of free-text data from 17,500 UK adults'. *BMC Public Health*, 22 (34), pp. 1–22.

124 Wright *et al.* (2021), pp. 1, 16–17.

125 Bargain, O. and Ulugbek, A. (2020). *Poverty and Covid-19 in Developing Countries*. Discussion Paper Series no. 13297. IZA Institute of Labor Economics, pp. 1–23; Blair, R.A., Morse, B.S., and Tsai, L.L. (2017). 'Public health and public trust: survey evidence from the Ebola virus disease epidemic in Liberia'. *Social Science & Medicine*, 172, pp. 89–97; Brodeur, A., Grigoryeva, I., and Kattan, L. (2020). 'Stay-at-home orders, social distancing and trust'. *Journal of Population Economics*, 34 (4), pp. 1321–54; Chan, H.F. *et al.* (2020). 'How confidence in health care systems affects mobility and compliance during the COVID-19 pandemic'. *PLoS ONE*, 15 (10), pp. 1–18; Han, Q. *et al.* (2021). 'Trust in government regarding COVID-19 and its associations with preventive health behaviour and prosocial behaviour during the pandemic: a cross-sectional and longitudinal study'. *Psychological Medicine*, 10 (1017), pp. 1–11; Nivette,

A.D. *et al.* (2021). 'Non-compliance with COVID-19-related public health measures among young adults in Switzerland: insights from a longitudinal cohort study'. *Social Science & Medicine*, 268, pp. 2–10; Olsen A.L. and Hjorth, F. (2020). *Willingness to distance in the COVID-19 pandemic*. Working paper. Department of Political Science and Center for Social Science Data: University of Copenhagen; Robinson, S.E. *et al.* (2021), 'The relevance and operations of political trust in the COVID-19 pandemic'. *Public Administration Review*, 81 (6), pp. 1110–19; Rubin, G.J., Amlôt, R., Page L, Wessely, S. (2009). 'Public Perceptions, Anxiety, and Behaviour Change in Relation to the Swine Flu Outbreak: Cross Sectional Telephone Survey'. *British Medical Journal*, 339 (2651), pp. 1–8; Schmelz, K. (2021). 'Enforcement may crowd out voluntary support for COVID-19 policies, especially where trust in government is weak and in a liberal society'. *Proceedings of the National Academy of Sciences*, 118 (1), pp. 1–8; Tang, C.S.-K. and Wong, C-Y. (2003). 'An Outbreak of the Severe Acute Respiratory Syndrome: Predictors of Health Behaviors and Effect of Community Prevention Measures in Hong Kong, China'. *American Journal of Public Health*, 93 (11), pp. 1887–88; Vinck, P. *et al.* (2019). 'Institutional Trust and Misinformation in the Response to the 2018–19 Ebola Outbreak in North Kivu, DR Congo: A Population-based Survey'. *Lancet Infectious Diseases*, 19 (5), pp. 529–36; Wright, L., Steptoe, A. and Fancourt, D. (2021). 'Predictors of self-reported adherence to COVID-19 guidelines. A longitudinal observational study of 51,600 UK adults'. *The Lancet Regional Health – Europe*, 4 (100061), pp. 1–8; Wright *et al.* (2022).

126 See for example: Barrios, J.M. *et al.* (2021). 'Civic capital and social distancing during the Covid-19 pandemic'. *Journal of Public Economics*, 193 (104310), pp. 1–11; Brouard, S., Vasilopoulos, P., and Becher, M. (2020) 'Sociodemographic and psychological correlates of compliance with the COVID-19 public health measures in France', *Canadian Journal of Political Science*, 53 (2), pp. 253–58; Guglielmi, S. *et al.* (2020), 'Public acceptability of containment measures during the COVID-19 pandemic in Italy: how institutional confidence and specific political support matter'. *International Journal of Sociology and Social Policy*, 40 (9–10), pp. 1069–85; Weinberg, J. (2022). 'Can political trust help to explain elite policy support and public behaviour in times of crisis? Evidence from the United Kingdom at the height of the 2020 coronavirus pandemic'. *Political Studies*, 70 (3), pp. 655–79; Woelfert, F.S. and Kunst, J.R. (2020), 'How political and social trust can impact social distancing practices during COVID-19 in unexpected ways'. *Frontiers in Psychology*, 11 (572966), pp. 1–16; Travaglino, G.A. and Moon, C. (2021), 'Compliance and self-reporting during the COVID-19 pandemic: a cross-cultural study of trust and self-conscious emotions in the United States, Italy, and South Korea', *Frontiers in Psychology*, 12 (565845), pp. 1–14.

127 Harper *et al.* (2021); Guglielmi *et al.* (2020).

128 Kooistra, E.B. and van Rooij, B. (2020). *Pandemic compliance: A systematic review of influences on social distancing behaviour during the first wave of the COVID-19 outbreak*. Research Paper No. 2022-29. Amsterdam Law School Legal Studies.

129 Seyd, B. and Bu, F. (2022). 'Perceived risk crowds out trust? Trust and public compliance with coronavirus restrictions over the course of the pandemic'. *European Political Science Review*, 14, pp. 155–170. See p. 157.

130 Ayres, I. and Braithwaite, J. (Eds.) (1992). *Responsive Regulation: Transcending the Deregulation Debate*. New York: Oxford University Press; Braithwaite, J. and Makkai, T. (1994). 'Trust and Compliance'. *Policing and Society: An International Journal*, 4 (1), pp. 1–12; Murphy, K. (2004). 'The Role of Trust in Nurturing Compliance: A Study of Accused Tax Avoiders'. *Law and Human Behavior*, 28 (2), pp. 187–209; Six, F. and Verhoest, K. (Eds.) (2017). *Trust in Regulatory Regimes*. Cheltenham: Edward Elgar.

131 Blair *et al.* (2017); Ruben *et al.* (2009); Tang and Wong (2003); Vinck *et al.* (2019).

132 Creaven (2023).

133 Creaven (2023), pp. 98–99, 108.

134 Seyd and Bu (2022), p. 167.

135 Harper *et al.* (2021), p, 1875.

136 Harper *et al.* (2021), pp. 1882–83.

137 Six, F. *et al.* (2021). 'What drives compliance with COVID-19 measures over time? Explaining changing impacts with Goal Framing Theory'. *Regulation & Governance* (7 October), pp. 1–19.

138 Six *et al.* (2021), pp. 4–5.

139 Lindenberg S., Six, F., and Keizer, K. (2021). 'Social Contagion and Goal Framing: The Sustainability of Rule Compliance'. Van Rooij, B. and Sokol, D.D. (Eds.) *Cambridge Handbook of Compliance*. Cambridge: Cambridge University Press.

140 Cava, M.A. *et al.* (2005). 'Risk Perception and Compliance with Quarantine during the SARS Outbreak'. *Journal of Nursing Scholarship*, 37 (4), pp. 343–47; Desclaux, A., Badji, D., Ndione, A.G., and Sow, K. (2017). 'Accepted Monitoring or Endured Quarantine? Ebola Contacts' Perceptions in Senegal'. *Social Science & Medicine*, 178, pp. 38–45; Webster, R.K. *et al.* (2020). 'How to Improve Adherence with Quarantine: Rapid Review of the Evidence'. *Public Health*, 182, pp. 163–69.

141 Bargain, O. and Ulugbek, A. (2020). *Poverty and Covid-19 in Developing Countries*. Bordeaux University: Bordeaux; Brouard, S., Vasilopoulos, P., and Becher, M. (2020). 'Sociodemographic and Psychological Correlates of Compliance with the COVID-19 Public Health Measures in France'. *Canadian Journal of Political Science*, 16 (4), pp. 1–6; Clark, C., Davila, A., Regis, M., and Kraus, S. (2020). 'Predictors of COVID-19 Voluntary Compliance Behaviors: An International Investigation'. *Global Transitions*, 2, pp. 76–82; Devine, D., Gaskell, J., Jennings, W., and Stoker, G. (2020). 'Trust and the Coronavirus Pandemic: What Are the Consequences of and for Trust? An Early Review of the Literature'. *Political Studies Review*, 19 (2), pp. 274–85; Jørgensen *et al.* (2021).

142 Six *et al.* (2021), p. 3.

143 Bogaert, S., Boone, C., and Declerck, C. (2008). 'Social Value Orientation and Cooperation in Social Dilemmas: A Review and Conceptual Model'. *British Journal of Social Psychology*, 47 (3), pp. 453–80. Boone, C., Declerck, C., and Kiyonari, T. (2010). 'Inducing Cooperative Behavior among Proselfs Versus Prosocials: The Moderating Role of Incentives and Trust'. *Journal of Conflict Resolution*, 54 (5), pp. 799–824.

144 Jørgensen *et al.* (2021); Pfattheicher, S. *et al.* (2020). 'The emotional path to action: empathy promotes physical distancing and wearing of face masks during the COVID-19 pandemic'. *Psychological Science*, 31 (11), pp. 1363–73.

145 Wright and Fancourt (2021), p. 5.

146 Oosterhoff, B. and Palmer, C. (2020). 'Psychological Correlates of News Monitoring, Social Distancing, Disinfecting, and Hoarding Behaviors among US Adolescents during the COVID-19 Pandemic'. *JAMA Paediatrics*, 174 (12), pp. 1184–90.

147 Six *et al.* (2021).

148 Six *et al.* (2021), p. 14.

149 Six *et al.* (2021), pp. 14–15.

150 Wilson, B. (2020). 'Off our trolleys: what stockpiling in the coronavirus crisis reveals about us'. *Guardian*. (3 April); O'Connell, M., de Paula, A., and Smith, K. (2020). *Preparing for a pandemic: spending dynamics and panic buying during the COVID-19 first wave*. Working Paper 2034 (October). London: Institute for Fiscal Studies.

151 Campbell, D. (2021). 'NHS staff abused by people seeking second Covid jab early for holiday'. *Guardian*. (10 July).

152 Durkheim, E. (1953). *Sociology and Philosophy*. London: Routledge. See esp. essays on 'The Determination of Moral Facts' (1906) and 'Value Judgements and Judgements of Reality' (1911). See also: Durkheim, E. (1961). *Moral Education: A Study in the Theory and Application of the Sociology of Education* [1925]. Glencoe Ill: The Free Press.

153 Durkheim (1953, 1961).
154 Durkheim (1985). See esp. 'Rules for the distinction of the normal from the pathological' (pp. 97–107). This was one of Durkheim's "functions" of crime – to clarify moral boundaries.
155 Elias, N. (2000). *The Civilizing Process: Sociogenetic and Psychogenetic Investigations*. (Revised edition). [1939]. Oxford: Blackwell; Elias, N. (1991). *The Society of Individuals*. Oxford: Basil Blackwell; Foucault, M. (1995). *Discipline and Punish: The Birth of the Prison*. [1975]. New York: Vintage.
156 Bauman, Z. (1989). *Modernity and the Holocaust*. Cambridge: Polity Press
157 ONS (2021). *Two-thirds of adults still plan to wear masks in shops and on public transport*. GOV.UK (online). (16 July).
158 ONS (16 July, 2021).
159 YouGov (2021). *Mask use among 18–24 year olds slumps following Freedom Day*. GOV.UK (online). (26 July).
160 Landler, M. and Castle, S. (2021). 'Britons, Unfazed by High Covid Rates, Weigh Their "Price of Freedom"'. *New York Times*. (31 August).
161 YouGov (2022).
162 Taylor, L. (2021). 'England's Rush to Reopen Is a Cautionary Tale for the U.S'. *Scientific American*. (16 August).
163 Landler and Castle (2021).
164 Da Silva, C. (2021). 'New variant? No masks? Here's what's driving the U.K.'s latest Covid surge'. *NBC News*. (23 October).
165 Allegretti, A. (2021). 'Ministers accused of putting staff at risk by not wearing masks in Commons'. *Guardian*. (18 August); *BBC News* (2021). 'Covid: Most Conservative MPs ditch masks as Commons returns'. (18 August); *BBC News* (2021). 'Tory MPs don't need masks as they know each other, says Rees-Mogg'. (21 October).
166 Glover, E. (2021). 'Chris Whitty on the three times we should still wear a mask after 19 July'. *Independent*. (5 July).
167 Creaven (2023).
168 YouGov (2022).
169 YouGov (2022).
170 YouGov (2022).
171 YouGov (2022).
172 YouGov (2022).
173 YouGov (2022).
174 YouGov (2022).
175 YouGov (2022).
176 Sachs (2021), p. 96.
177 Sachs (2021), p. 100.
178 Sachs (2021), pp. 96, 98.
179 YouGov (2021). *How good are Americans at following COVID rules, compared to other countries?* (online).
180 Sachs (2021), p. 98.
181 Sachs (2021), p. 93.
182 Nanda, S. and Ryan, J.M. (2022). 'The Importance of Culture in Understanding the COVID-19 Pandemic'. J.M. Ryan (Ed.) *COVID-19: Cultural Changes and Institutional Adaptations*. London and New York: Routledge.
183 Ryan, J.M. (2023a). 'COVID-19, Individual Rights, and Community Responsibilities'. J.M. Ryan (Ed.) *COVID-19: Individual Rights and Community Responsibilities*. London and New York: Routledge, p. 20.
184 Silova, I., Komatsu, H., and Rappleye, J. (2021). *Covid-19, Climate, and Culture: Facing the Crisis of (Neo) Liberal Individualism*. Network for international policies and cooperation in education and training (NORRAG).

185 Hofstede, G., Hofstede, G.J., and Minkov, M. (2010). *Cultures and Organizations: Software of the Mind* (3rd edition). New York: McGraw Hill.

186 Silova *et al.* (2021).

187 Sachs (2021), p. 100.

188 Silova *et al.* (2021).

189 Ryan (2023a), p. 18.

190 Silova *et al.* (2021).

191 Brouard, S., Vasilopoulos, P., and Becher, M. (2020). 'Sociodemographic and Psychological Correlates of Compliance with the COVID-19 Public Health Measures in France'. *Canadian Journal of Political Science*, 53, pp. 253–58. See also: Blagov (2020); Zajenkowski *et al.* (2020).

192 Bierwiaczonek, K., Kunst, J.R., and Pich, O. (2020). 'Belief in COVID-19 conspiracy theories reduces social distancing over time'. *Applied Psychology: Health Well-Being*, 12 (4), pp. 1270–85; Cowling, B.J. *et al.* (2010). 'Community psychological and behavioral responses through the first wave of the 2009 influenza A(H1N1) pandemic in Hong Kong'. *Journal of Infectious Diseases*, 202 (6) pp. 867–76; de Zwart, O., Veldhuijzen, I.K., Richardus, J.H., and Brug, J. (2010). 'Monitoring of risk perceptions and correlates of precautionary behaviour related to human avian influenza during 2006–2007 in the Netherlands: results of seven consecutive surveys'. *BMC Infectious Diseases*, 10 (114), pp. 1–15; Raude, J., Mccoll, K., Flamand, C., and Apostolidis, T. (2019). 'Understanding health behaviour changes in response to outbreaks: findings from a longitudinal study of a large epidemic of mosquito-borne disease'. *Social Science & Medicine*, 230, pp. 184–93; Springborn, M., Chowell, G., MacLachlan, M., and Fenichel, E.P. (2015). 'Accounting for behavioral responses during a flu epidemic using home television viewing'. *BMC Infectious Diseases*, 15 (21), pp. 1–14; van der Weerd, W. *et al.* (2011). 'Monitoring the level of government trust, risk perception and intention of the general public to adopt protective measures during the influenza a (H1N1) pandemic in the Netherlands'. *BMC Public Health*, 11 (575), pp. 1–12; YouGov (2022).

193 Fallov, M.A. and Blad, C. (Eds). (2018). *Social Welfare Responses in a Neoliberal Era: Policies, Practices and Social Problems*. Leiden: Brill; Howard, M. (1997). 'Cutting Social Security'. C. Walker and A. Walker (Eds.) *Britain Divided: The Growth of Social Exclusion in the 1980s and 1990s*. London: Child Poverty Action Group; Kus, B. (2006). 'Neoliberalism, Institutional Change and the Welfare State: The Case of Britain and France'. *International Journal of Comparative Sociology*, 47 (6), pp. 488–525; Pierson, P. (2002). 'Coping with Permanent Austerity: Welfare State Restructuring in Affluent Democracies'. *Revue Francaise de Sociologie*, 43 (2), pp. 369–406; Piven, F.C. (2015). 'Neoliberalism and the Welfare State'. *Journal of International and Comparative Social Policy*, 31 (1), pp. 2–9; Taylor-Gooby, P. (2013). *The Double Crisis of the Welfare State*. Basingstoke: Palgrave-Macmillan; Toynbee, P. and Walker, D. (2017). *Dismembered: How the Attack on the State Harms Us All*. London: Fabier; Toynbee, P. and Walker, D. (2017). 'Enemies of the State: The 40-year Tory project to shrink public services'. *Guardian*. (9 May).

194 Bradley, H., Erickson, M., Stephenson, C., and Williams, S. (2000). *Myths at Work*. Oxford: Blackwell; Cliff, T. and Gluckstein, D. (1996). *The Labour Party: A Marxist History*. 2nd edition. London: Bookmarks, pp. 345–48; Pyper, D. (2017). *Trade Union Legislation 1979–2010*. London: House of Commons Library. Briefing Paper 7882 (26 January).

195 Ball, S.J. (2012). *Global Education Inc.: New Policy Networks and the Neoliberal Imaginary*. London: Routledge; Barkawi, T. (2013). 'The Neoliberal assault on academia'. *Al Jazeera* (25 April); Callinicos, A. (2006). *Universities in a Neoliberal World*. London: Bookmarks; Carey, M. (2019). 'Some Ethical Limitations of Privatising and Marketizing Social Care and Social Work Provision in England for

Children and Young People'. *Ethics and Social Welfare*, 13 (3), pp. 272–87; Ferguson, I. (2014). 'Can the Tories abolish the welfare state?' *International Socialism*, 141 (Winter), pp. 13–36; Gilbert, N. (2002). *The Transformations of the Welfare State*. Princeton: Princeton University Press; Clarke, J., Smith, N., and Vidler, E. (2005). 'Consumerism and the reform of public services: inequalities and instabilities'. M. Powell, L. Bauld, and K. Clarke (Eds.) *Social Policy Review 7*. Cambridge: Polity Press; Giroux, H.A. (2014). *Neoliberalism's War on Higher Education*. London: Haymarket Books; Gosling, J. (2013). 'Privatising the NHS'. *International Socialism*, 139 (Summer), pp. 77–98; Hermann, C. (2010). 'The marketization of health care in Europe'. *Socialist Register*, 46, pp. 125–44; Himmelweit, S. (2014). 'The marketization of care before and during austerity'. Naples: IIPPE Annual Conference; Jones, A. (2015). 'The end game: The marketization and privatisation of children's social work and child protection'. *Critical Social Policy*, 35 (4), pp. 447–69; Krachler, N. and Greer, I. (2015). 'When does marketization lead to privatisation? Profit-making in English health care after the 2012 Health and Social Care Act'. *Social Science and Medicine*, 214, pp. 215–23; Lynch, K., Grummell, B., and Devine, D. (2012). *New Managerialism in Education: Commercialisation, Carelessness and Gender*. Basingstoke: Macmillan; MacDonald; Pollock, A.M. (2003). *NHS PLC. The Privatisation of Our Health Care*. London: Verso; Rikowski, G. (2006). *On the Capitalisation of Schools in England*. School of Education: University of Northampton; Whitfield, D. (2001). *Public Services or Corporate Welfare: The Nation State in the Global Economy*. London: Pluto Press; Whitfield, D. (2013). *UK Social Services: The mutation of privatisation*. European Services Strategy Unit (online).

196 Blakeley, G. (2018). 'Years of Austerity Have Created a Welfare State for the Middle Class'. *Vice*. (5 November); Butler, P. (2019). 'Social care chiefs: funding crisis puts tens of thousands at risk'. *Guardian*. (26 June); Butler, P. and Gentleman, A. (2013). 'Benefit cuts putting 200,000 children in poverty must be stopped, experts say'. *Guardian*. (27 March); Edminston, D. (2017). 'Welfare, Austerity and Social Citizenship in the UK'. *Social Policy and Society*, 16 (2), pp. 261–70; Gallagher, P. (2019). 'NSS and the health service: years of austerity hit the UK over the past decade with an ageing population'. *International Newsletter* (online). (30 December); Hastings, A. *et al.* (2015). *The Cost of the Cuts: The Impact on Local Government and Poorer Communities*. London: Joseph Rowntree Foundation; Kerasidou, A. (2019). 'Austerity measures and the transforming role of A&E professionals in a weakening welfare system'. *PLoS ONE*, 14 (2), pp. 1–18; Mendoza, K.A. (2015). *Austerity: The Demolition of the Welfare State and the Rise of the Zombie Economy*. Oxford: New Internationalist Publishers; Mueller, B. (2019). 'What is Austerity and How Has It Affected British Society?' *New York Times*. (24 February); Roberts, A., Marshall, L., and Charlesworth, A. (2012). *A Decade of Austerity: The Funding Pressures Facing the NHS from 2010/11 to 2021/22*. London: Nuffield Trust; Harris, J. (2012). 'The housing benefits cap means a wretched life for thousands in B & Bs. *Guardian* (16 September); Watkins, J. *et al.* (2017). 'Effects of health and social care spending constraints on mortality in England: a time trend analysis.' *BMJ Open*, 7 (11), pp. 1–9.

197 Brown, W. (2015). *Undoing the demos: Neoliberalism's Stealth Revolution*. New York: Zone Books; Clarke, J. and Newman, J. (1997). *The Managerial State: Power, Politics and Ideology in the Remaking of Social Welfare*. London: Sage; Dumenil, G. and Levy, D. (2004). *Capital Resurgent: Roots of the Neoliberal Revolution*. Harvard: Harvard University Press; Glyn, A. (2006). *Capitalism Unleashed: Finance, Globalization and Welfare*. Oxford: Oxford University Press; Harman, C. (2007). 'Theorising Neoliberalism'. *International Socialism* (117), pp. 87–122; Harvey, D. (2005). *A Brief History of Neoliberalism*. Oxford: Oxford University Press; Law, A., and Mooney, G.

(2007). 'Beyond New Labour: Work and Resistance in the "New" Welfare State'. G. Mooney and A. Law (Eds.) *New Labour, Hard Labour: Restructuring and Resistance inside the Welfare Industry*. Bristol: Policy Press; Leys, C. (2003). *Market-Driven Politics: Neoliberal Democracy and the Public Interest*. London: Verso; Stedman-Jones, D. (2012). *Masters of the Universe: Hayek, Friedman and the Birth of Neoliberal Politics*. Princeton: Princeton University Press.

198   Kaine *et al.* (2022), p. 3.
199   Kaine *et al.* (2022), p. 16.
200   Kaine *et al.* (2022), p. 17.
201   Wright *et al.* (2022), p. 18.
202   N'Konzi *et al.* (2022) actually recommend this dilution of stringency of controls to prevent non-compliance. This is even though they acknowledge that stringency of NPIs is necessary to curb pandemics. Basically, their pragmatism takes as a given that people are unreformable because the culture that supports and nurtures narrow rights-based individualism is also taken as a given.
203   Park *et al.* (2013).
204   Ölcer *et al.* (2020), pp. 4–5.
205   Quoted in Cummings, E. (2020). 'A likely culprit in Covid-19 surges: People hell-bent on ignoring social distancing orders'. *Vox*. (2 July).
206   Ryan, J.M. and Nanda, S. (2023a). 'Pandemic Politics and the Politics of the Pandemic'. Ryan (Ed.) *Individual Rights*, p. 107.
207   Griffiths, A.M., Albinsson, P.A., and Perera, B.Y. (2023). 'Balancing Rights with Responsibilities: Citizens' Responses to Expert Systems COVID-19 Infodemics'. Ryan (Ed.) *Individual Rights*, p. 29.
208   Sachs (2021), p. 100.
209   Ölcer *et al.* (2020), p. 6
210   Ganslmeier *et al.* (2022), p. 3.
211   Nanda, S. (2021). 'Inequalities and COVID-19'. J.M. Ryan (Ed.) *COVID-19: Global Pandemic, Societal Responses, Ideological Solutions*. London and New York: Routledge, pp. 112–14.
212   Nanda (2021), p. 119.
213   Nanda (2021), pp. 117–19.
214   Nanda (2021), p. 115.
215   Krekel, C., Swanke, S., De Neve, J-E., and Fancourt, D. (2020). *Are Happier People More Compliant? Global Evidence From Three Large-Scale Surveys During Covid-19 Lockdowns*. Discussion Paper Series: No. 13690. IZA Institute of Labour Economics; Wright, Steptoe, and Fancourt (2021).
216   Merton, R.K. (1938). 'Social structure and anomie'. *American Sociological Review*, 3 (5), pp. 672–82. See also: Agnew, R. (1992). 'Foundation for a general strain theory of crime and delinquency'. *Criminology*, 30 (1), pp. 47–87; Agnew, R. (2001). 'Building on the foundation of General Strain Theory: specifying the types of strain most likely to lead to crime and delinquency'. *Journal of Research in Crime and Delinquency*, 38 (4), pp. 319–61; Merton, R.K. (1964). 'Anomie, Anomia and Social Interaction: Contexts of Deviant Behaviour'. M.B. Clinard (Ed.) *Anomie and Deviant Behaviour*, New York: Free Press; Messner, S.F. and Rosenfeld, R. (2001). *Crime and the American Dream* (2nd edition). Belmont CA: Wadsworth; Messner, S.F. (1988). 'Merton's "social structure and anomie": the road not taken'. *Deviant Behaviour*, 9 (1), pp. 33–53; Rosenfeld, R. (1989). 'Robert Merton's contributions to the sociology of deviance'. *Sociological Inquiry*, 59 (4), pp. 453–66.
217   Travis Hirschi's social bonds theory. Hirschi, T. (1967). *Delinquency Research*. London: Collier-Macmillan; Hirschi, T. (1969). *Causes of Delinquency*. Berkeley: University of California Press; Gottfredson, M.R. and Hirschi, T. (1990). *A General Theory of Crime*. Stanford CA: Stanford University Press.

218 Ölcer *et al.* (2020), p. 6.
219 Robert Brenner has shown how government assistance in the US to manage the economic shocks caused by lockdown was heavily skewed towards the "too big to fail" (Brenner, 2020, p. 5) corporations. This included

> a giant rescue of non-financial corporations amounting to half a trillion dollars. That $500 billion was to be reserved entirely for companies with at least 10,000 employees and revenues of at least $2.5 billion per year. The Act set aside $46 billion to be shared between passenger airlines ($25 billion), cargo airlines ($4 billion) and "businesses necessary for national security", a code name for Boeing ($17 billion), leaving no less than $454 billion for the political authorities to distribute to the fortunate corporate recipients they would select. Yet even this huge sum turned out to be just the tip of the iceberg. The actual payday for the US's greatest non-financial companies would be of a different order of magnitude entirely (Brenner, 2020, pp. 6–7).

> Indeed, as Brenner tells, transfers to financial and non-financial corporations and industries in the first lockdown topped $7.7 trillion (Brenner, 2020, p. 5). At the same time, assistance was not extended to "endangered home-owning mortgage borrowers, to whom the bailed-out financial institutions had been lending" (Brenner, 2020, pp. 5–6). The result was that many big capitals actually prospered from the crisis with bonanza profits. This was as the poorer commonfolk struggled to cope financially owing also to furlough subsidies that were delivered patchily and which provided for bare safety-net compensations. By contrast with the trillions spent bailing out the corporate big players, "just $603 billion in total was allocated for direct cash payments to individuals and families ($300 billion), extra unemployment insurance ($260 billion), and student loans ($43 billion)", despite "soaring unemployment" (Brenner, 2020, p. 7). See Brenner, R. (2020). 'Escalating Plunder'. *New Left Review*, 123 (May/June), pp. 5–22.

220 Headline repeated breaches in the UK included those by health minister Matt Hancock, SAGE adviser Neil Ferguson, Johnson's chief adviser Dominic Cummings, and housing minister Robert Jenrick. See *Sky News* (2020). 'Lockdown: They told us to stay home – then went out. The political figures who broke the rules'. (23 May); *Al Jazeera* (2020). 'UK health chief caught in embrace that broke COVID rules'. (25 June).
221 Butler, P. (2020). 'Cummings trips damaged UK lockdown unity, study suggests'. *Guardian*. (30 July). Wright *et al.*'s (2021, 2022) research found a weak association between diminishing trust in the UK government and increased non-compliance with NPIs by people in high places.
222 Olsen and Hjorth (2020); Seale *et al.* (2020); Van Rooij *et al.* (2020); Rasul and Giuliano (2020).
223 This is established by a large range of studies in the UK and worldwide. For UK data and analysis see for example: Mishra, V. *et al.* (2021). 'Health Inequalities During COVID-19 and Their Effects on Morbidity and Mortality'. *Journal of Healthcare Leadership*, 13, pp. 19–26; Mathur, R. *et al.* (2021). 'Ethnic differences in SARS-CoV-2 infection and COVID-19-related hospitalisation, intensive care unit admission, and death in 17 million adults in England: an observational cohort study using the OpenSAFELY platform'. *Lancet*, 397 (10286), pp. 1711–24; ONS (2020). *Deaths involving COVID-19 by local area and socioeconomic deprivation: deaths occurring between 1 March and 17 April 2020.* (1 May); ONS (2020). *Deaths involving COVID-19 by local area and socioeconomic deprivation: deaths occurring between 1 March and 31 July 2020.* (28 August); ONS (2020). *Coronavirus (COVID-19) related deaths by ethnic group, England and Wales: 2 March 2020 to 15 May 2020.* (19 June); Stafford, M. and Deeny, S. (2020). *Inequalities and deaths involving COVID-19: What the links between inequalities tell us.* Health Foundation (online). (21 May); Local Government Association (2020). *Health Inequalities: Deprivation and Poverty and COVID-19.* LGA (online).

(April); PHE (2020). *Disparities in the risk and outcomes of COVID-19.* GOV.UK (online). (August).
224 Jaspal, R. and Breakwell, G.M. (2023). 'The Significance of Ethnicity in Vaccination Uptake: Social Psychological Aspects'. J.M. Ryan (Ed.) *COVID-19: Surviving a Pandemic.* London and New York: Routledge, pp. 139–40.
225 Research in the US has shown that low-income workers were three times less likely than high-income workers to be able to work from home and were four times more likely to run out of money due to the pandemic within three months of its start. See Yasenov, V. (2020). *Who Can Work from Home?* Research Paper Series: No 13197. IZA Institute of Labor Economics; Schaner, S. and Theys, N. (2020). *Individuals with Low Incomes, Less Education Report Higher Perceived Financial, Health Threats from COVID-19.* Leonard D. Shaeffer Center for Health Policy and Economics. (online). (1 April).
226 This is also evidenced by research carried out in the US. This issue does not seem to have motivated much research interest in the UK, however. But one study found that BAME people were not less inclined than White people to comply with physical distancing restrictions during the pandemic. See Garnier, R., Benetka, J.R., Kraemer, J., and Bansal, S. (2020). *Socio-economic disparities in social distancing during the COVID-19 pandemic in the United States.* NCBI: PMC (online). (9 November); Raisi-Estabragh, Z. *et al.* (2020). 'Greater risk of severe COVID-19 in Black, Asian and Minority Ethnic populations is not explained by cardio-metabolic, socioeconomic or behavioural factors, or by 25(OH)-vitamin D status: study of 1326 cases from the UK Biobank'. *Journal of Public Health*, 42 (3), pp. 451–60.
227 Lang *et al.* (2021); Plohl and Musil (2021); Seale *et al.* (2021); Shumway *et al.* (2021).
228 Barrios *et al.* (2020); Olsen and Hjorth (2020); Seale *et al.* (2020); Van Rooij *et al.* (2020); Rasul and Giuliano (2020).
229 Kamenidou *et al.* (2020).
230 Sachs (2021), p. 100.
231 Travaglino, G.A. and Moon, C. (2021). 'Compliance and Self-Reporting During the COVID-19 Pandemic: A Cross-Cultural Study of Trust and Self-Conscious Emotions in the United States, Italy, and South Korea'. *Frontiers in Psychology*, 12 (565845), pp. 1–14.
232 Travaglino and Moon (2021).
233 Blake, A. (2020). 'Trump's Most Belittling Comments About the Coronavirus'. *Washington Post.* (1 April); Gabbatt, A., and Evelyn, K. (2020). 'US Reports Daily Case Record of 52,000 After Trump Says Covid-19 Will "Disappear"'. *Guardian.* (1 July); Mangan, D. (2020). 'Trump dismissed coronavirus pandemic worry in January – now claims he long warned about it'. *CNBC.* (17 March); Paz, C. (2020). 'All the President's Lies About the Coronavirus'. *Atlantic.* (2 November).
234 Viglione, G. (2020). 'Four ways Trump has meddled in pandemic science – and why it matters'. *Nature.* (3 November); Victor, D., Serviss, L., and Paybarah, A. (2020). 'In His Own Words, Trump on the Coronavirus and Masks'. *New York Times.* (2 October); Wolfe, D. and Dale, D. (2020). '"It's Going to Disappear": A Timeline of Trump's Claims That Covid-19 Will Vanish'. *CNN.* (31 October); Wu, N. and Jackson, D. (2020). 'Trump: CDC Recommends Voluntary Use of Face Masks for Public to Stem Spread of Coronavirus'. *USA Today.* (3 April).
235 Brzezinski, A., Kecht, V., Van Dijcke, D., and Wright, A. (2021). 'Science skepticism reduced compliance with COVID-19 shelter-in-place policies in the United States'. *Nature of Human Behaviour*, 5, pp. 1519–27.
236 Paz (2020). See also: Egan, L. (2020). 'Trump Calls Coronavirus Democrats' "New Hoax"'. *NBC News.* (29 February); Rupar, A. (2020). 'Eric Trump Used His Latest Fox News Appearance to Push an Absurd Conspiracy Theory About Covid-19'. *Vox.* (18

May); Ingraham, L. (2020). 'Left fearmongering over COVID despite new data'. *Fox News*. (12 June). O'Connell, F. (2020). 'How Democrats Will Weaponize Coronavirus to Beat Trump'. *Washington Examine*. (26 February).

237 Rasul and Giuliano (2020). See also: Allcott, H. *et al.* (2020). *Polarization and Public Health: Partisan Differences in Social Distancing during the Coronavirus Pandemic*. National Bureau of Economic Research (NBER). (August). Working Paper 26946; Barrios, J.M. and Hochberg, Y. (2020). *Risk Perception Through the Lens of Politics in the Time of the COVID-19 Pandemic*. Working Paper 27008. (April). National Bureau of Economic Research (NBER); Gadarian, S.K., Goodman, S.W., and Pepinsky, T.B. (2020). 'Partisanship, Health Behavior, and Policy Attitudes in the Early Stages of the COVID-19 Pandemic'. Social Science Research Network (SSRN). (30 March).

238 Cheng, K.K., Lam, T.H., and Leung, C.C. (2020). 'Wearing face masks in the community during the COVID-19 pandemic: altruism and solidarity'. *Lancet*, 399 (10336), pp. 39–40; Pfattheicher, S. *et al.* (2020). 'The emotional path to action: empathy promotes physical distancing and wearing of face masks during the COVID-19 pandemic'. *Psychological Science,* 31 (11), pp. 1363–73; Jones, K.L. *et al.* (2018). 'Liberal and conservative values: what we can learn from congressional tweets'. *Political Psychology,* 39 (2), pp. 422–43; Vuolo, M., Kelly, B.C., and Roscigno, V.J. (2020). 'COVID-19 mask requirements as a workers' rights issue: parallels to smoking bans'. *American Journal of Preventative Medicine.* 59 (5), pp. 764–67; Capraro, V., and Barcelo, H. (2020). 'The effect of messaging and gender on intentions to wear a face covering to slow down COVID-19 transmission'. *Journal of Behavioral Economics for Health,* 4 (2), pp. 45–55; Finkelstein, J. *et al.* (2020). *COVID-19, Conspiracy and Contagious Sedition: A Case Study on the Militia-Sphere*. Rutgers University, Miller Center for Community Protection and Resilience; Shepherd, K. (2020). 'Tensions Over Restrictions Spark Violence and Defiance Among Protesters as Trump Pushes States to Reopen'. *Washington Post.* (13 May); Siegler, K. (2020). *Across America, Frustrated Protesters Rally To Reopen The Economy*. National Public Radio. (18 April); Thomson, S., and Ip., E.C. (2020). 'COVID-19 emergency measures and the impending authoritarian pandemic'. *Journal of Law and the Biosciences*, 7 (1), pp. 1–33; Capraro, V. and Barcelo, H. (2020). 'The effect of messaging and gender on intentions to wear a face covering to slow down COVID-19 transmission'. *Journal of Behavioral Economics for Policy*, 4 (2), pp. 45–55.

239 Kemmelmeier, M. and Jami, W.A. (2020). 'Mask Wearing as Cultural Behavior: An Investigation Across 45 U.S. States During the COVID-19 Pandemic'. *Frontiers in Psychology*, 12 (648692), pp. 1–24. (See p. 3).

240 Kemmelmeier and Jami (2020), p. 5.

241 Ryan and Nanda (2023a), p. 106. The authors also note a polarization of public attitudes to the pandemic along party-political lines more generally. Fewer Republican affiliates viewed the virus as harmful or dangerous to public health than Democrat affiliates. Fewer were worried than were Democrats about catching it, or about family members catching it, or being harmed by it.

242 Kemmelmeier and Jami (2020), p. 4.

243 Kemmelmeier and Jami (2020), p. 19.

244 Kemmelmeier and Jami (2020), p. 16.

245 Solomon, H. *et al.* (2022). 'Adherence to and enforcement of non-pharmaceutical interventions (NPIs) for COVID-19 prevention in Nigeria, Rwanda, and Zambia: A mixed-methods analysis'. *PLoS Global Public Health* 2 (9), pp. 1–18.

246 Solomon *et al.* (2022), p. 2.

247 Anon (2020). 'COVID-19 in Africa: no room for complacency'. *Lancet* (Editorial), 395 (10238), p. 1; Ihekweazu, C. and Agogo, E. (2020). 'Africa's response to COVID-19'. *BMC Medicine*, 18 (151), pp. 1–3; Ohia, C., Bakarey, A.S., and Ahmad, T. (2020).

'COVID-19 and Nigeria: putting the realities in context'. *International Journal of Infectious Diseases*, 95, pp. 279–81.

248 Solomon *et al.* (2022), pp. 2–3.
249 Massinga Loembe´, M. *et al.* (2020). 'COVID-19 in Africa: the spread and response'. *Nature Medicine*, 26, pp. 999–1003.
250 Hartwich, F. and Hedeshi, M (2020). *COVID-19 effects in sub-Saharan Africa and what local industry and governments can do.* United Nations Industrial Development Organization (UNIDO). (April); Ihekweazu and Agogo (2020); Massinga Loembe' *et al.* (2020)
251 Solomon *et al.* (2022), p. 3.
252 A similar story could be told for the poorest countries of Central Asia and Latin America. The story is well told by Serena Nanda (2021, pp. 110–12, 116, 117, 118), who presents a review of the impact of the pandemic and NPIs on the world's least developed countries and their poorest communities.
253 *Lancet* (Ed.) (2020); Abdalla, S. and Galea, S. (2020). 'Africa and Coronavirus – Will Lockdowns Work? *Think Global Health* (online). (16 April); Sun, N. and Zilli, L. (2020). 'COVID-19 Symposium: The Use of Criminal Sanctions in COVID-19 Responses – Enforcement of Public Health Measures' (3 April). *Opinio Juris* (online).
254 Ihekweazu and Agogo (2020); *Lancet* (Ed.) (2020).
255 Solomon *et al.* (2022), p. 3.
256 Solomon *et al.* (2022), pp. 1, 8–9.
257 Solomon *et al.* (2022), p. 2.
258 Solomon *et al.* (2022), p. 13.
259 Solomon *et al.* (2022), p. 12.
260 Solomon *et al.* (2022), p. 13.
261 Solomon *et al.* (2022), p. 11.
262 Creaven (2023), pp. 166–71.
263 Public Accounts Committee (2021). *COVID-19: Test, track and trace (part 1)*. GOV. UK (online). (18 January).
264 Fraser, C. and Briggs, A. (2021a). *NHS Test and Trace performance tracker*. Health Foundation (online). (13 May).
265 Fraser and Briggs (2021a).
266 UK Health Security Agency (2022). *NHS Test and Trace statistics (England): methodology*. GOV.UK (online). (18 May).
267 Smith, L. *et al.* (2021). 'Adherence to the test, trace, and isolate system in the UK: results from 37 nationally representative surveys'. *British Medical Journal*, 372 (608), pp. 1–13. See p. 4.
268 Fraser, C. and Briggs, A. (2021b). *What have we learned from a year of NHS Test and Trace?* Health Foundation (online). (3 June).
269 Smith *et al.* (2021), p. 6.
270 Fraser and Briggs (2021b).
271 UK Parliament (2021). *Test and Trace update: Twenty-Third Report of Session 2021–22*. Public Accounts Committee. (27 October), pp. 5–6.
272 Fraser and Briggs (2021b).
273 Briggs, A. and Fraser, S. (2020). 'Is NHS Test and Trace exacerbating COVID-19 inequalities?' *Lancet*, 396 (10267), pp. 1–2.
274 Sachs (2021), p. 102.
275 Chen, E. (2021). *Vaccine hesitancy: More than a pandemic*. Harvard University: The Graduate School of Arts and Sciences (online). (29 June).
276 Freeman, D. *et al.* (2020). 'COVID-19 vaccine hesitancy in the UK: the Oxford coronavirus explanations, attitudes, and narratives survey (Oceans) II'. *Psychological Medicine*, 52 (14), pp. 1–15.

277 Freeman *et al.* (2020), p. 5.

278 Freeman *et al.* (2020), p. 1.

279 Freeman *et al.* (2020), p. 8.

280 Denford, S. *et al.* (2022). 'Exploration of attitudes regarding uptake of COVID-19 vaccines among vaccine hesitant adults in the UK: a qualitative analysis'. *BMC Infectious Diseases*, 22 (407), pp. 1–14.

281 NIHR (2022). *People were hesitant rather than opposed to the COVID-19 vaccine, study finds.* Health Protection Research Unit in Behavioural Science and Evaluation at University of Bristol (online). (10 May).

282 Denford *et al.* (2022), p. 7.

283 Denford *et al.* (2022), pp. 5–6.

284 Denford *et al.* (2022), pp. 4–5.

285 Denford *et al.* (2022), p. 5.

286 Denford *et al.* (2022), p. 1.

287 Denford *et al.* (2022), pp. 9–10.

288 Chaudhuri, K. *et al.* (2022). 'COVID-19 vaccine hesitancy in the UK: a longitudinal household cross-sectional study. *BMC Public Health*, 22 (104), pp. 1–13. See also: Butter, S., McGlinchey, E., Berry, E., and Armour C. (2021). 'Psychological, social, and situational factors associated with COVID-19 vaccination intentions: A study of UK key workers and non-key workers'. *British Journal of Health Psychology*, 27 (1), pp. 13–29; Freeman, D. *et al.* (2021). 'Effects of different types of written vaccination information on COVID-19 vaccine hesitancy in the UK (OCEANS-III): a single-blind, parallel-group, randomised controlled trial'. *Lancet: Public Health*, 6 (6), pp. 416–27.

289 ONS (2021). *Coronavirus and vaccine hesitancy, Great Britain: 13 January to 7 February 2021.* GOV.UK (online). (8 March).

290 ONS (2021). *Coronavirus and vaccine hesitancy, Great Britain: 9 August 2021.* GOV. UK (online). (9 August).

291 Cited in McIntyre, N. and Thomas, T. (2021). 'As many as 6 million eligible Britons may not have had a Covid jab. Who are they?'. *Guardian*. (7 December).

292 ONS (2022). *Coronavirus and vaccination rates in people aged 18 years and over by socio-demographic characteristic and occupation.* GOV.UK (online). (20 January). England8 December 2020ecember 2021

293 GOV.UK (2022). *Coronavirus (COVID-19) in the UK: Vaccinations in England* (online). Accessed: 30 September 2022.

294 Cited in Wise, J. (2022). 'Covid-19: MPs call for greater efforts to reach the unvaccinated and partially vaccinated'. *British Medical Journal*, 378 (1743), p. 1. See also: Roberts, M. (2022). '3m adults in England still have no Covid vaccine'. *BBC News*. (13 July).

295 Tapper, J. (2022). 'Only 7% of 5–11s in England have had Covid jab as parents hesitate'. *Guardian*. (14 May).

296 Wise (2021), p. 1.

297 Ryan, J.M. and Nanda, S. (2023b). 'Vaccines: Are We Really in This Together?' Ryan (Ed.) *Surviving a Pandemic*, p. 179.

298 A link between vaccine hesitancy, indeed between anti-vax ideology, and right-wing anti-establishment politics and populist party affiliations, has also been reported for the UK, Italy, France and Greece (Jaspal and Breakwell, 2023, pp. 138–39. See Jaspal, R. and Breakwell, G.M. (2023). 'The Significance of Ethnicity in Vaccination Uptake: Social Psychological Aspects'. Ryan (Ed.) *Surviving a Pandemic*.

299 Cascini, F. *et al.* (2021). 'Attitudes, acceptance and hesitancy among the general population worldwide to receive the COVID-19 vaccines and their contributing factors: A systematic review'. *EClinicalMedicine* (online), 40, pp. 1–14.

300 Chaudhuri *et al.* (2022), p. 2. These studies included: Institute of Global Health Innovation (2021). *Covid-19: Global attitudes towards a COVID-19 vaccine.* Imperial College London (January); Robinson, E., Jones A., Lesser, I., and Daly, M. (2021).

'International estimates of intended uptake and refusal of COVID-19 vaccines: A rapid systematic review and meta-analysis of large nationally representative samples'. *Vaccine*, 39 (15), pp. 2024–34; Neumann-Böhme, S. *et al.* (2020). 'Once we have it, will we use it? A European survey on willingness to be vaccinated against COVID-19'. *European Journal of Health Economics*, 21, pp. 977–82; Caserotti, M., Girardi, P., Rubaltelli, E., Tasso, A., Lotto, L., and Gavaruzzi, T. (2021). 'Associations of COVID-19 risk perception with vaccine hesitancy over time for Italian residents. *Social Science & Medicine*, 272 (113688), pp. 1–9; Kourlaba, G. *et al.* (2021). 'Willingness of Greek general population to get a COVID-19 vaccine'. *Global Health Research Policy*, 6 (3), pp. 2–10; Feleszko, W., Lewulis, P., Czarnecki, A., and Waszkiewicz, P. (2021). 'Flattening the Curve of COVID-19 Vaccine Rejection – An International Overview'. *Vaccines*, 9 (44), pp. 2–8.

301 Lazarus, J.V., Wyka, K., White, T.M., *et al.* (2022). 'Revisiting COVID-19 vaccine hesitancy around the world using data from 23 countries in 2021'. *Nature Communications*, 13 (3801), pp. 1–14.

302 Khubchandani, J. *et al.* (2022). 'COVID-19 Vaccine Refusal among Nurses Worldwide: Review of Trends and Predictors'. *Vaccines*, 10 (2), pp. 1–13.

303 Lazarus, J.V., *et al.* (2023). 'A survey of COVID-19 vaccine acceptance across 23 countries in 2022'. *Nature Medicine*, 29 (2), pp. 366–75.

304 Results reported in Jarvis, H. (2022). *Vaccine hesitancy hardens in richer countries.* Brunel University London (online). (31 May). This estimates a much higher percentage of unvaccinated persons in the UK than the other studies I have cited. For the full survey see John *et al.* (2022).

305 John, P. *et al.* (2022). *Overcoming Barriers to Vaccination by Empowering Citizens to Make Deliberate Choices.* The British Academy (online) (May).

306 Jarvis (2022).

307 John *et al.* (2022).

308 Chaudhuri *et al.* (2022), p. 2.

309 Robinson, E., Jones, A., and Daly, M. (2021). 'International estimates of intended uptake and refusal of COVID-19 vaccines: A rapid systematic review and meta-analysis of large nationally representative samples'. *Vaccine*, 39 (15), pp. 2024–34.; ONS (2021). *Coronavirus and the social impacts on Great Britain.* GOV.UK (online). (29 January); ONS (2021). *Coronavirus and the social impacts on Great Britain.* GOV. UK (online). (19 February); ONS (2021). *Coronavirus and vaccination rates in people aged 70 years and over by socio-demographic characteristic, England: 8 December 2020 to 11 March 2021.* GOV.UK (online). (29 March); ONS (2021). *Coronavirus and vaccination rates in people aged 50 years and over by socio-demographic characteristic, England: 8 December 2020 to 12 April 2021.* GOV.UK (online). (6 May); ONS (2021). *Coronavirus and vaccination rates in people aged 70 years and over by socio-demographic characteristic, England: 8 December 2020 to 9 May 2021.* GOV.UK (online). (7 June); Morgan, W. (2021). 'Poor vaccine take-up in BAME communities is not just down to hesitancy'. *Conversation.* (1 March); Local Government Association (2021). *A Review of research into vaccine uptake in the UK.* LGA (online). (12 June); Razai, M.S., Osama, T., McKechnie, D.G.K., and Majeed, K. (2021). 'Covid-19 vaccine hesitancy among ethnic minority groups'. *British Medical Journal*, 372 (513), pp. 1–2.

310 Hussain, B. *et al.* (2022). 'Overcoming COVID-19 vaccine hesitancy among ethnic minorities: A systematic review of UK studies'. *Vaccine*, 40 (25), pp. 3413–32.

311 ONS (2021). *Coronavirus and vaccine hesitancy, Great Britain: 9 August 2021.* GOV. UK (online). (9 August). This was the final report in this series to date (mid-July 2022).

312 ONS (2021). *First dose vaccinations rates in people aged 40 years and over by socio-demographic characteristic, 8 December 2020 to 15 May 2021, England.* GOV.UK (online). (10 June).

313 ONS (8 March, 2021).

314 ONS (8 August, 2021).

315 ONS (20 January, 2022).

316 Wise (2022).

317 ONS (20 January, 2022).

318 See Ministry of Housing, Communities and Local Government (2020). *People living in deprived neighbourhoods*. GOV.UK (online). (16 June); DWP (2020). *Ethnicity facts and figures: Income distribution*. GOV.UK (online). (29 September). Whereas 42 percent of White households are in the two highest income quintiles (that is, within the wealthiest 40 percent of households), only 15 percent of Bangladeshi, 11 percent of Pakistani, and 25 percent of Black households are in these higher earnings brackets. Almost 20 percent of Black people reside in the most severely economically deprived areas of the UK – that is, in the poorest tenth of neighbourhoods. More than 26 percent of Bangladeshi-Asian adults do. But the ethnic minority group suffering the highest levels of economic marginalization are Pakistani-Asians – 31 percent of whom live in the most income-deprived neighbourhoods. By contrast, less than nine percent of White people are resident in the poorest ten percent of neighbourhoods.

319 Becares, L., Shaw, R., Nazroo, J., and Irizar, P. (2022). *Understanding the fundamental role of racism in ethnic inequities in COVID-19 vaccine hesitancy*. (Runnymede/CoDE Covid Briefings). Runnymede Trust and Centre on the Dynamics of Ethnicity (CoDE). The authors estimate that, in the UK, racism in its various forms explains 50 percent of the vaccine hesitancy of Black people, 30 percent of the vaccine hesitancy of Pakistani and Bangladeshi people, and 23 percent of the vaccine hesitancy of Indian and mixed ethnicity people. However, it is not clear that the "domains of racism" they hold accountable are not also "domains of classism", so the hesitancy is shaped by both.

320 As a SAGE report put it, when reflecting on the gloomy findings of the UK Household Longitudinal Survey. See Geddes, L. (2021). 'Covid vaccine: 72% of black people unlikely to have jab, UK survey finds'. *Guardian*. (16 January). Events would show that these were huge underestimates of vaccine compliance. Nonetheless, the problem of non-compliance was real enough.

321 Razai (2021), p. 1.

322 As, again, SAGE put it. Cited in Geddes (16 January, 2021).

323 Razai (2021), p. 1.

324 Razai (2021), p. 1.

325 Naqvi, M. *et al*. (2022). 'Understanding COVID-19 Vaccine Hesitancy in Ethnic Minorities Groups in the UK'. *Frontiers in Public Health*, 10 (917242), pp. 1–10.

326 Naqvi *et al*. (2022), p. 3.

327 Naqvi *et al*. (2022), pp. 3–4.

328 ONS (8 March, 2021).

329 ONS (8 August, 2021).

330 Home Office (2018). *Ethnicity facts and figures: age groups*. GOV.UK (online). (28 August).

331 ONS (2021). *COVID-19 vaccine refusal, UK: February to March 2021: Exploring the attitudes of people who are uncertain about receiving, or unable or unwilling to receive a coronavirus (COVID-19) vaccine in the UK*. GOV.UK (online). (7 May). For the full report see IFF Research (2021). *COVID-19 vaccines refusal study, UK: February – March 2021*. ONS (online). (6 May).

332 Also included were some parents. There were 50 participants in all, 30 of whom were interviewed in depth.

333 ONS (7 May, 2021), pp. 2–3.

334 IFF Research (2021). The lockdowns were sometimes mooted as conspiratorial government experiments in how people coped with the suspension of freedoms. COVID-

19 symptoms were sometimes attributed to the impact of 5G wi-fi masts. The pandemic was sometimes seen as exaggerated in order to justify lockdowns that protected people from the greater danger posed by these 5G installations. Scepticism over the pharmaceutical industry was encouraged by reports that one of the companies had been granted legal immunity from prosecution in the event that its vaccine made recipients seriously ill. Fears were expressed that the vaccines would cause genetic mutations in the body or infertility or was responsible for deaths in care homes that were hushed-up by the government. Some respondents based their understanding of the virus and the vaccines on social media, disregarding mainstream news, because they were sceptical of the objectivity of the corporate media.

335 ONS (7 May 2021), pp. 3–5.
336 Relevant US studies include Latkin, C.A. *et al.* (2021). 'Trust in a COVID-19 vaccine in the U.S.: A social-ecological perspective'. *Social Science and Medicine*, 270 (113684), pp. 1–8; Doherty, I.A. *et al.* (2021). 'COVID-19 Vaccine Hesitancy in Underserved Communities of North Carolina. *PLoS ONE*, 16 (11), pp. 1–14; McCabe, S. *et al.* (2021). 'Unraveling Attributes of COVID-19 Vaccine Hesitancy in the U.S.: A Large Nationwide Study. *BMJ Yale* (online). (4 May).
337 Ryan and Nanda (2023b), p. 180.
338 Jaspal and Breakwell (2023), p. 140.
339 Ryan and Nanda (2023b), p. 179.
340 Ryan and Nanda (2023b), p. 179.
341 Abba-Aji, M., Stuckler, D., Galea, S., and McKee, M. (2022). 'Ethnic/racial minorities' access to COVID-19 vaccines: A systematic review of barriers and facilitators'. *Journal of Migration and Health*, 5 (100086), pp. 1–13.
342 Abba-Aji *et al.* (2022), p. 1.
343 Abba-Aji *et al.* (2022), p. 1.
344 Lazarus *et al.* (2022), p. 1
345 Khubchandani *et al.* (2022), p. 1.
346 IFF Research (2021).
347 Creaven (2023).
348 To be clear, this argument is not that minorities and the poor are less "civilized" than others. Rather, it is that decivilizing mechanisms at work in society as a whole interact with the harms of systemic racism and classism to generate a higher prevalence of vaccine hesitancy among oppressed minorities and the socially excluded.
349 This is a more significant factor in explaining hesitancy amongst racial and other oppressed minorities (that is, among LGBTQ groups) in the US. Also in the US, vaccine hesitancy is especially common among migrant populations owing to fears of deportation. See Ryan and Nanda (2023b), pp. 179–80
350 Only one minority participant expressed misgivings that there was perhaps insufficient trialling of the vaccines in non-White populations specifically, though she also was concerned that there was not enough testing in general. One other (non-minority) participant referred to the Thalidomide scandal as a "legacy" example of corporate irresponsibility by the pharmaceutical industry in fast-tracking an unsafe drug that could be repeated with the COVID vaccines. A majority of participants said they trusted the scientific experts with regard to the pandemic. Others were more sceptical, saying they respected their views but did not see them as necessarily having an objective view on the COVID vaccines, or their views as being decisive. Only a small minority said they disregarded the scientists. But this was not because they were seen as untrustworthy or biased. Rather, it was because they were difficult to understand and disagreed with each other, which was confusing. See IFF Research (2021).
351 ONS (7 May, 2021), p. 5.
352 Jarvis (2022).
353 Creaven (2023), pp. 151–56.

354 See for example: Dingwall, R. (2022). 'Lockdown caused this wave of avoidable deaths'. *Telegraph.* (20 August); Le, B.Y. (2022). 'Did So-Called "Johns Hopkins Study" Really Show Lockdowns Were Ineffective Against Covid-19?'. *Forbes.* (6 February); McKie, R. (2022). 'Britain got it wrong on Covid: long lockdown did more harm than good, says scientist'. *Observer.* (2 January).

355 As exemplified by the so-called Great Barrington Declaration. See PA Media (2020). 'Herd immunity letter signed by fake experts including "Dr Johnny Bananas"'. *Guardian.* (19 October).

356 Woolhouse, M. (2022). *The Year the World Went Mad: A Scientific Memoir.* London: Allen Churchill.

357 McKie (2022).

358 Khan, N. (2023). 'Pandemic Eugenics: The Delta Variant, Child Mortality, and the New Racism'. Ryan (Ed.) *Surviving a Pandemic.* As Khan tells, school reopenings during the delta wave were accompanied by the failure of most state authorities to require mask-wearing in schools, and the decision of several to actually ban it, which basically left children without protection. As Khan also shows, children from lower-income and oppressed minority cohorts had much higher mortality and hospitalization rates than those among the better-off White cohorts.

359 Khan (2023), p. 58.

360 Creaven (2023), pp. 165–71.

361 Creaven (2023), Ch.1.

362 Creaven (2023), Ch.1, Ch. 4.

363 Irfan, F.B. *et al.* (2022). 'Coronavirus pandemic in the Nordic countries: Health policy and economy trade-off'. *Journal of Global Health,* 12 (05017), pp. 1–13. See pp. 8–9. The researchers also show that Sweden gained no discernible economic benefit in comparison with the other Nordic countries in embracing this "Swedish exceptionalism". As they conclude (p. 1): "There was no trade-off between public health policy and economy during the COVID-19 pandemic in the Nordic region. Sweden's relaxed and delayed COVID-19 health policy response did not benefit the economy in the short term, while leading to disproportionate COVID-19 hospitalizations and mortality".

364 Dewan, A. (2021). 'Covid-19, Nordic trust and collective denial: Sweden and Norway compared'. *Coronatimes.* (21 January).

365 WHO (2022). *Global excess deaths associated with COVID-19, January 2020–December 2021* (online). (May).

366 The Lockdown Files Team (2023). 'Jeremy Hunt: Britain has "a lot to learn" from Swedish approach to Covid rules'. *Telegraph.* (11 March).

367 Anon (2021). 'Did Sweden's Covid-19 experiment pay off in the end?' *Week.* (8 September).

368 Irfan *et al.* (2022), p. 2.

369 Dewan (2021).

370 Bendix, A. (2021). 'A year and a half after Sweden decided not to lock down, its COVID-19 death rate is up to 10 times higher than its neighbors'. *Insider* (21 August); Diderichsen, F. (2021). 'How did Sweden Fail the Pandemic?' *International Journal of Health Services,* 51 (4), pp. 417–22.

371 Irfan *et al.* (2022), pp. 3, 9–10.

372 Diderichsen (2021), p. 417.

373 Anon (2021). See also: Dewan (2021); Hiltzik, M. (2022). 'Did Sweden beat the pandemic by refusing to lock down? No, its record is disastrous'. *Los Angeles Times.* (31 March).

374 Dewan (2021).

Conclusion

In this book, I have presented a political critique and sociological analysis of the international political response to the novel coronavirus outbreak. In doing so, I have sought to grasp the inadequacies of state policymaking with regard to COVID-19 as the result of neoliberal politics and ideology, the protection of corporate interests, and the constraints imposed on state actors by mega-capitalism and interstate (including imperial) rivalries in the "global" age.

The power of the world market and of corporate capital to shape national and international politics is rarely questioned in the contemporary social sciences, owing to the near-hegemony of globalization theory. However, the reverse power of the nation-state system (and of the most powerful nation-states within that system) to shape economic orders and limit and facilitate capitalist enterprise is rather less recognized, and for the same reason. But, as I have shown in this book, states, nations, and nationalisms matter. Indeed, they matter as much as they ever did. If the pandemic lockdowns and border closures and bailouts of the corporate sector are not evidence enough of this, the point may be further substantiated by considering briefly the power of citizenship (or rather who exercises power over it) in our COVID-stricken times.

Contrary to fashionable concepts of "post-nationalism", "de-nationalism", and "trans-nationalism", which contend that globalization is generating or has generated deterritorialized or world citizenries, the pandemic forces us to confront the fact that the opposite is true. It has punctured this particular myth. This is because the border closures and national lockdowns that governments brought in to combat the spread of COVID-19 show us that (as much as ever before) citizens are made by nations and that non-citizens have few rights. For, when the borders closed and the stay-at-home orders were issued, non-nationals who were trapped willingly or otherwise within their host countries found they were not entitled to unemployment benefits or rental waivers or public healthcare or the compensations of furloughs, just as others outside those borders with visas or residence permits were refused entry or re-entry. These people found that they were non-citizens, without entitlements, because they were non-nationals.[1]

When this happened, as it did to millions across the world, where were the "globalist" organs of juridical or political authority (such as the UN) that lamented or challenged this state of affairs? As Atefeh Ramsari rightly says:

DOI: 10.4324/9781003437208-6

While new – postnational, transnational – formulations were introduced to relocate citizenship beyond the boundaries of the nation-state, the COVID-19 pandemic pulls the concept back within these boundaries even more explicitly. States have been the only legitimate site for the regulation of citizenship, although some supranational institutions strive to take decisions concerning regional or global issues. The problems raised by the pandemic have challenged the postnational claim, which argues that membership is transcending national borders to become global and that international human rights norms guarantee individual rights all around the world. During the pandemic, the nation-state has reappeared as the only locus for the allocation of rights and has mobilized citizenship as a means of control and distribution of resources.[2]

Whether or not Ramsari regards this present state of affairs as the resurgence or restoration of the nation-state's role in allocating and upholding rights (and the corresponding reversal of the cause of universal human rights under "globalization") or as business as usual is unclear. The former is suggested by her talk of the "reappearance" of this role of the state and by the title of her book chapter (referring to "the decline of global citizenship"). However, I am inclined towards the latter view.

Yes, of course, universal human rights are enshrined in the UN Charter. Yes, of course, there is such a thing as international law, including human rights law. But these rights and laws (and whatever penalties and sanctions for breaching them are mandated by the UN) are never applied in or on behalf of the actual interests of oppressed peoples. Nor are they utilized to punish states that violate human rights if those states happen to be allies or partners of the US or the West – Israel and Saudi Arabia being the obvious examples. They certainly are not applied to uphold human rights law or to censure human rights violations in the West or in the North – such as those meted out by the US state's fondness for mass incarceration (especially of poor Black and Latino minorities)[3] or by the current UK government's plan to dispatch asylum-seekers and refugees, except Ukrainians, to Rwanda.[4]

Rather, these are applied selectively, for political rather than moral or humanitarian purposes. That is, they are applied to "outlier", "rogue", "opposed", or "failed" states, in order to secure strategic or economic goals. To be clear, it is not that human rights are unimportant for the leading state-power actors, or for the supranational institutions of international governance that serve their interests. Even politicians are human beings. It is just that there are always more important matters (economic growth, capitalist profits, political stability, international security) to attend to so that rights on their own (divested of these other concerns) cannot warrant the investment of resources or expenditure of concerted diplomatic energies.

Now, in this book, I have argued not only that "states matter" – and matter a lot – in world affairs but that they have been absolutely central to the management and mismanagement of the pandemic. International organizations were, for the most part, bystanders. To add another example to those already offered, it was the bankrolling of the pharma companies by the wealthiest nation-states that allowed the speedy development of the vaccine fix. Moreover, as I have shown, it was asymmetrical power relations in the interstate system that mostly determined (and is still determining) the distribution of vaccine supplies worldwide – who got what, who got it first, and who hardly got anything.

The structure of international relations in relation to the world capitalist economy, as I have shown it, renders the interstate system as one organized for competition rather than for cooperation, and this also establishes global political economy as an imperial order. This is in the sense that interstate competition is asymmetric, rooted as it is in unequal exchange in "free" markets so that certain states dominate (those mainly of the Global North), with one of these (the US) exercising hegemony over the others. This is why vaccine competition between nations (vaccine nationalism) was and is also vaccine imperialism – to the advantage of the "developed" countries and to the disadvantage of the "developing" and "underdeveloped" ones. As I have argued, vaccine nationalism even threatened to seriously hamper the vaccine rollout in a large part of the "developed" world, that is, in Europe. This was owing to the UK–EU dispute over the allocation of supply, which risked perpetrating major harm on public health in Britain and across the mainland.

In this book, I have also sought to attribute the weaknesses of "community" or "people" responses to COVID-19, in terms of inconsistent adherence to NPIs and vaccine hesitancy, especially in certain parts of the world, and particularly among certain social groups, to the corrosive impact on civic society of certain cultures of individualism and of deepening class and "racial" class divisions in de-legitimizing political and other authorities (such as managerial science) in the neoliberal era. These social and cultural conditions, I have argued, seriously compromise the effectiveness of public health defence policies when faced with pandemic events such as COVID-19. This is an especially critical matter because, as I argue elsewhere,[5] our contemporary age is one of zoonotic accelerationism and of radicalized pandemic hazard.

My argument in this book has been developed by focusing critique around two key themes that seem to me to be integral to a sociology of pandemics in the "global" age. Firstly, the impacts of cultures of individualism and consumerism, and of pervasive and deeply entrenched social inequalities (that is, *decivilization*), in weakening the compliance of people with NPIs and in encouraging vaccine hesitancy that would protect communities from pandemics such as COVID-19. Secondly, how the primacy of interstate competition and imperial politics over interstate cooperation in international relations (which exists by virtue of the conversion of states under capitalism and neoliberalism into political allies of corporate interests) also undermined an effective international policy response to COVID-19. This was as universal human interests were subordinated to local national ones in the Global North and in the high-income countries.[6]

The companion volume to this undertaking, *Contagion Capitalism*, completes my analysis of pandemic risk by situating this in the capitalist world economy, corporate science, and consumer culture. This, as I have stated in the introduction to this book, mobilizes other resources of critique to explore new but related themes that are also fundamental, I think, to understanding global pandemics in the contemporary world. These are especially:

1. How the political mobilization of science and expertise as modes of legitimation for government policies compromised public health in the service of the interests of economic powerholders in the present pandemic.
2. How corporate mega-capitalism today has rendered human populations the world over increasingly vulnerable to the threat of viral and other pandemics.
3. How the accelerated risk of global pandemics in our contemporary age is integral to the ecological crisis of unsustainability of the capitalist mode of production in the "global" corporate age. Thus, epidemiological rift is an aspect of planetary rift.
4. How the instrumental mode of biomedical technoscience under capitalism not only obscures a sociological understanding of the roots of global pandemics (and thereby obstructs recognition of solutions that are possible only by recasting socioeconomic and sociopolitical orders) but also itself threatens public health and poses its own pandemic risks.

Taken together, these volumes attempt the rather ambitious (and perhaps overly so) project of locating or situating the COVID-19 crisis and indeed of global pandemics to come in the deep emergent structures – cultural, political, and economic – of our contemporary civilization of capital. Indeed, the purpose of this enterprise is to mobilize the tools of social theory in order to show how and why such crises throw into stark relief the profoundly anti-human, anti-social, and anti-ecological trajectory of this civilization of ours. They (pandemics and the manner in which they are addressed by powerholders) function as beacons or flares that re-expose all of the manifold inequities, injustices, and dysfunctions of the social systems that convey them and that otherwise are in danger of being normalized under conditions of "business as usual". That is, they throw into stark relief the systemic inhumanity of our modern civilization. If there is hope for humanity in the present crisis, it may lie in the capacity of these negative dialectics to demystify our age, and hence reenergize popular movements for a world based on justice and equality.

Admittedly, though, there are, as of yet, few signs that the pandemic is challenging the mutually reinforcing global orders of neoliberalism, nationalism, imperialism, and corporate capitalism, which are incompatible with a universal humanism, despite the role of these in the failures of public health protection internationally. On the contrary, the evidence is suggestive that these have not been undermined by the crisis, at least in the short term. Indeed, there is even a case for thinking that these have been emboldened by it.

Nationalism certainly has been strengthened by the border closures, travel restrictions, vaccine wars, export bans on PPE, and the opportunities allowed by the crisis for nationalist politicians and populist opinion-formers to cast various non-national Others as internal or external threats to national health or security (including as bearers of viral hazard). So, for Donald Trump, COVID-19 is the "Chinese disease", whereas for Boris Johnson it is "kung flu". These processes have reinvigorated a sense of embattled collective nationhood for many, providing a further boost to neo-conservative populism, and reinforcing social divisions and inequalities, which are both exposed and also exacerbated by the pandemic.[7] The pandemic has provided new opportunities for neocons, nationalists, and state authorities to cast people as strangers in our midst and at our door (migrants, guest workers, refugees, etc.), as potential enemies within, and to withhold from them entitlements that are associated with citizenship.[8] As for imperial rivalries, these have arguably been intensified by the economic fallout from the pandemic and lockdowns and have taken new forms, notably "vaccine diplomacy". Is it simply a coincidence that Russia's war in Ukraine is prosecuted in the shadow of the plague archipelago?

And what of neoliberalism and the corporate world that it serves? Undoubtedly, the world economy has taken a major hit, on all indicators (output growth, GDP performance, levels of trade, sales and investment, etc.), so that international capitalism as a whole is in the doldrums. But the biggest corporations and the global corporate elite that run them have largely evaded the economic impacts of the crisis so far, having weathered initial stock market wobbles, as smaller businesses have gone to the wall and millions have lost their jobs. Indeed, many corporations have profited from the crisis, cosseted by astronomical government subsidies under emergency measures, recording record shareholder values, as the "real" economy and those who staff it have suffered the loss and endured the hardship.

As Michael Ryan puts it, "the usual millionaire-class vultures who make their fortunes on the distress of others have been able to reap trillions in profit – both through market speculation as well as through taxpayer-funded government bail-outs".[9] One of these vultures, pharma capitalism, has of course sucked up billions of taxpayers' money to fund the development of the vaccines only then to appropriate as wholly private property the massive profits from their global sales. "Virtual" capitalism too has massively grown its profits from the expansion of internet services and platforms to service pandemic-induced home-working, home-shopping, home-entertainment, and home-based social interactions.[10] As for neoliberalism, this has its rationale and mandate for the indefinite perpetuation of austerity, welfare retrenchment, retrogressive taxation, and the squeezing of the incomes of the working poor and the common folk to recover the massive public debts generated by its corporate bankrolling. If neoliberalism has its way, we can expect a further hardening of wealth and income disparities worldwide.

The necessity of socialism

By way of a conclusion, I will settle for making some observations. These are those which are merely suggestive of remedies or alternatives to our current predicament. These arguments are developed in greater detail in my *Contagion Capitalism*.

If our world economy and corresponding mode of political governance was based on utility, public ownership, and social or associative enterprise rather than on commodity exchange, private property, and corporate enterprise, it would, I contend, be robust enough to manage a pandemic such as the present one without drawing upon itself serious material and social harms. One reason for this would be that, under these social forms, expert advice to government ministers would not be so much skewed by a perceived need to weigh up public health benefits against negative economic collaterals. This, however, is not the political world in which government scientific advisers and public health experts operate. Rather, they operate within the structural constraints and imperatives imposed by corporate-capitalist relations of production on an international scale as mediated by greater-or-lesser forms of national-level neoliberal governance.

In a world in which economic stability and prosperity depend simply on the security of tangible material use values rather than on the maximization of revenues from exchange, policymakers would also have made a much better fist of protecting their communities and peoples from the present pandemic. This is because, in such a world, risk-taking or gambling with public health protection would not be the default position, as it is under our present political and economic arrangements.

However, George Ritzer has suggested that the failures of public health policy were perhaps not those stemming from governments taking unreasonable, unwarranted risks with public safety in the service of corporate profits. Rather, for him, the US government's and indeed the world's lack of advance preparations for the pandemic may be interpreted through the lens of his McDonaldization theory – a case of the "irrationality of rationality"[11]:

> In the era of the McDonaldization of society, one might have expected the world, especially the United States, to at least have in place a rationalized plan to deal with such a pandemic ... Had such a plan been in existence early in the outbreak, the pain (in terms of number of illnesses and deaths, magnitude of the economic disaster, etc.) from the pandemic would have been reduced significantly. However, there was no plan at the beginning of 2020. One reason may have been that it would have seemed inefficient to engage in those preparations just in case there was a pandemic.

Under McDonaldization, then, a "just-in-time" rather than a "just-in-case" system to manage the pandemic may be considered by powerholders as rational, which is why most of the world adopted that approach. Under the former, "what would be needed in a pandemic would be produced and arrive just in time to deal with it". This would mean relying on "systems that had little or no slack, underutilized resources, or excessive inventory", in contrast to a just-in-case system that would have more slack, a stockpile of resources, and a bigger inventory.[12] Ritzer's point is that the rationality of the just-in-time system was established by the fact that the alternative would have been irrational (that is, inefficient, costly, wasteful) if there had been no pandemic. The balance of probabilities on any newly emergent disease "going viral", so to speak, would always be low so that a just-in-time system would be a better use of resources.

From a critical Marxist standpoint, however, Ritzer's application of the concept of the "irrationality of rationality" that establishes the "reasonableness" of a just-in-time system of pandemic management may be interrogated – and found wanting. What in fact was rational about it? Governments the world over knew that the risk of a major global pandemic was a real and growing one. This is what their scientific advisers and public health experts had been telling them for years. These scientific advisers and public health experts had also been telling them for years that they needed to prepare in advance for a pandemic, that is, prepare just-in-case systems to deal with one. Moreover, they had been telling them exactly what these just-in-case systems should look like.[13]

Thus, even from the narrow instrumental logic of cost-benefit analysis, however unlikely it is that any specific zoonotic disease will pose pandemic harm, sooner or later one will come along that will. This shows us, I suggest, that lack of pandemic pre-preparedness, is therefore less a story of governments such as those of the US and UK self-consciously adopting the wrong system (that is, just-in-time rather than just-in-case) and is more a case of reckless endangerment of public health motivated by the neoliberal prioritization of profits over people. On the eve of the pandemic, there was no alternative to a so-called just-in-time system (in reality, a "rather-too-little-and-too-late" policy) because decades of retrenchment and austerity had stripped away the public resources to support anything else.

COVID-19, when it arrived on the scene, was regarded by the experts as potentially a very serious matter, but only *potentially* so. This legitimized powerholders in their equivocation or fence-sitting on matters of public health protection against the virus because they wished to avoid economic (that is, business) harms unless the necessity of these for protection was proven. By contrast, where policymaking is bound within the framework of a de-commodified (that is, socialist) world economy, the default position when faced with such uncertainties would always be "safety first", that is, proactive planning and prompt maximal action on the basis of worst-case-scenario planning. I contend that policymakers under socialism much more than those under capitalism would be incentivized to avoid subordinating issues of public health to purely economic considerations.

This is because the harms caused by a pandemic such as COVID-19 to a "real economy" (that is, one based on use value) would be far less than those it must cause to our actual "money economy" (based on exchange value). For sure, under capitalism, exchange value depends on use value. But exchange value, not use value, is the motive force of capitalist production; capitalist profitability and shareholder value are parasitic upon a real economy of use value. This is how capitalism transcends and indeed partially undermines an economy of need in the service of an economy of want or desire, indeed of induced or manufactured desire.[14] A commodified economy, I contend, must radically weaken the capacity of governments to act decisively and robustly in prioritizing public health protection at the expense of "business as usual".

Such is especially the case given the longstanding zombification of the world economy under the sway of corporate-capitalist ownership and of failed neoliberal remedies to reverse the system's tendencies towards declining profits, stagnation, and recession. The paradox of capitalism today is that the incomes of the rich and super-corporations have never been greater just as the system itself has rarely been less stable or prone to slowdown and generalized crises. Zombie capitalism not only pressurizes neoliberal governments and business-friendly states to eschew "safety first" policies with regard to public health faced with pandemic events (owing to its structural predominance in the world economy and its corresponding radical economic fragility) but also is especially vulnerable to being tipped into tumultuous recessionary crises by such events. Zombie capitalism not only ferments zoonoses with pandemic potential but also lacks the basic resilience to cope with their economic fallout when they arrive.

An international commonwealth of countries sharing a socialist world economy also offers the prospect of a much more joined-up or internationally coordinated policy response to pandemics-in-the-making than is possible under the present imperially based competitive international state system. This is simply because a socialist *commonwealth* – as the name implies – is based on cooperation rather than competition between countries and peoples (in the latter case rendered necessary by the competition of capitals in the marketplace), including the sharing of resources on the basis of solidarity and equality. National competition in sport and games may serve the purpose of entertainment value (and here it has no other consequence), but this is radically disadvantageous in matters of importance to most people globally. People's lives and livelihoods are too important to be decided by a tug-of-war for financial advantage among a tiny elite of corporate CEOs and property owners.

The present global organization of politics as interstate competition and imperial rivalries discussed in this book serve the goals of the world capitalist economy. This is inasmuch as this offsets or obstructs the development of a critical anti-capitalist, pro-socialist working-class consciousness across the world. Universal humanity is undermined by nationhood because this means that rights of citizenship substitute for rights of personhood, that is, for *human* rights. This occurs, as I have argued, because nationalities or nationhoods confer these exclusively on those contained within their borders and withhold them from others. These then become rather like privileges of club membership that bind people to the citizenship-conferring state and that detach them from others.

Naturally, then, citizenship places obstacles (that is, those of national allegiances and national chauvinism) in the path of "workers of the world uniting"[15] in pursuit of their common interests. Class struggles and social movements in different places are split off from each other because they are sequestered within national borders where they encounter in relative isolation the condensed political power of the local state. National states are in turn, as I have argued, bound by a relationship of structural interdependence to their home-grown or home-based capitals so that their primary function is ensuring the competitive success of these enterprises in the market *vis-à-vis* those of their overseas rivals. Because there are *rival* capitals there are *rival* states. And because there are *rival* states there are *rival* peoples.

Under socialism, by contrast, nationality as such, and with it citizenship, is done away with. There are instead communities and countries of place and common rights of personhood that are universal. Governments are no longer tied to serving the cause of capital accumulation since the economic security of those they serve is no longer dependent on success in market competition. This means that governments under socialism (as opposed to socialist governments under capitalism – a contradiction in terms, unless that government is working to abolish capitalism) are much more divested of motives and opportunities to compete rather than cooperate with each other when faced with matters of international concern – such as an impending or unfolding pandemic.

What would this mean in practice? I will offer three examples. Firstly, under socialism, internationalism would have had a much better chance of prevailing in the vaccination rollout to defeat COVID-19, rather than vaccine nationalism and imperialism carrying the day. As we have seen, the latter has generated monstrous asymmetries in the worldwide distribution of jabs, costing hundreds of thousands of lives, especially in the Global South. Secondly, under socialism, proactive collaborative border defence policies to minimize the export and import of the disease would not have given a fillip to national chauvinism or a politics of racialized blame-mongering for the crisis. This has inevitably been the case, as things stand, because our world is one of rival states and rival firms, which needs to mobilize people as competitors in the service of capital and which relates people to each other as rivals for the leftovers from the corporate table. Finally, because under socialism there are no citizens (of nations) but rather people who own universal rights, the possibility of discrimination against migrants (or other visitors – such as guest workers and students) in any country where there are border closures under emergency conditions, such as those of a pandemic, would be undermined. Such discrimination has been a distressing feature of the present pandemic.[16]

Is this a utopia? Perhaps. What is clear is that progressive politics need utopias to guide them. But there is progressive or liberatory potential at least in the radicalized negative dialectics of the present conjuncture, whether or not this is realized. As Michael Ryan rightly says:

> The current situation is indeed presenting an "us" vs. "them" scenario. But it is also presenting humanity … with an opportunity to do something. One option is to sit back and continue to let "them" take advantage of a global pandemic to increase "their" profits, power, and discriminatory ideologies. Another is to encourage, nay demand, that our fellow citizens, political leaders, and global institutions enforce an honest version of "we". The first choice leads to a world of even greater othering and inequality. The second leads us to a world where a global humanity comes together as a larger community and begins to measure its successes by the well-being of the worst off among us. So far we have largely made the wrong choice. It isn't too late to make the right one.[17]

Now, Scott Schaffer draws our attention to what he calls the "necroethics" of neoliberal capitalism that the pandemic has thrown into sharp relief.[18] These are ethics that deemed those workers who could not work from home during the lockdowns (disproportionately workers on lower incomes, in lower status jobs, of minority ethnic membership) as "essential" workers so that they were required to carry on as usual in the eye of the pandemic storm, placing themselves and their families at risk from the disease, which those higher up the socioeconomic scale evaded. These essential workers as defined by neoliberal authorities were not simply key workers by any sensible definition. In fact, these included workers in

> food and agriculture; emergency services; transportation, warehouse, and delivery; industrial, commercial, and residential facilities and services; health care; government and community-based services; communications and IT; the financial sector; the energy sector; water and wastewater management; the chemical sector; and critical manufacturing industries. In the United States, that amounts to over 55 million workers, as opposed to 86 million who worked in nonessential industries, with the proportion roughly the same in Canada.[19]

The pandemic has thus reminded us that, even from the perspective of neoliberal powerholders, it is the massed ranks of the manual industrial and post-industrial working class that are essential to the reproduction of capitalism, whereas others are rather less so. As importantly, the pandemic also shows us that, from the perspective of neoliberalism, those workers who are essential are not particularly those who are placed in the service of supporting or caring for other people (though these are included in their number). Rather, these are those who are placed in the service of supporting or nurturing "resources" – the subordination of people to resources, the sacrifice of people to profits. Thus,

> we can understand the "essential workers" here as expendable, fodder to keep the global capitalist system going, which US Treasury Secretary Steven Mnuchin has said cannot be stopped, even if it takes hundreds of thousands of deaths. And our willingness to expose these groups of people to the dangers presented by the pandemic demonstrates that a central component of late capitalism is an ethics of expendability, one that makes the death of Others easily conceivable if we validate them as heroes and temporarily raise their meager earnings by two dollars per hour.[20]

This, I think, is at the centre of the negative dialectics of our pandemic-ravaged present, from which a critical global consciousness may emerge. Schaffer himself concedes the possibility:

> Perhaps by bringing this liberal-democratic capitalist necroethics into the light, we can show that it's not triage for the sake of saving others but culling human beings, members of our society, for the sake of saving the resources of a few. Perhaps this will also be the historical moment at which this ethos ends, and we can transform the death-worlds we have enabled to be created into worlds that give all people life.[21]

There is, in short, still hope.

Sean Creaven

12 July 2022 (updated May 2023)

Notes

1 Ramsari, A. (2021). 'The Rise of the COVID-19 Pandemic and the Decline of Global Citizenship'. J.M. Ryan (Ed.) *COVID-19: Global Pandemic, Societal Responses, Ideological Solutions*. London and New York: Routledge.
2 Ramsari (2021), p. 102.
3 Sentencing Project (2021). Trends in U.S. Corrections: U.S. State and Federal Prison Population, 1925–2019, Washington DC: Sentencing Project. See also: Chambliss, W.J. (1994). 'Policing the ghetto underclass: the politics of law and law enforcement'. *Social Problems*, 41 (2), pp. 177–94; Parenti, C. (2000). *Lockdown America: Police and Prisons in the Age of Crisis*, London: Pluto Press; Reiman, J. (2007). *The Rich Get Richer and the Poor Get Prison: Ideology, Class and Criminal Justice*, 8th edition, New York: Macmillan; Wacquant, L. (2001). 'The Penalisation of Poverty and the Rise of Neo-Liberalism'. *European Journal on Criminal Policy and Research*, 9 (4), pp. 401–12.
4 Walsh, P.W. (2022). *Q&A: The UK's policy to send asylum seekers to Rwanda*. University of Oxford: The Migration Observatory. (10 June).
5 Creaven, S. (2024). *Contagion Capitalism: Pandemics in the Corporate Age*. London and New York; Routledge. (Forthcoming).
6 Hence the politics of vaccine nationalism and vaccine imperialism that has risked the lives of tens of millions worldwide.
7 Ryan, J.M. (2021). 'The Blessings of COVID-19 for Neoliberalism, Nationalism, and Neoconservative Ideologies'. Ryan (Ed.) *Global Pandemic*.
8 Nanda, S. (2021). 'Inequalities and COVID-19'. Ryan (Ed.) *Global Pandemic*
9 Ryan (2021), p. 80.
10 Ryan (2021), p. 85.
11 Ritzer, G. (2021). 'McDonaldization in the Age of COVID-19'. Ryan (Ed.) *Global Pandemic.*
12 Ritzer (2021), p. 24.
13 I discuss elsewhere how this has unfolded in the UK. See Creaven, S. (2023). *The Pandemic in Britain: COVID-19, British Exceptionalism, and Neoliberalism*. London and New York: Routledge, pp. 30–31.
14 Sklair, L. (2002). *Globalisation: Capitalism and Its Alternatives*, 3rd edition. Oxford: Oxford University Press (Ch. 7: 'Culture-ideology of Consumerism').
15 Marx, K. and Engels. F. (1967). *The Communist Manifesto* [1848]. Harmondsworth: Penguin, p. 121.
16 Nanda (2021); Ramsari (2021).
17 Ryan (2021), p. 91.
18 Schaffer, S. (2021). 'Necroethics in the time of COVID-19 and Black Lives Matter'. Ryan (Ed.) *Global pandemic.*
19 Schaffer (2021), p. 47.
20 Schaffer (2021), p. 48.
21 Schaffer (2021), p. 51.

Index

For Product Safety Concerns and Information please contact our EU
representative GPSR@taylorandfrancis.com
Taylor & Francis Verlag GmbH, Kaufingerstraße 24, 80331 München, Germany

www.ingramcontent.com/pod-product-compliance
Lightning Source LLC
Chambersburg PA
CBHW061623220326
41598CB00026BA/3854